ON FLINCHING

On Flinching

Theatricality and Scientific Looking from Darwin to Shell Shock

TIFFANY WATT SMITH

OXFORD
UNIVERSITY PRESS

OXFORD
UNIVERSITY PRESS
Great Clarendon Street, Oxford, OX2 6DP,
United Kingdom

Oxford University Press is a department of the University of Oxford.
It furthers the University's objective of excellence in research, scholarship,
and education by publishing worldwide. Oxford is a registered trade mark of
Oxford University Press in the UK and in certain other countries

First Edition published in 2014

Impression: 1

Published in the United States of America by Oxford University Press
198 Madison Avenue, New York, NY 10016, United States of America

British Library Cataloguing in Publication Data
Data available

Library of Congress Control Number: 2014932272

ISBN 978–0–19–870093–7

Printed and bound by
CPI Group (UK) Ltd, Croydon, CR0 4YY

To Michael Hughes,
with gratitude

Acknowledgements

I would like to thank the Arts and Humanities Research Council and the British Academy, whose generous financial support over the last five years allowed me to develop this project and see it through to publication. I am also grateful for funds made available by the School of English and Drama at Queen Mary University of London to facilitate my attendance at conferences over the years possible, and the Wellcome Trust for their ongoing support of the Queen Mary Centre for the History of the Emotions.

This project grew out of doctoral research undertaken at Queen Mary's School of English and Drama and Centre for the History of the Emotions. I am indebted to Nicholas Ridout and Thomas Dixon who supervised my PhD with unsparing generosity, acuity, and humour. Their differing intellectual styles and creative approaches animated my research from the beginning, and working with them has been a great pleasure. I would also like to thank Steven Connor and Jim Davis who acted as examiners for the thesis, and whose thought-provoking suggestions have proved invaluable as I continued to work on it. A whole range of scholars shared their ideas with me, and read or listened to mine, offering encouragement and suggesting other avenues to explore. I would particularly like to thank Sally Shuttleworth, Carolyn Burdett, Helen Rodgers, Ruth Livesey, Paul White, Kirsten Shepherd-Barr, Isobel Armstrong, Catherine Maxwell, and all the anonymous peer reviewers of my work. There have been countless others whose passing comments at conferences, seminars, and trips to the pub have entered the slipstream of my thinking too.

The Centre for the History of the Emotions at Queen Mary continues to provide me with a stimulating and congenial environment for research, and I would like to thank all my fellow centre members, particularly Rhodri Hayward and Fay Bound Alberti, as well as the many scholars who have visited over the years. Among all my wonderful colleagues at the School of Drama, I'd particularly like to thank Jen Harvie, Caoimhe McAvinchey, and Michael McKinnie for their patient and judicious advice at various tentative and panicky stages, Sarah Thomasson for her diligent work as a research assistant, and David Wright for kindly creating the film stills reproduced in Chapter Four. I am grateful to Jacqueline Baker, my editor at Oxford University Press, and her team who steered this book through to publication.

It is extraordinarily lucky for cultural historians of the nineteenth century that so many of the resources we need have been digitized. I would like to acknowledge all those unsung heroes whose hours of scanning nineteenth-century newspapers and obscure psychological texts save us so much time and labour. But archival research remains an immensely important and satisfying part of our work, offering unique sensory experiences, and with them, unforeseen insights. I am particularly grateful to the archivists at the Wellcome Library, the Cambridge University Library, and the Royal College of Physicians Heritage Centre for their help identifying the relevant materials, as well as to all the staff at the British Library.

The germ of the idea for the book came when I watched my husband Michael Hughes imitate a pose in a painting. Over the years I've worked on this project, he has provided unstinting practical and emotional support, intellectual fellowship, and writerly guidance, and it is to him that this book is dedicated. My always supportive parents, Ursula and Ian, brothers Tom and Dan, and my many in-laws and friends have also been magnanimous comrades on this journey: for their kindness and patience, I am truly thankful.

In preparing this book, I have drawn on earlier published material. Parts of Chapter One previously appeared as 'Darwin's Flinch: Sensation Theatre and Scientific Looking in 1872', *Journal of Victorian Culture*, 15 (2010), 101–18 (Winner, 2009 Graduate Essay Prize Competition), and a version of the material in Chapter Three appeared as 'Henry Head and the Theatre of Distractions' in *19: Interdisciplinary Studies in the Long Nineteenth Century*, 12 (2011), 1–17. Some of the ideas explored in the introduction also appear in 'Cardboard, Conjuring and "A Very Curious Experiment"', *Interdisciplinary Science Reviews*, 38, 4 (2013), 306–20. I am grateful to the editors of these publications for their permission to reproduce this material.

Contents

List of Illustrations

Introduction: Playing at Looking, Playing at Being Seen

> Each gesture is an event—one might even say, a drama—in itself.
>
> Walter Benjamin, 'Franz Kafka. On the Tenth Anniversary of his Death' (1934), reprinted in *Illuminations*.[1]

One Tuesday afternoon, about five years ago, M. and I decided to visit the National Gallery in London. We were standing in front of Caravaggio's *Salome Receives* the *Head of Saint John the Baptist*, where I was knowledgably imparting some half-remembered facts about chiaroscuro, when I turned round to discover my audience had abandoned me. M. had wandered off to the other side of the empty gallery, where, standing before a small gilt-framed painting in the corner, he was attempting to contort his body into a most peculiar pose. Extending his hands, as if to protect himself from something lurching from the canvas before him, he hunched up his left shoulder and turned his torso and face aside. Then, checking back at the painting, he adjusted the angle of his limbs, widened his eyes so that they seemed to bulge, and opened his mouth in a silent gasp. I performed a well-rehearsed wince of my own (I am easily embarrassed, and M. is given to embarrassing demonstrations in public) but as there was no one around to notice, I abandoned the theatrics and crept up behind him to see what he was doing.

He was attempting to imitate another performance, a pose struck in the canvas before him. It was a portrait by Caravaggio, *Boy Bitten By A Lizard* (1596) depicting a rosy-cheeked young Roman street boy recoiling, in shock, or perhaps pain, from the surprise attack of an angry reptile (Figure 1). The painting captures the drama, the visceral force, of

[1] Walter Benjamin, 'Franz Kafka. On the Tenth Anniversary of his Death' (1934), repr. in *Illuminations*, trans. Harry Zohn (London: Pimlico, 1999) pp. 108–35 (p. 117).

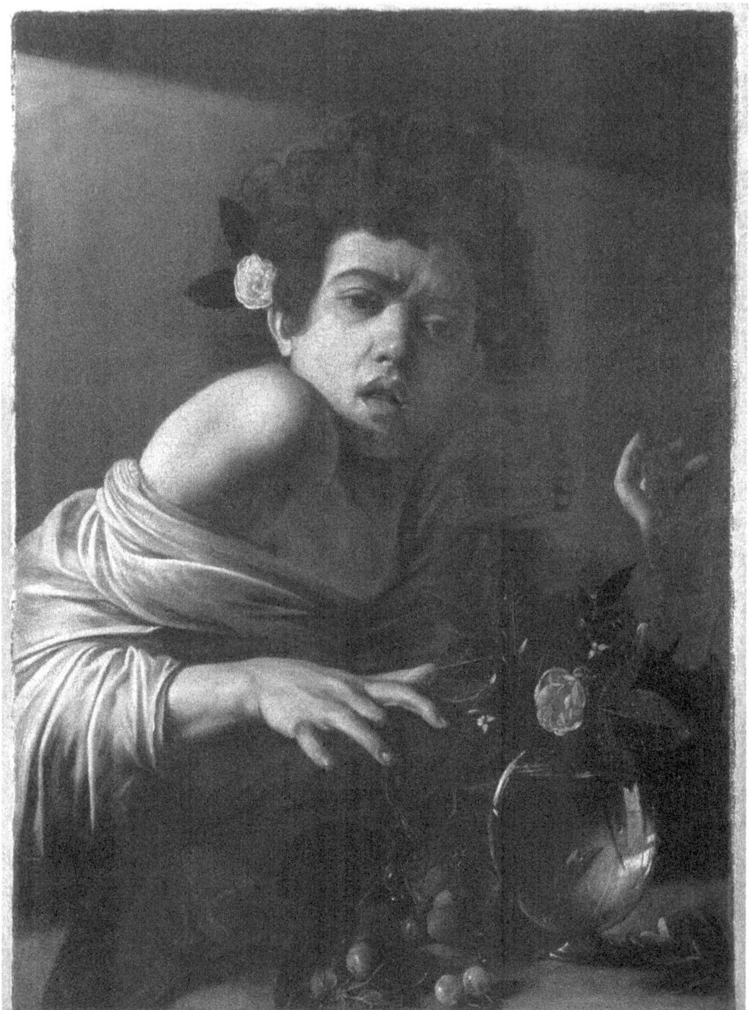

Fig. 1. *Boy Bitten By A Lizard*, Michaelangelo Caravaggio (*c*. 1596).

Bought with the aid of a contribution from the J. Paul Getty Jr. Endowment Fund, 1986. © The National Gallery, London

an involuntary flinch. But watching M. attempt to mimic the boy's pose also brought to mind the experience of the model, his aching muscles frozen in a carefully choreographed attitude of alarm. I had usually consigned flinching to the realm of automatic movements, regarding it to be merely an involuntary reflex for self-protection. But confronted with this nested series of imitations—M., the painting, the posing model—I wondered about the times recoiling and cringing are self-consciously enacted responses too. My own cringe in the empty gallery was certainly rhetorical, a gesture performed with an imaginary audience in mind. Moreover, though M.'s posing was clearly self-conscious, it also seemed to be a way for him to engage with the experience depicted on the canvas, his gaze flicking back and forth between his own muscles and those of the boy in the painting. Was imitating the boy's gesture a way of entering into a felt complicity with the scenario in the painting? Were M.'s contortions a kind of self-experiment in looking, a deliberate attempt to invoke in his own body the ghostly ripples of another's emotions? It was a curious puzzle. Because if by flinching M. was leaning into the painting, sampling its sensory world, he was only able to do so by recoiling from it, by turning aside, averting his eyes and protecting himself from its encroaching horrors.

FLINCHES, WINCES, CRINGES AND STARTS: 1872–1918

During a backstage tour of the circus on Drury Lane, at some point in the 1830s, Queen Victoria and her retinue paused before a cage containing a tiger. The fearsome beast, gnawing a hunk of bloody meat between its paws, looked up at his audience. Suddenly, he sprang forwards with a tremendous roar, rattling the bars of the cage. 'The boldest of the royal suite splendidly retreated', wrote the actor-manager Alfred Bunn. But according to a different account written twenty-five years later by the politician John Hobhouse 'the youthful Queen never moved face or foot. With look undiverted, and still more deeply riveted, she continued to gaze on the novel and moving spectacle.'[2] In her unflinching demeanour—which was almost certainly more rhetorical than real—the monarch was attributed with an emotional self-mastery usually only associated with men in the Victorian period. Jumping startled into the air, retreating and turning aside, or other forms of recoiling, shrinking, wincing, and flinching were habitually linked to intrinsic cowardice, feminized sensitivity, or attention-seeking theatrical performers. To stand unmoved before a ferocious creature, mastering Nature with a sustained and controlling 'gaze', was behaviour more befitting the man of science.

[2] Alfred Bunn, *The Stage: Both Before and Behind the Curtain*, iii, 3 vols. (London: Bentley, 1840); John Hobhouse, *Recollections of a Long Life* (London: W. Clowes & Sons, 1865). Both quoted in Richard Schoch, *Queen Victoria and the Theatre of Her Age* (Basingstoke: Palgrave Macmillan, 2004) p. 125.

By the second part of the nineteenth century, expressions of horror, disgust, and surprise were appearing with increasing frequency on the pages of newspapers, novels, and scientific tracts. Pedestrians cringed as express trains hurtled past them and winced from the clanging cymbals of street hawkers. Audiences jumped out of their seats as horses crashed onto the stage in theatres, or recoiled in delighted shock at the latest electromagnetic phenomenon on display in London's galleries of practical science. Both an embarrassing liability and a visceral pleasure, flinches and winces were part and parcel of the era's restless technological advances and burgeoning mass entertainment culture. At the same time, the 'startle reflex'—recoiling from danger, jumping backwards, turning the head away, and raising the hands—was fast becoming an important object of scrutiny for physiologists, neurologists, and psychologists alike. The second part of the nineteenth century was a critical time for the ways flinching, wincing, and shrinking came to be understood. Where before the nineteenth century, doctors, philosophers, and religious authorities had spoken of the 'moral passions' and the 'affectations of the soul', Victorian physiologists turned their attention to the newly secular category of 'the emotions'. Measuring raised pulses, horripilation, and dilated pupils, they re-framed fear, horror, and disgust in the language of nerves, reflexes, and evolution. For these men of science, the flinch was less a moral failure or sympathetic gesture than the centerpiece of a new physiological framework for understanding perception and emotion. Involuntarily recoiling was symptomatic of an alarming new condition: as Thomas Dixon has put it, during the nineteenth century the emotional subject fell from a state of 'extensive voluntary control' over her feelings, to one of 'enslavement' to the vagaries of the impulsive body and its 'useless physical urges'.[3]

In the fifty-year period addressed by this book, a transformation occurred in the way the recoiling body was understood. Beginning with Darwin's portrait of a vestigial body, whose flinches were forged over millennia to ensure the survival of the species, and concluding with the shell-shocked soldiers who returned from the First World War trembling and recoiling from imagined dangers, this book tells the story of an emotional body seen as increasingly malleable and unreliable. During this period, the idea that flinching exemplified the body's uniform and predictable reflex responses, gave way to the notion that our cringes and starts were prey to illusion, and that the body's perceptual and emotional machinery could be manipulated from without. At the same time, the period between 1872 and 1918 also witnessed profound changes in the scientific practices used to

[3] Thomas Dixon, *From Passions to Emotions: The Creation of a Secular Psychological Category* (Cambridge and New York: Cambridge University Press, 2003) p. 176.

measure and represent this emotionally responding body. New technologies were deployed, such as the sphymograph, pneumograph, photograph, and cine-camera, which allowed men of science to measure and represent the body's most fleeting, delicate movements without recourse to their own unreliable human eyes. Such technologies helped articulate the idea that emotional responses were observable physical events, but they also drew attention to the potentially disruptive presence of the scientific observer himself. As Lorraine Daston and Peter Galison have described, these self-recording machines ushered in a new model of dispassionate and objective scientific looking, compelling human observers to restrain themselves and their emotions so as not to interfere with the phenomena they studied. Objectivity included an ethical injunction, with scientists aspiring to 'the self-discipline of saints', required to 'foreswear judgement, interpretation, and even the testimony of [their] own senses'.[4] As Michel Foucault put it, the paradigm for this new ideal of looking was the scientific 'gaze': the 'gaze' 'refrains from intervening' he wrote, 'it is silent and gestureless. Observation leaves things as they are.'[5]

It might be a surprise, then, to discover that while these 'silent and gestureless' scientific observers provoked and measured flinches in their animal and human subjects, they could also be passionate performers, cringing, wincing, and flinching during their experiments too. If feelings of shock, pain, and disgust were a much-studied part of their subjects' affective and perceptual machinery, experimenters experienced them too. At times their flinches were a surprise even to themselves, as when they were startled by an unexpected noise, or recoiled from the stab of a needle. At other times, their winces were self-consciously induced, for example, when they attempted to measure their own compulsion to shrink in fear, or compared their startle-reflex to those of the chimps and children they studied. On occasion, flinching was part of an elaborate, even theatrical, choreography of looking when the scientist, fearful of disrupting the scene he observed, recoiled behind doors to hide from his subject. These flinches were by no means obscured in the official discourse. On the contrary, they appeared in the books, articles, and lectures in which the scientist described his experiments and the feats of looking they required. But even greater evidence for them can be found among the traces of the fleeting, intangible, day-to-day experimental practices which linger in laboratory notebooks, love-letters, and the scribbles on the back of

[4] Lorraine Daston and Peter Galison, 'The Image of Objectivity', *Representations*, 40 (1992) 81–128 (pp. 82–3).

[5] Michel Foucault, *The Birth of the Clinic*, trans. A. M. Sheridan (London and New York: Routledge, 2009) p. 131.

photographs. Rather than seeing these emotional gestures as aberrations in the late nineteenth-century culture of objectivity, this book argues that the scientist's flinches highlight a distinctive pattern of passionate and self-conscious looking that was already circulating widely in this period. It was a motif of embodied and emotional spectatorship that can best be understood through the techniques and problems it shared with that other cornerstone of Victorian culture—the theatre.

This book argues that alongside the sphymograph and rotary recorder, theatre itself was a key apparatus used in scientific experiments in the late nineteenth century. This is not simply to claim that public scientific displays in this period had a certain theatrical flair about them, although this was certainly true. As historians of science, James Secord, Bernard Lightman, and Iwan Rhys Morus among them, have argued, these spectacular public demonstrations and the theatrical spaces that facilitated them were part and parcel of the way Victorians created their scientific knowledge.[6] For their part, historians of theatre including Joseph Roach, Kirsten Shepherd-Barr, and Stanton Garner, have described the ways scientific discoveries and techniques impinged on theatre in this period, and in particular, on the rise of naturalism in the latter part of the century.[7] However, this book goes further in claiming that the worlds of Victorian science and theatre were even more intimately entwined than existing scholarship credits. In the nineteenth and early twentieth centuries, science did not only inform theatrical innovations, and theatre did not only emerge at points when scientists made spectacles of themselves and their discoveries, but more surprisingly, theatricality was deep within the scientific experiment and a key part of the emergence of objective looking itself.

It is worth noting that the words 'scientist' and 'theatricality' were introduced to the English language within a few years of each other. William Whewell invented the word 'scientist' in 1834, to describe the vocation

[6] For an overview of the relationship between experimentation and spectacular scientific demonstrations in the nineteenth century, see: Iwan Rhys Morus, 'Placing Performance', *Isis*, 101 (2010) 775–8. See also: James Secord, 'Extraordinary Experiment: Electricity and the Creation of Life in Victorian England', in *The Uses of Experiment: Studies in the Natural Sciences*, ed. David Gooding, Trevor Pinch, and Simon Schaffer (Cambridge: Cambridge University Press, 1989) pp. 337–73; Iwan Rhys Morus, '"More the Aspect of Magic than Anything Natural": The Philosophy of Demonstration', in *Science in the Marketplace, Nineteenth-Century Sites and Experiences*, ed. Aileen Fyfe and Bernard Lightman (Chicago and London: University of Chicago Press, 2007) pp. 337–70; Bernard Lightman, *Victorian Popularizers of Science* (Chicago and London: University of Chicago Press, 2007).

[7] Joseph R. Roach, *The Player's Passion: Studies in the Science of Acting* (Michigan: University of Michigan Press, 2001); Stanton B. Garner, Jr., 'Introduction: Is There a Doctor in the House? Medicine and the Making of Modern Drama', *Modern Drama*, 51, 3 (2008) 311–28; Kirsten Shepherd-Barr, *Science on Stage: From* Doctor Faustus *to* Copenhagen (Princeton, NJ: Princeton University Press, 2006).

of those who rejected the fantastical claims of metaphysics and theology, and pursued instead the rigours of experimental proof.[8] Three years later in 1837, Thomas Carlyle coined 'theatricality' to describe an inauthentic sort of posturing, the opposite of sincerity and truth.[9] At first glance, it might seem impossible to fully reconcile these two worlds and their competing epistemological demands. Yet, even as the modern ideal of scientific objectivity was taking shape, theatrical techniques such as directing fictional scenarios, acting, and eliciting emotional responses from spectators were used by scientists in their pursuit of knowledge about the emotional body. In turn, scientists found themselves beset by theatre's problems—its excesses, its emotional contagions, and most of all its queasy slippages between seeming and being which troubled any easy assertion that a particular feeling or action was truly *there*. How scientists, like theatrical audiences, negotiated these failures of transparency became an important part not only of their day-to-day laboratory practice, but also left traces in the conceptual ideas about the body they produced.

This affinity between scientific observers and theatrical audiences came clearly into focus when both groups of spectators flinched. How might the moments when scientists found themselves becoming a spectacle, when they turned aside and skittered backwards, their steady gaze interrupted in a moment of visceral recoil, raise the possibility of thinking about scientific looking as a type of emotional performance, as even a theatrically self-conscious act? This book argues that, even in the age of objectivity, scientists continued to participate in a wider culture of passionate and demonstrative looking that was firmly linked to theatrical audiences in this period. In detecting a distinctive pattern of looking, *On Flinching* builds on existing scholarly debate about how Victorians understood the ways they encountered the world, recognising that their acts of spectatorship were not only limited to their visual sense, but also included hearing, touching, feeling, and performing too.[10] Theatrical audiences were

[8] William Whewell first used the word in print in 1834, reporting that he had suggested the idea of introducing the word 'scientist' to replace 'philosopher' at a meeting of the British Association for the Advancement of Science the previous year. The word, however, was not in general use until the turn of the century. William Whewell, 'Mary Somerville's *On the Connexion of the Physical Sciences*', *Quarterly Review*, 51, 101 (1834), 54–68 (p. 59).

[9] 'By act and word he strives to do it; with sincerity, if possible; failing that, with theatricality' wrote Thomas Carlyle. Quoted in Tracy C. Davis, 'Theatricality and Civil Society', in *Theatricality*, ed. Thomas Postlewait and Tracy C. Davis (Cambridge: Cambridge University Press, 2003) pp. 127–55 (p. 130).

[10] Two recent edited collections which illustrate the breadth of work currently taking place on this topic are: Luisa Calè and Patrizia Di Bello (eds.) *Illustrations, Optics and Objects in Nineteenth-Century Literary and Visual Cultures* (London: Palgrave, 2010); Colette Colligan and Margaret Linley (eds.), *Media, Technology, and Literature in the Nineteenth Century: Image, Sound, Touch* (Farnham: Ashgate, 2011).

extremely important for those who thought and wrote about spectatorship in the long nineteenth century, their techniques of looking debated by novelists, theatre-critics, actors, philosophers, and psychologists alike. There was, of course, no such thing in this period as 'the theatre audience' or 'the theatre spectator'. Even putting to one side the notorious difficulty of re-constructing the actual affective experiences of historical theatregoers, audiences were also discursively produced in multiple and often contradictory ways. At one extreme, there were audiences who attended the sensation melodramas of the 1860s and 1870s, whose raucous and overexcited responses were considered part of the show itself. At the other were those middle-class audiences of The Drama, a category of increasingly naturalistic theatre which emerged in the 1880s, who were expected neither to be seen nor heard. Somewhere in the middle were fashionable audiences with their view-obscuring matinee hats and affected yawns, the distracting programme-rustlers, the critics who could watch and simultaneously monitor their own feelings, and the spectators who found themselves entranced, even hypnotized, by the actors on stage. But in these many different visions of theatre-watching, one question kept recurring: how did audience members negotiate *their own theatricality*?

Then, as now, being part of an audience involved participating in a live encounter, one marked not only by the co-presence of spectators and performers, but also by the social experience of sitting amidst a group of other audience members too. Spectators' own emotional performances were not simply understood as part of the spectacle; they also played a vital role in how theorists explained the ways how audiences made sense of what they were watching and developed a shared experience. It was their knowingness about the effects they produced as performers themselves, in addition to their capacity to negotiate the slippery fictions of the theatrical world and perform alongside them, which marked out theatre audiences as a distinctive breed of observers. Theatrical looking, however, was not confined to the playhouse. As those Victorians who worried about looking made clear, the idea of a passionately performing spectator wandered beyond the auditorium, to emerge in lecture halls and law courts, laboratories, and museums of medical curiosities. Perhaps most surprisingly, its found its way into the heart of the human experiment too.

Each of the four chapters of this book centres on a single scientific experiment, each teasing out connections running between the act of scientific observation and the passionate performances of theatregoers. Chapter One takes a self-experiment performed by Charles Darwin in the London Zoological Gardens in 1872 as its starting point. To illustrate the efficacy of our evolved, involuntary reflexes, Darwin pressed his nose up against the glass tank of a puff adder—and when the snake lunged, the man of science quickly drew back. But in its self-conscious emotionality, Darwin's experiment also recalled the behaviour of audiences of 'sensation theatre' who enjoyed their own winces and starts at life-like spectacles of destruction. Chapter Two explores the emotional interactions between the neurologist David Ferrier and his experimental monkey F, at University College London between 1881–2. Attempting to locate the centre for hearing in the brain, Ferrier repeatedly tried to startle the monkey to see whether or not he had suppressed her ability to hear. In this chapter, the neurologist's efforts to conceal himself, flinching and recoiling in an attempt to hide from his subject, are compared to similar attempts made by theatre spectators who learnt to hide behind an imaginary 'fourth wall' when naturalism emerged in the 1880s. The third chapter investigates neurologist Henry Head's flinches and winces during a self-experiment in nerve regeneration that he performed with the psychologist W. H. R. Rivers. After severing his radial nerve, Head measured the slow and painful return of sensation to his left hand between 1903–7, undergoing tests which often made him wince with pain. To report his sensations, Head entered into a trance-like state, out of which he was often startled by sudden noises outside. This chapter compares Head's winces and starts to those of spectators in the avant-garde theatre of the early 1900s, where both actresses and audiences were startled from their reverie by the whispers and shuffles of their fellow audience members. The final chapter addresses Arthur Hurst's experimental treatment of shell-shocked soldiers recorded in his medical film *War Neuroses* (1917–18). Hurst approached the treatment as a theatrical endeavour, persuading patients and doctors to perform as both actors and audiences for the camera. Drawing attention to the range of spectators solicited by Hurst's cure, this chapter argues that theatrical looking persisted even with the introduction of film in medical experiments.

In these interdisciplinary readings, the flinches, winces, starts, and recoils of scientific observers and their subjects perform three interlocking roles. Firstly, they form a history of the recoiling body as itself an object of investigation. How was the startled subject understood in the period between 1872 and 1918? What new meanings did flinching accrue, what old ones did it retain, and what was the significance of starting and wincing for wider scientific and cultural debates about the emotionally responsive body at this time? Secondly, moments when scientific observers recoiled in their experiments are starting points for this book's interdisciplinary approach, which draws attention to the theatricality in the encounter between experimental subject and scientific observer. Pointing up how scientific experimenters drew on theatrical techniques and negotiated theatrical problems in their efforts to map and understand the responsive body, this part of the analysis also highlights the often overlooked emotional and embodied dimensions of experimental practice. Finally, close readings of the flinches performed by scientific observers and theatre audiences open out into this book's larger theme of spectatorship in the nineteenth century. Each flinch reveals a moment of 'double perspective', in which audience members both watched, and watched themselves. This motif of self-reflexive looking suggests that a passionate and performed spectatorship was one of the ways late Victorians thought about their looking. Not least, thinking about flinching extends the reach of what we might mean by spectatorship. The recoiling body shields itself from contamination, at the same time as becoming caught up in the transmissions of visceral affects, it is simultaneously a reflex jerk and a self-reflexive, relational gesture. At once self-protective, demonstrative, and participatory, flinching reminds us that looking involves not only gazing towards, but becoming aware of oneself as watched, and watching, too.

TWITCHY LIMBS, MORAL TEMPERAMENTS

When Thomas Carlyle published his prophetic *The Signs of the Times* in 1829, he characterized 'Old England' as a land captured by 'frenzies and panics' in which a 'State of Danger' would become the 'condition of things'.[11] The industrialized landscape, with its shrieking trains and clanking machines, and in particular, London, replete with strident hawkers and street musicians, provided plenty of opportunities for the unsuspecting passer-by to be startled. As Charles Dickens, one of the great chroniclers of what Victorians called the 'age of 'auscultation', put it, even at night, when noises faded and merged 'into a distant ringing hum', an explosion, perhaps a gun shot, could make 'the few foot-passengers start, stop and stare about them', arouse the dogs, make cats scamper, and the church clocks, 'as if they were startled too', begin to strike.[12] Embracing the hazards of the technological age, during the 1860s theatregoers enjoyed a vogue for sensation theatre, in which train crashes, shipwrecks, and burning buildings were staged with alarming verisimilitude, to 'hold the spectator breathless, to harrow up his soul, to excite him', leaving him 'thrilled and startled'.[13] While some found pleasure in the city's incessant shocks, others became inured to them, and others still grew so sensitive as to imagine

[11] Thomas Carlyle, 'The Signs of the Times' (1829), in *Critical and Miscellaneous Essays* (Boston: Phillips, Sampson and Company, 1858) pp. 187–95 (p. 187).

[12] John M. Picker, *Victorian Soundscapes* (Oxford and London: Oxford University Press, 2003) p. 6; Charles Dickens, *Bleak House* (1853) (London: Penguin, 1996) p. 749.

[13] Anon., 'Sensational Dramas', *The Era*, 22 January 1881; Anon., 'Theatres', *The Graphic*, 19 March 1881.

dangers omnipresent. The question of why one flinched—from sudden movements in darkened alleyways, from drawn shotguns, loud noises, or vivid hallucinations—was one conceived both in the language of moral temperaments and nervous dispositions. Each gesture, as Benjamin knew, opens up to a 'drama'.

Interest in the 'instinctive movements' of the limbs can be traced back to the writings of Aristotle (384–322 BCE) and Galen (129–216 CE), who believed that parts of the body, even if they were not anatomically connected, could act upon each other through sympathy.[14] In the seventeenth century, René Descartes (1596–1650) argued that it was life-giving 'animal spirits', bouncing rapidly along the muscles and nerves like reflected light (*réfléchi*), which caused him to instinctively withdraw from danger. Using the example of a man who accidentally stepped in a fire, Descartes explained that some of the animal spirits travelled 'to muscles which serve to pull the foot away from the fire, some to muscles which turn the eyes and head to look at it, and some to muscles which make the hands move and the whole body turn in order to protect it'.[15] In 1753, the German physiologist Albrecht von Haller (1708–77) initiated the modern experimental tradition for understanding involuntary recoils and flinches. Placing a lighted taper on the hind leg of a decapitated frog, he noticed that the frog's leg automatically twitched away from the heat. This suggested to Haller that an immaterial soul substance (usually located in the brain, and not normally attributed to frogs) was not necessary to explain automatic gestures. Rather, he argued that power of 'instinctive' movement lay in the muscles themselves, a phenomenon he termed muscular 'irritability'. Less than ten years later, Robert Whytt (1714–66) attempted to disprove Haller's heresy, by showing that a decollated frog, even if it withdrew from painful stimuli, ceased its movements when the marrow was removed from its spine. Whytt had intended to show that muscles alone were not capable of producing involuntary movement, but that a soul or spiritual substance was also required. However, in the process he accidentally provided the first tentative evidence for the existence of a simple spinal reflex.[16]

Sixty years later, in a paper given to the Royal Society of London in 1833, Marshall Hall (1790–1857) gave the first full description of the

[14] Edwin Clarke and L. S. Jacyna, *Nineteenth-Century Origins of Neuroscientific Concepts* (Los Angeles and London: University of California Press, 1987) p. 102.

[15] René Descartes, 'Treatise on Man', trans. John Cottingham, Robert Stoothoff, and Dugald Murdoch, *The Philosophical Writings of Descartes*, i, ed. Cottingham, Stoothoff, and Murdoch (Cambridge: Cambridge University Press, 1985) pp. 99–108 (p. 101–2).

[16] Clarke and Jacyna, *Nineteenth-Century Origins of Neuroscientific Concepts*, p. 105.

spinal reflex system. Replacing the terminology of 'sympathetic', 'instinctive', or 'automatic' reactions with the mechanistic language of the 'reflex arc', he set out what would prove the defining physiological paradigm of the nineteenth century.[17] In a series of experiments on animals including turtles, frogs, snakes, rabbits, and hedgehogs, Hall backed up Whytt's observation that animals could continue to perform automatic responses after being decapitated, but were 'no longer obedient to stimuli' when their spinal marrow was drawn 'gently out of its canal'.[18] The explanation Hall gave was a purely physiological one: impulses were conducted along the spinal cord (*Medulla Spinalis*) to and from the brain stem (*Medulla Oblongata*), in turn producing responses in the peripheral nerves. In his account of the simple spinal system, the body's responses were uniform and predictable, operating as smoothly as a machine. There was no individual agency, and certainly no soul: the body merely responded on its own. However, as the nineteenth century drew on, physiologists became interested in the ways this reliable simple reflex could become corrupted by environments, habits, and even emotions, leaving the body vulnerable to deception and prone to mis-performance.

With the publication of the *Descent of Man* in 1871, and *The Expression of the Emotions in Man and Animals* the following year, Charles Darwin (1809–82) described the human body as subject to a painstakingly slow but perpetual process of transformation. Flinches, he argued, had evolved as a protective mechanism, but at the same time, they were not always reliable responses to the environment. Rather, they could also be the result of the 'vividness of the imagination' and strength of fear: he noted that 'after one violent start' both horses and children are 'very apt to start again'.[19] At the same time as Darwin was writing the *Expression*, the neurologist John Hughlings Jackson (1835–1911) investigated the causes of seizures at the London's National Hospital for Paralysis and Epilepsy. Linking the starting points of his patients' seizures with lesions found in distinct parts of the brain discovered in post-mortem examinations, Hughlings Jackson found evidence that suggested brain injury or disease might affect the smooth operation of even the most simple spinal reflex.[20] In 1906, Charles Scott

[17] Ruth Leys, *From Sympathy to Reflex: Marshall Hall and His Opponents* (New York and London: Garland Publishing, 1990) p. 169.

[18] Marshall Hall, 'On The Reflex Function of the Medulla Oblongata and Medulla Spinalis', *Philosophical Transactions of the Royal Society of London*, 123 (1833) 635–65 (p. 644; p. 646).

[19] Charles Darwin, *The Expression of the Emotions in Man and Animals* (London: Murray, 1872) p. 38.

[20] John Hughlings Jackson, *Clinical and Physiological Researches on the Nervous System* (London: Churchill, 1875).

Sherrington (1857–1952) building on Hughlings Jackson's clinical work, argued that rather than understanding our reflexes to be organized solely around a discrete spinal arc, they should be seen as integrated, with no part of the nervous system capable of responding without also affecting other parts too. Envisaging a pulsing network of stimuli, nerves, muscles, and brain, Sherrington understood that an involuntarily recoil did not only respond to, but could itself be transformed by its environment.[21] The First World War, with its devastating parade of shell-shocked casualties, their hearing heightened and their 'flinch-reflexes' alarmingly exaggerated, provided ample evidence of the malleability of the body's involuntary reactions under stress. Even a movement as simple as withdrawing one's body from sudden danger—one of the most seemingly predictable involuntary acts—could be warped through the persistent fear that characterized life in the trenches. The discovery that the basic reflexes were themselves flexible and able to be 're-educated' gave rise to Ivan Petrovich Pavlov's (1849–1936) stimulus-response experiments on the 'psychic secretions' of dogs begun in the 1890s, and in 1920 to the classical conditioning experiments of John B. Watson and Rosalie Rayner in America.[22] The latter were particularly unnerving for their attempts to condition 'fear reactions' in a toddler Little Albert by striking a hammer against a suspended metal bar each time the child was shown a toy rabbit. Eventually, the 'child started violently' upon seeing the rabbit, 'his breathing was checked and the arms were raised in a characteristic manner'.[23] Within a hundred years of Hall's depiction of a stable and reliable reflex arc, then, physiologists, neurologists, and psychologists had come to believe that involuntary movements could render the body unfamiliar even to its owner, the outside environment capable of distorting even those perceptions and emotions we most take for granted.

Physiological investigations dominated nineteenth-century thinking about flinching. However, this did not mean the gesture was entirely bleached of its older moral associations. Where flinching hardened into an important universal physiological category, it also retained earlier links with cowardice, vacillation, and betrayal. Though it is wordless—although perhaps accompanied by an expletive or cry—a flinch, as any gesture, enjoys what Clifford Geertz called 'thick meanings', signifying as

[21] Charles Scott Sherrington, *Integrative Action of the Nervous System* (New Haven, CT: Yale University Press, 1906).

[22] Ivan Petrovich Pavlov, *Conditioned Reflexes: An Investigation of the Physiological Activity of the Cerebral Cortex*, trans. G. V. Anrep (London: Oxford University Press, 1927).

[23] John B. Watson and Rosalie Rayner, 'Conditioned Emotional Reactions', *Journal of Experimental Psychology*, 3, 1 (1920), 1–14 (p. 2).

a 'speck of behaviour, a fleck of culture'.[24] From the Old French *flenchir, flainchir* ('to turn aside'), according to the *OED* the earliest recorded use of the word 'flinch' or 'flinche' in English appears in John Lyly's proto-novel *The Anatomy of Wit* (1578). For Lyly, to flinch was to turn aside or from someone in an act of treachery or deceit. When a friend steals the hero's fiancée, the latter demands to know: 'if thou wast minded to love me, why dost thou flinche at the last?'[25] Sixteen years later, Thomas Nashe in *The Unfortunate Traveller* (1594) connected flinching to disloyalty and cowardice. Caught trying to sidle off the battlefield, Jack Wilton vociferously denies all wrongdoing, declaring that 'he would not flinch a foot, but make his withered body a buckler, to bear off any blow that should be advanced against him'.[26] One might withdraw through a collapse of valour or resolve, but it was the sorts of people involved in shady dealings who were seen as most liable to flinch from the bonds of subterfuge. In the anonymous comic poem *Dobson's Drie Bobbes* (1607) a group of servants, who have been bunking off in the hayloft and witnessed their mistress cavorting there with her lover (and worse, one of them has accidentally 'pist into hir mistris necke unknowne to hir'), vow to keep their secret until the grave. 'Let us stand to it like frindes', they swear. 'Let them flinch that feares.'[27]

In his earliest incarnations then, the flincher was a disloyal, untrustworthy figure 'who hangs back or gives way, especially in times of crisis' (*OED*). This meaning lingered throughout the nineteenth century. Among the thieves of Victorian London, being unflinching betokened steely inscrutability. 'There was no flinching about the girl' observes Fagin in *Oliver Twist* (1837–8) when he meets Nancy for the first time, and scrutinizes her 'narrowly' for signs of treachery.[28] Almost three hundred years after the hayloft pact, Arthur Conan Doyle described a gang of plotting criminals striking an unscrupulous deal in *The Sign of Four* (1890). 'We have sworn it. The four of us must always act together', one claims. To which his co-conspirator replies, 'You see, Morstan... Small is a man of his word. He does not flinch from his friends. I think we may very well trust him.'[29]

[24] Clifford Geertz, 'Thick Description: Toward an Interpretative Theory of Culture', *The Interpretation of Cultures* (New York: Basic Books, 1973) pp. 3–32 (p. 3).

[25] John Lyly, *Euphues, The Anatomy of Wit; and, Euphues and his England* (1578), ed. Leah Scragg (Manchester: Manchester University Press, 2003) p. 77.

[26] Thomas Nashe, *The Unfortunate Traveller, and Other Works*, ed. John Barry Steane (Harmondsworth: Penguin, 1972) p. 261.

[27] George Dobson, *Dobsons Drie Bobbes. A Story of Sixteenth Century Durham*, ed. Ernest Alan Horsman (London: Oxford University Press, 1955) p. 98.

[28] Charles Dickens, *Oliver Twist* (1838) (London: Penguin, 2003) p. 161.

[29] Arthur Conan Doyle, *The Sign of Four* (1890) (London: Penguin, 2001) p. 112.

It was at the end of the seventeenth century that flinching took on the additional meaning of a sudden movement, in which we 'recoil from something in alarm or repugnance' (*OED*). Wincing (to make 'an involuntary shrinking movement in consequence of or in order to avoid pain') and cringing ('to contract the muscles of the body usually involuntarily', to 'shrink', to 'cower') started to be used interchangeably with 'flinch'. The significance of such movements became most conspicuous through their absence. Children were criticized for their tendency to wince in fear and shock, leading John Locke to advise parents that 'enduring Children gently to suffer some degrees of Pain without shrinking' would give 'firmness to their Minds', courage and resolve—although he also warned that only very trusting children can 'be accustomed to bear very painful and rough usage from you without flinching'.[30] While inured children might over time become unflinching, only women with exceptional courage and self-mastery could manage the task. During her backstage visit to the circus, Queen Victoria moved neither face nor foot when the tiger pounced. Bathsheba Everdene, likewise, wins special praise because she manages, during her brief career as a knife–thrower's assistant in *Far From the Madding Crowd* (1874), not to move a muscle as the blades land around her: 'Bravely born!' says Troy. 'You didn't flinch a shade's thickness. Wonderful in a woman!'[31] To flinch was so closely linked to femininity, that for a man to do so would humiliatingly call his gender into question. Thus, as Thomas Hardy put it in his description of visiting a particularly vigorous hairdresser in *The Return of the Native* (1878), 'to flinch, exclaim, or move a muscle' at the 'scarifications of the neck by the comb, would have been thought a gross breach of good manners' pronouncing you 'no man at once.'[32]

Examples of pathological or excessive flinching reflected these cultural associations. Exaggerated starting was conventionally diagnosed as a female complaint. For example, in 1850 a dictionary of symptoms of the 'disposition, mind and head', prescribed a herbal remedy *Kali Carbonicum* for patients 'easily startled at the least touch'. As the description of the symptoms continues, it becomes clear that women were the archetype for this illness: 'she starts with a loud cry at an imaginary occurrence (e.g. as if a bird flew towards the window).'[33] The degenerate, the insane, the

[30] John Locke, *Some Thoughts Concerning Education* (1693) (London: Churchill, 1712) p. 177.

[31] Thomas Hardy, *Far from the Madding Crowd* (1874) (London: Penguin, 2003) p. 162.

[32] Thomas Hardy, *The Return of the Native* (1878) (London: Penguin, 1999) p. 169.

[33] R. E. Dudgeon, *The Pathogenetic Cyclopaedia: A Systematic Arrangement and Analysis of the Homeopathic Materia Medica, Part I: Containing the Symptoms of the Disposition, Mind and Head* (London: Samuel Highley, 1850) p. 37.

so-called 'primitive' were also seen to be prone to excessive displays of flinching. In 1880, the American neurologist George Miller Beard (1839–83) happened upon a French-Canadian lumberjack community in the Moosehead region of Maine, all of whose members shared a compulsion to start excessively at the least noise. Moreover, their shrieks and recoils were contagious, and did not subside with familiarity to the stimuli (today, the condition is called 'hyperekplexia'). Emphasizing their alterity, and as if describing a novelty circus act, Beard named the community the 'Jumping Frenchmen of Maine.'[34]

While sustaining her gaze was seen as part of Queen Victoria's noble character, and recoiling too readily, a degenerate weakness, flinching and resisting it, was also linked to the unreliable world of theatrical pretence. In Henry Mayhew's account of life in the London slums, first published in 1851, the young boys, as we might imagine, associated recoiling with femininity. 'It is called "plucky" to bear pain without complaining', Mayhew reported. 'To flinch from expected suffering is scorned, and he who does so is sneered at and told to wear a gown, as being more fit to be a woman.' But for Mayhew himself, the boys' unflinching demeanour was something fake rather than a faithful expression of inner resilience. The boys 'show a disregard for pain' and 'delight in tattooing their chests and arms with anchors, and figures of different kinds', he wrote. 'During the whole of this painful operation the boy will not flinch but laugh and joke with his admiring companions as if perfectly at ease.'[35] Far from lamenting the desensitization of the slum-dwellers, Mayhew presented them as inauthentic: they talk '*as if* they were perfectly at ease' (my italics). In a similar vein, the opening pages of George Eliot's *Daniel Deronda* (1876) find Gwendolen wondering about the appropriate response on turning over her hand during a game of roulette. Aware she is being scrutinized by a strange man, she decides that 'she should not flinch'—as, no doubt, she usually does in an appealing girlish display—'but go on playing as if she were indifferent to loss or gain'.[36] When Deronda's unnerving presence causes Gwendolen to quite consciously adapt her female affectations, her flinches emerge as part of a theatrical repertoire of social graces.

Two contexts in which the unreliability of flinches came into focus were the clinic and the theatre. In doctors' surgeries, faking a wince could be a lucrative business. In 1864, the *Medical Times and Gazette* reported on

[34] George Miller Beard, 'Experiments with the Jumpers or Jumping Frenchmen of Maine', *The Journal of Nervous and Mental Disease*, 7 (1880), 487–90.

[35] Henry Mayhew, *London Labour and the London Poor* (1851) (Oxford: Oxford University Press, 2010) p. 24.

[36] George Eliot, *Daniel Deronda* (1876) (London: Penguin 1995) p. 11.

an insurance trial in which a man claimed to have been injured aboard a South–Western Railway train (Mr Ingham was the judge; the witness, an apparently rather gullible doctor):

> MR INGHAM: Did you see him again on the subject?
> WITNESS: Yes, I did about two days afterwards. He complained of great pain in the back. I examined his back, and on pressing the part he seemed to have a great deal of pain.
> MR INGHAM: How did he show it?
> WITNESS: He flinched when I touched him. There was no external mark.

When the man's claim was revealed to be a scam, the judge scolded the physician:

> MR INGHAM: Of course, if a man is shamming illness, he will flinch when you attempt to touch him. I should advise you to be a little more cautious another time.[37]

At the same time in the theatre, a start or recoil was an important part of the repertoire of gestures learnt by actors in the nineteenth century, a rehearsed 'point' through which the performer made visible moments of sudden perception or crises of recognition. As the depiction of 'Terror' in Johann Jacob Engel and Henry Siddons's *Practical Illustrations of Rhetorical Gesture and Action* reveals, jumping away, or shrinking, crouched in horror, were two favoured methods of making fear visible for the audience (Figure 2).[38] If flinching's earliest associations were to deviousness or treachery, then, even the most apparently involuntary of winces and cringes could retain a sheen of insincerity, making those who witnessed them wonder about how reliably outer appearances testified to the remote terrain of inner feelings.

Yet, even if flinching could be a deliberate performance, it could also, to quote Brian Massumi, 'unmake sense by scrambling significations already in place'.[39] Involuntarily starting could create uncanny feelings, estranging the flincher from her own body. In the 1850s, a journalist compared the entire population of China following the Taiping Rebellion of 1850, to a startled person who became 'suddenly conscious through every limb

[37] 'Medical Certificates', *Medical Times and Gazette, 20* (August 1864) repr. in *A Journal of Medical Science Literature, Criticism and News*, ii (London: John Churchill, 1864) p. 200.

[38] Johann Jacob Engel and Henry Siddons, *Practical Illustrations of Rhetorical Gesture and Action, Adapted to the English Drama*, trans. Henry Siddons (London: Richard Phillips, 1807) p. 91.

[39] Brian Massumi, *Parables for the Virtual: Movement, Affect, Sensation* (Durham: Duke University Press, 2002) p. 1.

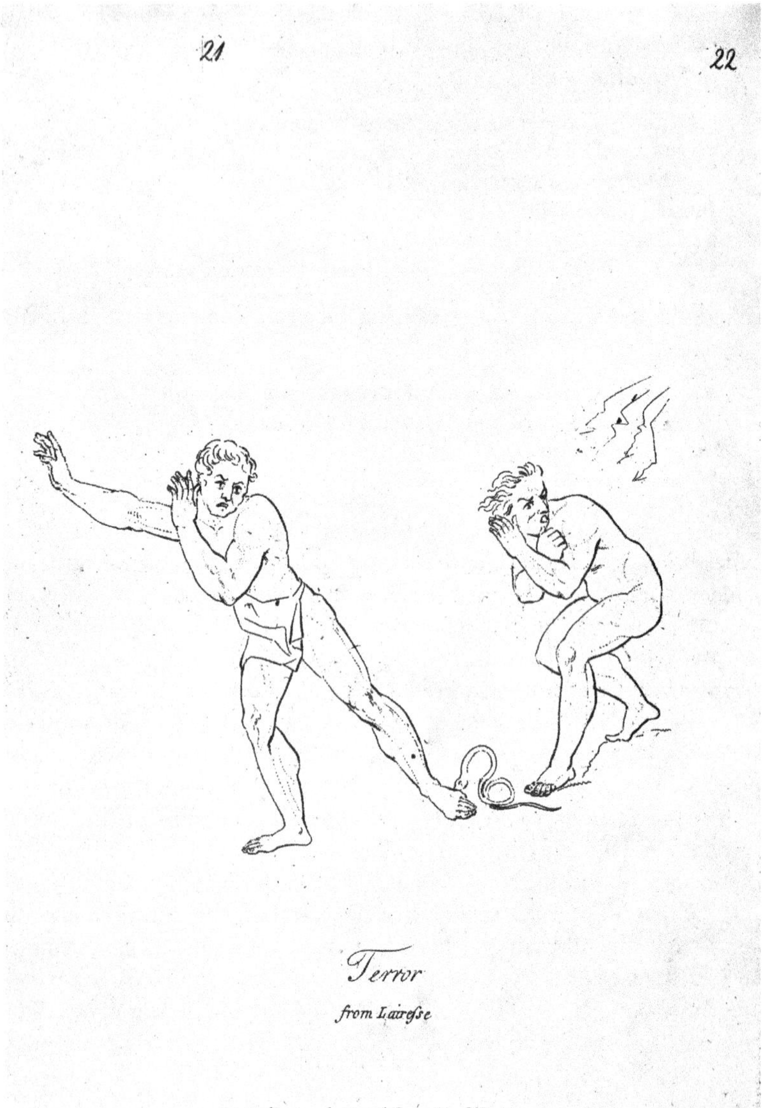

Fig. 2. *Terror*, figs. 21 and 22, Johann Jacob Engel and Henry Siddons, *Practical Illustrations of Rhetorical Gesture and Action, Adapted to the English Drama*, trans. Henry Siddons, 2nd edn. (London: Sherwood, Neely, and Jones, 1822) p.102.

and nerve of a living power' it had 'never dreamt of exercising'.[40] If such quasi-electrical surges of attention might feel unfamiliar, the strength of a person's response to fear or shock could also rattle a person's sense of themselves as an intentional, purposeful being. In 1890, the psychologist William James recalled seeing a young boy startled by a passing train:

> The other day I was standing at a railroad station with a little child, when an express-train went thundering by. The child, who was near the edge of the platform, started, winked, had his breathing convulsed, turned pale, burst out crying, and ran frantically towards me and hid his face. I have no doubt that this youngster *was almost as much astonished by his own behaviour as he was by the train.* (my italics)

To feel 'one of these explosions' for the first time, wrote William James, was 'an entirely novel experience'. While the next time the child encountered a similarly frightening train, he might be able to 'foresee' his own conduct, each flinch or start would nonetheless always be as 'involuntary and uncontrollable' as the first.[41] For James, as we shall see in the first chapter, such emotional responses foregrounded the idea that subjective emotional feelings followed on from the body's reflex responses, rather than preceding them. In the work of those who reflected on theatre-going in the 1860s and 70s, a similar dislocation of inner feeling and outward, visceral affects can be detected. For audiences of this period's so-called 'sensation theatre', being 'thrilled and startled' by its thunder machines and collapsing scenery was an indispensible part of the spine-tingling pleasures of the evening. Yet, such visceral pleasures were also seen to be shallow. Not only did audiences feed 'their eye with an empty picture', but in flinching, they entered an economy of surfaces in which 'empty' bodily reflexes rather than profound emotional experiences were enjoyed.[42] In flinches discussed in both theatrical and psychological contexts, then, the relationship between inner feelings and outward performances was rearranged.

Flinches may heighten our senses, making us alert and defensive. Yet, they can also transgress our boundaries, transmitted like viruses among crowds, or performed in bodily sympathy as when we wince from another's pain. While a flinch enfolds, protects, and betrays, it also suggests porous ways of being, pointing up visceral co-experience and the wandering of bodily affects. We might recoil *from* a sudden noise or dangerous sight in defence and self-protection, but we also wince *with*, in fellowship.

[40] 'The Revolution in China', *The Eclectic Magazine of Foreign Literature, Science and Art*, 31 (New York: Bidwell, 1854) p. 91.

[41] William James, *The Principles of Psychology*, ii, 2 vols. (New York: Holt, 1890) p. 487–8.

[42] Anon., 'Theatres', *The Graphic*, 19 March 1881.

The flinch James described emphasized the way emotions protected for the purposes of survival. But throughout the nineteenth century, flinching also came to exemplify the vicarious feelings associated with sympathy and later, empathy. The eighteenth-century moralist Adam Smith made sympathetic flinching a cornerstone of his *Theory of Moral Sentiments*: 'when we see a stroke aimed, and just ready to fall upon the leg or arm of another person, we naturally shrink and draw back our own leg or our own arm', he wrote, 'and when it does fall, we feel it in some measure, and are hurt by it as well as the sufferer.'[43] For Smith, our capacity to imaginatively put ourselves in the position of another underpinned our moral sense. During the nineteenth century, the link between wincing and intimate sympathy continued. For William Godwin in *Fleetwood, or, the New Man of Feeling* (1805), vicarious flinches spoke of innate fellowship: 'if there is a being who feels the blow under which I flinch, in whom my sensations are by a kind of necessity echoed and repeated, that being is a part of myself.'[44] Wincing at another's pain usually testified to kindness and compassion, but could also betray the flincher, reconfiguring the gesture's already established links to treachery. In Elizabeth Barrett Browning's translation of Aeschylus's *Prometheus Bound* (1897), the errant god is forced to witness the horrifying spectacle of a battle between mankind and Zeus's army. He cringes as the humans are defeated:

STRENGTH: Dost thou flinch again
  And breathe groans for the enemies of Zeus?
  Beware lest thine own pity find thee out
HEPHAESTUS: Thou dost behold a spectacle that turns
  The sight o' the eyes to pity.[45]

It is, of course, only because Hephaestus's flinches are themselves so visible that his sympathy endangers him. Through his involuntary performance before the pitiful show, the watching God makes a spectacle of himself too.

While throughout the nineteenth century, recoiling spectators shirked and avoided, demonstrating their womanish fear or working-class spinelessness, they also found ways of experiencing each other's feelings through viscerally felt complicity. If the uncanny automatism of involuntarily flinching could unnerve and disrupt, flinches could also be learnt responses, carefully choreographed with an audience in mind. In all cases, however, like Hephaestus, by virtue of their virtuoso muscular displays, flinchers did not only watch, but found themselves part of the show. The

[43] Adam Smith, *The Theory of Moral Sentiments* (1759) (London: Millar, 1761) p. 4.

[44] William Godwin, *Fleetwood, or, the New Man of Feeling* (1805) (London: Bentley, 1853) p. 179.

[45] Elizabeth Barrett Browning, *Poetical Works* (London: Elder, 1897) p. 142.

implications of thinking of flinchers as simultaneously affective and performative may come into focus through recourse to a distinctive German model of spectatorship: *Schaulust.*

SCHAULUST

In the history of flinching audience members, the tale of Leontius, told by Socrates in Plato's *The Republic*, is something of a foundational myth. Among Athenians it was a famous story—'yes I've heard the story too', says Glaucon.[46] One day Leontius was walking back to Athens from the Peiraeus, when, outside the city's walls, he saw an executioner. At the executioner's feet lay several corpses, about to be shunted off the edge of the ravine, to rot or be pecked by vultures. 'On the one hand', says Socrates, Leontius, 'experienced the desire to see them.' But at the same time 'he felt disgust and averted his gaze' ('he tried to divert himself from it' according to a different translation, 'he tried to turn aside' according to a third).[47] At first glance, Leontius's recoil appears to spring from overwhelming feelings of disgust, and his flinch seems to contain him: his hands clamped over his eyeballs, his body crumpled in on itself, he holds himself together against the deformation threatened by corpses. For Socrates, the tale of Leontius warns of the dangers of flinching at scenes of horror, for such visceral and overpowering responses loosen the mind's grip on itself, compromising a cornerstone virtue of the Athenian *polis*, one's self–possession (one's *sophrosyne*, or *saophrosynê*). Variously translated as 'self–knowledge', 'soundness of mind', 'sobriety', and 'knowing one's place' *sophrosyne*, was, as Helen North points out, a politically invested concept. Usurpers, Persians, and other luxurists—Achilles, for example, who as Socrates complains, is portrayed 'as generally weeping and wailing' (3.388.a–b)—are distinctly un–*sophrosyne*; suppliant maidens and demure youths such as Odysseus's son Telemachus, have *sophrosyne* in spades.[48] The dangerous over-emotionality of wincing and cringing gave Socrates at least one reason for censoring all the 'horrifying and frightening' plays and poems. 'We must get rid, too of all the ghosts and corpses, and all other things of this

[46] Plato, *The Republic*, trans. Desmond Lee (Harmondsworth: Penguin, 1988), IV 439e–440a, pp. 215–16. Hereafter all citations will be to this translation, unless otherwise specified, and will appear as book, section, and line number in parentheses in the text.

[47] Plato, *The Republic*, p. 216; Plato, *The Republic*, trans. A. D. Lindsay (London: Dent and Sons, 1906) p. 128; Plato, *The Republic*, trans. John Llewelyn Davies and David James Vaughan, ed. Andrea Tschemplik (Oxford: Rowman and Littlefield 2005) p. 159.

[48] Helen North, *Sophrosyne: Self-Knowledge and Self-Restraint in Greek Literature* (New York: Cornell University Press, 1966) p. 3.

kind, whose very names are enough to make everyone who hears them shudder' (3.387.c). Leontius's flinch before the corpses incurs a loss of self-possession—and points up the threat of being possessed by others too.

In her passionately argued essay *Regarding the Pain of Others* (2003), Susan Sontag invokes Leontius's predicament, arguing that his flinch symbolizes an embattled consciousness, a struggle between a desire to see, and his obedience to an injunction to turn aside.[49] Because of his guilt-ridden morbid fascination, Sontag describes Leontius as a voyeur. Yet, if Leontius is a voyeur, he does not spy secretively on a forbidden scene, like peeping Tom—who in Alfred Tennyson's poem *Godiva* (1840) bore 'a little auger-hole in fear' to spy on the naked noblewoman.[50] Nor does he, like the cinematic voyeur imagined by the film theorist Laura Mulvey in the 1970s, sit hidden in the dark, with the illusion of being both alone and of 'looking in on a private world'.[51] Leontius is not alone, but is watched silently by the executioner, who perhaps stands in for the readers of *The Republic* themselves. At the edge of the ravine, having turned corpses into spectacles, Leontius turns himself into theatre too. His performance of 'will I, won't I look?' enthralling for those who watch him, also seems to provide Leontius with more enjoyment than the corpses alone promise. Leontius is overexcited: his pleasure resides not so much in peering *at* corpses, 'subjecting them to a controlling and curious gaze', as in flinching from them.[52] In this way, he participates in a curious kind of spectatorial game. While for Sontag, Leontius's flinch signifies an inner turmoil, she also recognizes the contradictory gratifications of the visceral movement itself. 'There is the satisfaction of being able to look at the image without flinching,' she observes, but there is also 'the pleasure in flinching'.[53] Just as M. fashioned a flinch in the art gallery before the self-consciously recoiling boy in the painting, and in turn was watched by me, so Leontius became both a performer and audience member. Alongside the executioner and the dead bodies, Leontius entered into what Jacques Rancière has called a 'choreographic community, where no one remains a static spectator', but rather deciding where to watch is to participate.[54]

[49] Susan Sontag, *Regarding the Pain of Others* (London: Hamish Hamilton, 2003) pp. 86–7.

[50] Alfred Tennyson, 'Godiva' (1842) repr. in *The Poetical Works of Alfred Tennyson* (Boston: Ticknor and Fields, 1860) p. 196–8 (p. 198).

[51] Laura Mulvey, 'Visual Pleasure and Narrative Cinema' (1975), in *Visual and Other Pleasures* (London: Macmillan, 1989) pp. 14–28 (p. 17).

[52] Mulvey, 'Visual Pleasure and Narrative Cinema', p. 17.

[53] Sontag, *Regarding the Pain of Others*, p. 37.

[54] Jacques Rancière, *The Emancipated Spectator*, trans. Gregory Elliott (London and New York: Verso, 2009) p. 5.

The term used by Mulvey to describe the voyeur's pleasure—'scopophilia'—is a word used widely in Anglophone psychoanalytic literature. It is a Greek translation of the German *Schaulust*, the word first used by Freud to describe the 'perversion' of voyeurism in the *Three Essays on the Theory of Sexuality* (1905).[55] In fact, 'scopophilia'—or 'scoptophilia' as it was originally spelt—is a neologism, and its coinage was the result of an intriguing translation blunder. James Strachey, who oversaw the translation of Freud's complete works in the 1920s, admitted in 1962 that 'the Glossary Committee disgraced itself lamentably' over the question of 'how to translate *Schaulust*—the pleasure in looking. Greek terminology was all the rage, and the word "scoptophilia" was accepted with acclamation.' He continued:

> You might have imagined we should have remembered telescopes and microscopes and so have suspected that the Greek root for looking was something like 'scop.' Actually there is a Greek root 'scop' but what it means is 'to make fun of.' And so to this day you may still come upon references to the component sexual instinct of pleasure in derision.[56]

The mis-translation opens up a suggestive alternative to the voyeur's solitary, silent, and mastering gaze. Perhaps it is through its proximity to the Greek word *scotophilia*, or love of darkness, that *scoptophilia* has become synonymous with fantasies of separateness and hiding, of gazing in on a private world. The original German *Schaulust*, however, evoked a broader range of spectatorial pleasures, ones that resonate with the unintended meaning of *scopophilia*: the *Schaulustige* makes fun of—or perhaps, makes fun out of—looking.

Whilst in anglophone psychoanalytic literature *Schaulust* is often translated as 'the sexual pleasure in looking', the etymology of the word enjoys wider meanings.[57] *Lust*, which can mean desire or appetite, also designates less forceful enjoyment: to have *Lust* (*Lust haben*) is to feel like doing something (*ich habe Lust, diesen Film zu sehen*, I feel like watching this film; *ich habe Lust, in den Park zu gehen*, I fancy going to the park). And while the *schau* in *Schaulust* is the root of the German verb *schauen* to see, *die Schau* is a show: *eine Schau machen*, to put on a show, *etwas zur Schau tragen*, to make a show of something, to make something into a show.

[55] Sigmund Freud, 'Three Essays on the Theory of Sexuality' (1905), trans. and ed. James Strachey, *The Standard Edition of the Complete Psychological Works of Sigmund Freud*, vii, 24 vols. (London: Hogarth Press, 1974) pp. 123–231 (p. 157).

[56] James Strachey, 'Obituary of Joan Riviere, 1883–1962', *International Journal of Psycho-analysis*, 44 (1963) 228–30 (p. 229).

[57] Acknowledging the difficulty of translating *Schaulust*, Bruno Bettelheim suggested a translation along the lines of 'the sexual pleasure in looking'. Bruno Bettelheim, *Freud and Man's Soul* (London: Chatto & Windus, 1982) p. 91.

Thus, the *schau/Schau* in *Schaulust* brings together the activities of watching and being seen, and a *Schaulustige* may be thought of as someone who wants to look, but who also performs their looking for others to watch. It is a double meaning that recalls the German word for a theatrical performance or play, *das Schauspiel—spielen*, to play, *schauen* to watch, *die Schau*, that which is there to be seen—so that the pleasures of theatre-going, like the pleasures of *Schaulust*, may involve playing at looking, and playing at being seen looking. A *Schaulustige*, therefore, might be one who, like M., participates in the spectacle they observe by performing alongside it. Or who like Leontius, finds pleasure in their own emotional performance as much as in the show provided. Or one who—as did I whilst watching M. in the gallery—performs their winces and cringes self-consciously for the benefit of other audience members, making a show of their watching and turning the act of spectatorship into a kind of theatre itself.

The translation blunder is also interesting because it reminds us that the problem of looking Freud was engaging with was not altogether abstract, but born out of a very particular set of historical circumstances. When Freud chose the word *Schaulust* to describe the sexual instinct or drive (*Triebe*) of looking, he did so in the context of a public outcry over *Schaulust* in German-speaking countries. This was a debate about how to look that pitted the objective or studious gaze of the cultivated German against the visceral, overexcited pleasures of boisterous, uneducated, and working-class audiences. At the centre of the controversy were the *Völkerschau*—literally, 'people shows'; in Britain, these same pseudo-scientific exhibits of people from the African colonies were called 'Human Zoos'.[58] Part scientific exhibitions, part immersive theatrical spectacles in which men and women from Europe's colonies enacted 'primitive' rituals, the *Völkerschau* prompted public debate about the emotionality and suggestibility of their audiences. As Sierra A. Bruckner notes, 'in the eyes of the middle-classes the "objective" way of seeing of the cultivated German seemed to be giving way to *Schaulust*, the untutored "lust to look" and undisciplined behaviours of gawking spectators', leading the impresarios who organized the *Völkerschau* to employ scholars to certify that exhibitions served 'scientific purposes', and not entertainment ones.[59] The bodily excesses of the

[58] Nadja Durbach, 'London, Capital of Exotic Exhibitions from 1830–1860', in *Human Zoos: Science and Spectacle in the Age of Colonial Empires*, ed. Pascal Blanchard et al. (Liverpool: Liverpool University Press, 2008) pp. 81–8 (pp. 81–7).

[59] Sierra A. Bruckner, 'Spectacle of (Human) Nature: Commercial Ethnography between Leisure, Learning and *Schaulust*', in *Worldly Provincialism: German Anthropology in the Age of Empire*, ed. Penny H. Glenn and Matti Buzi (Ann Arbor: University of Michigan Press, 2003) pp. 127–55 (p. 129).

theatricalized audience, who flinched and cringed, pointed, laughed, and gawked were set against the 'silent and gestureless' ideal gaze of an educated scientific observer.[60] If the second part of the nineteenth century was a period in which scientific objectivity hardened into a distinctive way of looking, this change came hand in hand with a more clearly defined notion of its antithesis—the emotional, noisy, and theatrical audience member. Perhaps it is telling that in German-speaking countries, the problem of passionate looking emerged in the context of the public exhibition of scientific curiosities. In Britain too, scientific practices raised uncomfortable questions about the distinction between legitimate and illegitimate types of spectatorship, questions which emerged in irate letters to newspapers and anti-vivisection polemics as well as in the scientific articles, laboratory notebooks, and speeches from the heart of the scientific establishment itself. Despite the many attempts to tease them apart, *Schaulust* lingered in scientific looking, not always an opposition to an ideal and restrained gaze, but sometimes part and parcel of the very techniques that defined objectivity itself.

THEATRES OF SCIENCE

The past thirty years have witnessed an expansion of scholarly activity exploring the conduits of transmission and exchange between nineteenth-century scientific ideas and their wider culture. As Laura Salisbury and Andrew Shail have put it, scholars have unearthed reciprocal connections between science and fiction, poetry, painting, photography, and film-making which often run 'in unexpected directions'.[61] The mutually enfolding discourses of scientific writing and Victorian literature have been explored to great effect by Gillian Beer, Sally Shuttleworth, George Levine, Laura Otis, and David Amigoni and to name only a few.[62] Mapping

[60] Foucault, *The Birth of the Clinic*, p. 131.

[61] Laura Salisbury and Andrew Shail, 'Introduction', *Neurology and Modernity: A Cultural History of Nervous Systems 1800–1950* (Basingstoke: Palgrave Macmillan, 2010) pp. 1–41 (p. 9).

[62] There are far too many recent works to list here, but Laura Otis's introduction to *Literature and Science in the Nineteenth Century: An Anthology*, ed. Laura Otis (Oxford: Oxford University Press, 2002) p. 17–28, provides a useful overview, as does Salisbury and Shail's introduction to *Neurology and Modernity: A Cultural History of Nervous Systems 1800–1950*, ed. Salisbury and Shail, pp. 1–41. See also: Gillian Beer (ed.) *Open Fields: Science in Cultural Encounter* (Oxford: Clarendon Press, 1996); Sally Shuttleworth, *The Mind of the Child: Child Development in Literature, Science, and Medicine 1840–1900* (Oxford: Oxford University Press, 2010); George Levine, *Darwin* the *Writer* (Oxford: Oxford University Press, 2011); Laura Otis, *Networking: Communicating with Bodies and Machines in the Nineteenth Century* (Michigan: University of Michigan Press,

the relationship between the visual arts and practices of scientific imagery has also proved fruitful in showing how the nineteenth-century's iconography of nature was deeply embedded in aesthetic modes of representation.[63] Given how important this burst of interdisciplinary activity has been for our understanding of nineteenth-century culture, it is a surprise that the interactions between science and that cornerstone of Victorian entertainment, the theatre, has not been more closely studied. The role of theatricality in early modern science and medicine, with its alchemical theatres and mysterious transformations wrought on the body by the passions and humours, have yielded rich rewards for cultural historians. As Stanton Garner has argued, this was in part because in this period illness and its treatment were already 'so deeply implicated in the theatrical'. He continues that in the nineteenth century, the epistemological and practical concerns of science and theatre diverged; with their syphmographs, photographs, and cultivation of objectivity, science and medicine 'proceeded in less performative directions'.[64] Certainly, the influence of science on late nineteenth-century theatre has been part of a number of important studies, including Joseph Roach's examination of the influence of psychology on actor training, Stanton Garner's work on the impact of scientific objectivity on the naturalist aesthetic, Jane Goodall's investigation of the many surprising ways the idea of evolution found its way onto the popular stage, and Kirsten Shepherd-Barr's exploration of the ways playwrights have mined scientific ideas in both the thematic and formal aspects of their work.[65] However, the relationship between science and theatre explored in these works has largely been construed as unreciprocated.

Yet, it is not true to say that theatre played absolutely no role in nineteenth-century scientific life, or indeed that its contribution has been entirely overlooked. Public exhibitions were an important part of Victorian scientific and medical culture. At London's University College

2001); David Amigoni, *Colonies, Cults and Evolution: Literature, Science and Culture in Nineteenth-Century Writing* (Cambridge: Cambridge University Press, 2007); Anne Stiles, *Popular Fiction and Brain Science in the Late Nineteenth Century* (Cambridge: Cambridge University Press, 2012).

[63] See: Jonathan Smith, *Charles Darwin and Victorian Visual Culture* (Cambridge: Cambridge University Press, 2006); Barbara Larson and Fae Brauer (eds.) *The Art of Evolution: Darwin, Darwinisms, and Visual Culture* (Lebanon: Dartmouth College Press, 2009); Colette Colligan and Margaret Linley, *Media, Technology, and Literature in the Nineteenth Century: Image, Sound, Touch* (Farnham: Ashgate, 2011).

[64] Stanton B. Garner, Jr., 'Introduction: Is There a Doctor in the House?' pp. 315–16.

[65] Stanton B. Garner Jr., 'Artaud, Germ Theory, and the Theatre of Contagion', *Theatre Journal*, 58, 1 (2006) 1–14; Joseph Roach, *The Player's Passion*; Jane Goodall, *Performance and Evolution in the Age of Darwin: Out of the Natural Order* (London: Routledge, 2002); Kirsten Shepherd-Barr, *Science on Stage*.

Hospital in the 1850s, epileptic and hysterical patients undergoing astonishing personality changes under mesmeric influence were paraded before experts to show the efficacy of the treatment. In France in the 1880s, Charcot's Tuesday demonstrations of hysterical women at the Salpêtrière, were carefully crafted theatrical extravaganzas which proved enduringly popular with medical students. As Georges Didi-Huberman, Elaine Showalter, and Alison Winter among others have argued, these theatrical shows had far-reaching consequences for treatment, not least because framing hysterical patients as actresses called into question the authenticity of their illness and severity of their suffering.[66] At the same time, the latest scientific discoveries proved an enduring attraction for novelty-seeking Victorians. Travelling fairground shows depicting 'wonders of the natural world'—among them, mermaids, giants, and learned animals—proved enduringly attractive. Meanwhile, in the cities, enterprising commercial galleries of practical science such as London's Adelaide Gallery and the Royal Polytechnic Institution, presented flash-bang demonstrations of electromagnetics and pyrotechnics alongside conjuring shows and dissolving views, further blurring the boundaries between entertainment and edification. Even at the Royal Institution, the home of elite science, celebrated lecturers Michael Faraday and John Tyndall were not immune from the lure of the spotlight: astonishing the public with experiments in physics and chemistry, they acted as ringmasters 'pulling in crowds and amazing them with nature's secrets' to make 'science and its products real to their audiences'.[67]

As Bernard Lightman and Iwan Morus among others have argued, it is important to see these theatrical spectacles as part and parcel of the creation of scientific knowledge in the Victorian period.[68] Even after the emergence of the fully professionalized scientist working in university laboratories towards the end of the century, scientific enquiry continued to take place in heterogeneous spaces. The proximity of scientific enquiry and theatrical entertainment may itself call into question straightforward distinctions between the activities of experimentation and demonstration. There are many examples of popular theatrical exhibitions shaping the substance of

[66] Georges Didi-Huberman, *The Invention of Hysteria: Charcot and the Photographic Iconography of the Salpêtrière* (1982), trans. Alisa Hartz (Cambridge, MA and London: MIT Press, 2003); Elaine Showalter, *The Female Malady: Women, Madness and English Culture 1830–1980* (London: Virago Press, 1985); Alison Winter, *Mesmerized: Powers of Mind in Victorian Britain* (Chicago: University of Chicago Press, 2000).

[67] Morus, "More the Aspect of Magic than Anything Natural", p. 337.

[68] Iwan Rhys Morus, 'Worlds of Wonder: Sensation and the Victorian Scientific Performance', *Isis*, 101 (2010) 806–16; Bernard Lightman, *Victorian Popularizers of Science* (Chicago and London: University of Chicago Press, 2007).

scientific discoveries, as when the Hunterian museum purchased the skeletons of dead circus attractions for anatomical investigations, or experimenters devised ever-more elaborate technologies to meet the voracious demands of the general public eager to be astonished by new scientific inventions. For some observers, attending a scientific demonstration felt like being part of, or at least present at, the making of new knowledge. As Morus has discussed, a journalist from *The Times* who witnessed a demonstration of Professor Pepper's Great Induction Coil in 1869, spoke of the machine, with its 'effects, beautiful or terrible, such have never been seen before', as 'an instrument of discovery as much as demonstration'. Morus concludes that 'looking at events such as this one and the sites where they took place should therefore provoke us to re-examine conventional distinctions... between backstage experimentation and public exhibition' and encourage us to pay further attention to the role of theatre and performance in the 'process of constructing Victorian science'.[69]

However, Morus's suggestion that scholars pay heed to the role of theatre in Victorian experiments should be read in the context of a larger 'performative turn' in the history, sociology, and philosophy of science. It has been almost twenty-five years since the word 'performance' started to appear in articles and books which sought to emphasize the importance of experiments in creating scientific knowledge. Instead of celebrating the contemplative acts of lone heroic discoverers, a new vanguard of philosophers such as Ian Hacking and Andrew Pickering drew attention to the communal endeavour of scientists, and the way their discoveries were shaped by multiple historical and cultural forces. For Pickering, the idiom of performativity brought into focus the agency of bustling networks of practices, people, and machines.[70] Experimental techniques performed repeatedly, whether by precision instrument or a laboratory technician, could do more than simply 'represent' reality, they might 'intervene' in it too.[71]

It is important to note, however, that the word 'performance' typically appears in discussions of experiments. Words like 'theatre', 'stage', and 'showmanship' are freely used to describe the scientist's flamboyant encounters with the general public, but in relation to the relative solitude of the laboratory, talk of 'performance' prevails.[72] The diverse meanings

[69] Morus, "More the Aspect of Magic than Anything Natural", p. 337.

[70] Andrew Pickering, *The Mangle of Practice: Time, Agency, and Science* (Chicago: University of Chicago Press, 1995) p. 7.

[71] Ian Hacking, *Representing and Intervening: Introductory Topics in the Philosophy of Natural Science* (Cambridge: Cambridge University Press, 1983). See also: David C. Gooding, 'Experiment', in *A Companion to the Philosophy of Science*, ed. W. H. Newton-Smith (Oxford: Blackwell, 2000) pp. 117–26 (p. 124).

[72] For a further discussion of this point, see: Tiffany Watt Smith, 'Cardboard, Conjuring and "A Very Curious Experiment"', *Interdisciplinary Science Reviews*, 38, 4 (2013), 306–20.

accrued by the terms 'performativity' and 'theatricality', and the relationship between them, has been the subject of intense debate among performance theorists.[73] In science studies, the implications of thinking in terms of performativity stands in opposition to the representative demands of theatre: while 'the representational idiom casts science as…an activity that seeks to represent nature, to produce knowledge that maps, *mirrors, or corresponds* to how the world really is' (my italics), approaching scientific culture as a network of performances circumvents 'fears about the adequacy' of these representations.[74] In such a context, the paradigm of performativity is, as the theatre scholar Nicholas Ridout tantalizingly puts it, 'more innocent' than that of theatre. 'Theatre is guilty and it knows it', writes Ridout. It is guilty of emotional excess and mis-performance, over-dramatization and pretence, of deceptions, illusions, and representations.[75] By focusing more neutrally on *things done*, rather than more guiltily on *things being pretended to be done*, talk of performativity can skirt over the more problematic dimensions of theatricality, providing a sometimes anaemic version of embodied scientific encounters.

Morus is right to say that there was 'no unidirectional trajectory from laboratory to theatre' in the nineteenth century, 'but rather, a complex interplay', and his suggestion that thinking about performances may help us to understand both the 'relatively private acts' of experiments and 'the relatively public ones of cajoling and persuading an audience' is important.[76] However, it only goes so far. Aside from acknowledging that Victorian science was always already implicated in its wider theatrical culture, it remains unclear how exactly this would have shaped the 'relatively private' acts of scientific practice and discoveries. This book makes a stronger claim. It argues that while we might expect theatricality to characterize the moments science overtly 'showed-off' before paying crowds, its guilty charades also lurked around the processes of devising and enacting experiments, using instruments, making observations, collating results, phrasing ideas, and forging new concepts. Though its argument takes place against a backdrop of already theatricalized scientific culture, this book focuses on experiments where the scientist performed for none other than

[73] See: Tracy C. Davis and Thomas Postlewait 'Theatricality: An Introduction' in *Theatricality*, ed. Tracy Davis and Thomas Postlewait (Cambridge: Cambridge University Press, 2003) pp. 127–55; Erika Fischer-Lichte, 'Theatricality: A Key Concept in Theatre and Cultural Studies', *Theatre Research International*, 20, 2 (1995) 85–9 (p. 85).

[74] Pickering, *The Mangle of Practice*, p. 5.

[75] Nicholas Ridout, *Stage Fright, Animals, and Other Theatrical Problems* (Cambridge: Cambridge University Press, 2006) p. 4.

[76] Morus, 'Worlds of Wonder', p. 814.

himself, his collaborators, or his experimental monkeys. Moreover, whilst Morus invokes a very general notion of Victorian theatre, *On Flinching* takes very seriously the idea that historically specific theatrical problems and techniques were part of the performativity of everyday 'relatively private' acts of nineteenth-century experimental scientific practice.

In the four experiments discussed in this book, experimenters utilized a range of distinctive theatrical techniques, producing recognizably theatrical interactions between their own bodies and those they observed. In so doing, these men of science found themselves straying close to the condition of theatrical audiences, and in turn, were tormented by the problems of theatrical representation in their pursuit of objective looking. Extending the arguments of Pickering, Morus, and Lightman, then, this book should also act as a counterpoint to the emphasis placed by Daston and Gallison on the role of mechanical or self-recording technologies in the cultivation of scientific objectivity in the period, with by arguing that alongside the photograph and sphymograph, theatre continued to be used as an apparatus for making the emotional body visible. Moreover, by focusing on the theatricality of experiments, this book suggests unexpected ways for exploring the easy-to-overlook embodied and affective aspects of scientific looking, what Christopher Lawrence and Steven Shapin have called 'the embodied form and vicissitudes' of scientific ideas.[77] With its sleight of hand and misdirection, its missed connections between form and content, its emotionality, dissimulation, and queasy slippages between seeming and being, the untrustworthy world of theatre, once it had wandered into the space of experimentation, brought forth many feelings, among them uncertainty, amusement, and embarrassment. Through these emotional experiences, the scientific observer became acutely aware of his own presence as a passionate actor in the experimental encounter. In turn, when we explore these performances alongside those of his theatrical counterparts, a distinctive motif of looking in the late nineteenth and early twentieth century comes into view.

LOOKING, EMOTION, AND THEATRICALITY

There are aspects of human experience that until a few decades ago would not have seemed worthy subjects of academic study. The body, its sensations and emotions have become hot topics, and histories of the senses,

[77] Christopher Lawrence and Steven Shapin, 'Introduction: The Body of Knowledge', in *Science Incarnate: Historical Embodiments of Natural Knowledge*, ed. Lawrence and Shapin (Chicago and London: University of Chicago Press, 1988) pp. 1–21 (pp. 2–3).

including smelling, tasting, and touching, as well as studies of specific passions such as fear, laughter, or boredom have yielded significant new ways of thinking about the past.[78] For those studying the nineteenth century, questions of looking and visuality have proved enduringly compelling. Jonathan Crary, Kate Flint, Isobel Armstrong, Chris Otter, and Martin Willis, among others, have shown how the nineteenth century's newly industrialized environments and its proliferation of new optical technologies transformed the way Victorians thought and wrote about the relationship of the perceiving subject to the perceived world.[79] In addition to spectacular new mass entertainment technologies such as the diorama and popular optical toys such as the stereoscope, Victorians also renegotiated their role as observers with each new medical discovery (such as the X-ray), architectural innovation (e.g. fully glazed buildings), or strategy for monitoring institutional spaces (such as prisons, schools, and libraries). Intellectual historians have approached these machines, practices, spaces, and objects as, to use Deleuze and Guattari's evocative phrase, '*assemblages*', networks through which metaphorical and material practices intersect.[80] As Friedrich Kittler has put it, we can begin to understand how that culture may have thought about themselves as observers,

[78] For an overview of the current work being done on the histories of Victorian senses see Colligan and Linley, *Image, Sound and Touch*. See also: *Alain Corbin, Odor and the French Social Imagination* (1982), trans. Aubier Montaigne (Oxford: Berg, 1986); David Howes, *Empire of the Senses* (Oxford: Berg, 2004); Constance Classen, *The Deepest Sense: A Cultural History of Touch* (Chicago: University of Illinois Press, 2012). For an overview of current work in the history of emotions, see Susan J. Matt, 'Current Emotion Research in History: Or, Doing History from the Inside Out', *Emotion Review* 3, 1 (2011) 117–24. See also: Patricia Meyer Spacks, *Boredom: The Literary History of a State of Mind* (Chicago and London: University of Chicago Press, 1995); Joanna Bourke, *Fear: A Cultural History* (London: Virago, 2005); William Reddy, *The Making of Romantic Love: Longing and Sexuality in Europe, South Asia, and Japan, 900–1200* (Chicago and London: University of Chicago Press, 2012).

[79] For the genealogy of current interest in nineteenth-century visuality, see Vanessa R. Schwartz and Jeannene M. Przyblyski, 'Visual Culture's History: Twenty-First-Century Interdisciplinarity and its Nineteenth-Century Objects' in *The Nineteenth-Century Visual Culture Reader*, ed. Schwartz and Przyblyski (London: Routledge, 2004) pp. 3–14. See also: Jonathan Crary, *Techniques of the Observer: On Vision and Modernity in the Nineteenth Century* (Cambridge, MA and London: MIT Press, 1992); Kate Flint, *The Victorians and the Visual Imagination* (Cambridge: Cambridge University Press, 2000); Isobel Armstrong, *Victorian Glassworlds: Glass Culture and the Imagination 1830–1880* (Oxford: Oxford University Press, 2008); Chris Otter, *The Victorian Eye* (Chicago: University of Chicago Press, 2008); Luisa Calè and Patrizia Di Bello (eds.) *Illustrations, Optics and Objects in Nineteenth–Century Literary and Visual Cultures*; Martin Willis, *Vision, Science and Literature, 1870–1920: Ocular Horizons* (Pickering and Chatto, 2011).

[80] Gilles Deleuze and Félix Guattari, *A Thousand Plateaus: Capitalism and Schizophrenia*, trans. Brian Massumi (London: Continuum, 2004) p. 504.

spectators, or audiences by exploring the networks of 'technologies and institutions that allow a given culture to select, store and process' their ideas about looking.[81] Some of the key models of spectatorship to emerge from such studies include the *flâneur*, the Panopticon, and the medical gaze: as both Flint and Otter have rightly reminded us, in the nineteenth century no single way of looking dominated, but the period was a field in which multiple and sometimes idiosyncratic patterns of visuality overlapped and intersected.[82]

In the context of this ongoing debate about looking, moments in which observers turned away from the spectacle in horror, surprise, or shock offer an intriguing counterpoint. On the one hand, they draw attention to the multi-sensory somatic aspects of perception: as Luisa Calè and Patrizia Di Bello have recently emphasized, it was not only the eyes which were involved when Victorians engaged with the world around them; sudden noises, strange smells, unpleasant tactile sensations, and, of course, unanticipated emotional responses, were also important aspects of spectatorship in the nineteenth century, modes of engagement which went 'against the rise of a nineteenth-century history of objectivity'.[83] On the other, shrinking away from a terrifying sight, turning away the face, covering the eyes or mouth, was also itself a highly visible gesture. Whether performed involuntarily or quite deliberately, flinching made the observer conscious of his or her own bodily performance, and in turn, made others aware of it too. In other words, flinching not only brought the multi-sensory and emotional aspects of looking to the foreground, but also the performed, and social dimensions of spectatorship too—a fact that many who wrote about watching and looking during the nineteenth century also realized. The flinches which appear in this book are the scraps of fleeting bodily practices which have lingered in letters, photographs, and films; at the same time, flinches also bring our attention to the role of emotion and performance in the period's written discourses about spectatorship. Tracing the flinches of scientific observers, and the ways they echoed the shrinking and wincing performances of theatre audiences, this study brings to the foreground the motif of multi-sensory, social, and self-conscious looking suggested by the German word *Schaulust*, arguing it may be positioned alongside patterns of spectatorship already identified by scholars of this period.

[81] Friedrich A. Kittler, *Discourse Networks 1800/1900* (Stanford: Stanford University Press, 1990) p. 369.

[82] Otter, *The Victorian Eye*, p. 21.

[83] Luisa Calè and Patrizia Di Bello, 'Introduction: Nineteenth-Century Objects and Beholders', in Calè and Di Bello (eds.) *Illustrations, Optics and Objects in Nineteenth-Century Literary and Visual Cultures*, pp. 1–24 (p. 1).

In her work exploring the interstices between nineteenth-century scientific writing and literature, Beer has described interdisciplinary methodologies as those which not only emphasize 'the circulation of intact ideas across a larger community', but also bring 'into question the methods and materials of differing intellectual practices and may uncover problems disguised by the scope of established disciplines'. One such 'intact idea' explored in this book is a motif of passionate and performed spectatorship which circulated across disparate cultural sites in the late nineteenth and early twentieth centuries. At the same time, this book attests to what Beer has called 'the transformations undergone when ideas enter other genres or different reading groups'.[84] In particular, it is the roles currently assigned to theatre audiences both among theatre historians and those investigating wider questions of nineteenth-century visuality, which a focus on flinching spectators may lead us to reconsider.

As Lynn M. Voskuil has suggested, late nineteenth-century audiences constitute something of a 'disciplinary blind spot' for historians of theatre.[85] Theatre audiences from the earlier part of the nineteenth century have been characterized as a highly vocal and volatile group, as oppositional and even subversive in the politically charged public space of the theatre. As Elaine Hadley has put it, they were seen as 'protestors with grievances to speak and public roles to play'.[86] By the end of the nineteenth century, however, the interaction and participation which had fostered this radicalism was seen to be on the wane. In part, this has been attributed to the technological changes of the late nineteenth-century playhouses, an effect of moving the working-class patrons, usually the most vociferous, from the pit area right in front of the stage to the upper gallery in 1880, for example, or introducing electric lighting the following year, which allowed the audience to sit in the dark for the first time. Hand in hand with these changes in infrastructure, a new naturalistic aesthetic emerged, with its fourth wall and prohibition on actors talking to—or even acknowledging—the audience. As Bertolt Brecht, whose critique of naturalism has had a powerful hold over theatre scholars eager to redeem theatre from its bourgeois late nineteenth-century conventions, put it, audiences of naturalism felt themselves to be simply 'looking through a key-hole' as if they

[84] Gillian Beer, 'Forging The Missing Link: Interdisciplinary Stories', in *Open Fields: Science in Cultural Encounter*, ed. Gillian Beer (Oxford: Clarendon Press, 1996) pp. 115–45 (p. 115).

[85] Lynn M. Voskuil, 'Feeling Public: Sensation Theatre, Commodity Culture, and the Victorian Public Sphere', *Victorian Studies* 44 (2002) 245–72 (p. 249).

[86] Elaine Hadley, *Melodramatic Tactics: Theatricalized Dissent in the English Marketplace, 1800–1885* (Stanford: Stanford University Press, 1995).

weren't *really there* at all.[87] For these reasons—and this is what the 'blind spot' is according to Voskuil—historians of theatre have tended to equate the late nineteenth century with an increased passivity and inertia among audiences, their gaze in many ways replicating the scientific observer who does not intervene in the scene played out before him, but simply monitors a world oblivious to his presence. Voskuil is making a general point, and whilst she has certainly identified a problem in the wider scholarly debate, it is also important to note that some scholars have challenged this dominant narrative of passivity. Jim Davis and Victor Emeljanow, for example, have cautioned against generic conceptions of audiences in the nineteenth century, reminding us that even if West-End houses had become more polite, 'batches of rampant hooting boys' remained very much part of the auditorium scene in the East End.[88] Ridout, on the other hand, exploring the affective dissonance of the auditorium, has emphasized the discomfort and self-consciousness which can be an unwelcome part of theatre-going, even at the point when the sociality and co-presence of the auditorium seems most powerfully obscured.[89] Nonetheless, the equation between late nineteenth-century theatre audiences and passivity as opposed to participation has gained some traction in other academic disciplines too.

The art historian Jonathan Crary's *Techniques of the Observer: On Vision and Modernity in the Nineteenth Century* has been one of the more influential accounts in the field of nineteenth-century visuality, although is not uncontested. Crary traces the conditions and forces that in the 1820s and 1830s 'produced a new kind of observer'.[90] His argument, simply put, is that in the early years of the nineteenth century the previously 'stable and fixed' relations (p. 3) between the observing subject and the outside world were radically transformed through a new set of cultural metaphors and technological practices that foregrounded the unreliability of vision. According to Crary, visuality in the seventeenth and eighteenth centuries was characterized by clarity and fixity, principles both constituted by and expressed through the optical device of the *camera obscura*. The *camera obscura*—in which the viewer, positioned inside a darkened chamber, observed an image of the outside world projected through a tiny hole onto

[87] Bertolt Brecht, *The Messingkauf Dialogues* (1942), trans. John Willett (London: Methuen, 1977) p. 51.

[88] Jim Davis and Victor Emeljanow, *Reflecting the Audience* (Iowa City: University of Iowa Press, 2001) p. 58.

[89] Ridout, *Stage Fright*, pp. 1–2.

[90] Crary, *Techniques of the Observer*, p. 3. Hereafter all citations will be to this edition, and will appear as page numbers in parentheses in the text.

a screen—manifested an observing subject whose interiority (expressed by the chamber) was distinct from the outside world. Thus, the *camera obscura* performed 'an operation of individuation' (p. 14), in which the viewer, isolated and enclosed in the darkness and gazing upon a delimited scene of the external world, became a 'knowing subject' in relation to a stable and unwavering outside world (p. 39). Importantly, the *camera obscura* prevented 'the observer from seeing his or her position as part of the representation' (p. 41), but rather insisted on a distinction between the corporeal and subjective self and the world he or she gazed upon (p. 70).

Crary contends that in the 1820s and 1830s this model of visuality was superseded by a different pattern, one which radically destabilized the relations between perceiver and the perceived world. This new model lodged the observer 'in another apparatus, within the unstable physiology and temporality of the human body' (p. 70). The emergence of optical toys, for example, the stereoscope, phenakistiscope, and the diorama, drew attention to the way visual experience was dependent on a subjective physiology, which was 'again and again shown to be defective, inconsistent, prey to illusion, and, in a crucial manner, susceptible to external procedures of manipulation and stimulation that have the essential capacity to *produce experience for the subject*' (p.92, original italics). As such the 'guarantees of authority, identity, and universality supplied by the *camera obscura*' were lost, and the relationship between the observer and observed world was becoming irrevocably mingled: 'the viewing body and its objects begin to constitute a single field on which inside and outside are confounded' (p. 73).

Crary's work has been critiqued for its technological determinism, its insistence on schism and rupture, its privileging of the eye, and its subsequent assumption of a 'dominant model' of an observer, most extensively, and sympathetically, by W. J. T. Mitchell, but also by Flint whose work aims, as a counterbalance, to explore 'the particularities of spectatorship', and Otter who instead proposes a 'multiplicity of overlapping, intersecting and contrasting perceptual "patterns" recurring throughout the nineteenth century'.[91] But Crary's depiction of the kind of looking which happened in nineteenth-century theatres also bears further interrogation. To be clear, theatres and their audiences—though they were undoubtedly a vital component of nineteenth-century daily life—are not the focus of any extended discussion in *Techniques of the Observer*. However, theatres do make occasional appearances in Crary's book, and when they do, they are habitually

[91] W. J. T. Mitchell, *Picture Theory: Essays on Verbal and Visual Representation* (Chicago: University of Chicago Press, 1995) pp. 19–23; Kate Flint, *The Victorians and the Visual Imagination*, p. 22; Chris Otter, *The Victorian Eye*, p. 21.

equated with pre-nineteenth-century styles of looking, in short, with the techniques of the *camera obscura*. Alongside 'linear perspective and the *camera obscura*', Crary points out that the Italian theatre incarnates fixed spectatorial relations (p. 12). In his discussion of Canaletto, he argues it was the artist's preoccupation with 'the theatricality' of Venice that led him to use the *camera obscura*, claiming that the intelligibility of the city as a stage depended on a 'precisely specified relation between a delimited point of view and a tableau' (pp. 52–3). The interior of the *camera obscura* is described as a space of 'theatre of representations' (p. 73). And the famous nineteenth-century illusion 'Pepper's Ghost', a phantasmagoric ghost produced for a production of Charles Dickens's *The Haunted Man* in 1862, was closer, writes Crary, to the spectatorial relations of the *camera obscura* than to the demystified optical devices of the 1830s and 1840s which made 'no claim that the real is anything other than a mechanical production' (p. 132). It is in his introduction that Crary makes his clearest statement about the sort of looking theatre makes possible: when nineteenth-century observers came to knowingly collude in creating a visual experience, the notion of being a 'passive onlooker at a spectacle, *as at an art gallery or theatre*' (p. 5, my italics) was overthrown.

On Flinching interrogates the equation between theatrical audiences and passivity by arguing that embodied and affective audience performances may be understood as a form of interactivity and participation in the live event. Unlike the stereoscope, the phenakistiscope, and the zootrope, theatre was, of course, not inherently a technology of nineteenth-century modernity. But it did undergo its own modernizing processes, absorbing the latest technological inventions and pioneering others. More importantly, however, the theatre auditorium was a space around which questions about looking—and particularly, about the collective, affective, and visceral aspects of spectatorship—were raised and contested. The possibility that theatres offered a distinctive nineteenth-century space both for looking and being visible has begun to be acknowledged. For example, in *Victorian Glassworlds*, Isobel Armstrong has drawn attention to the mirrored curtain that hung between the stage and auditorium in the Coburg Theatre (now London's Old Vic) in the 1820s. The shimmering curtain, which fragmented and distorted the reflections of the audience who looked at it, became emblematic of the experience of moving through a city newly furnished with glass. As Armstrong puts it, 'the externalized body repeatedly returns to the looker from the environment, often as a moving palimpsest in the cityscape, overwritten by other images'.[92] One

[92] Isobel Armstrong, *Victorian Glassworlds*, p. 96.

of the reasons Armstrong's analysis of the Coburg curtain is suggestive for this study, is that it reminds us that becoming self-conscious, or aware of one's own role in the visual experience, was an important component of theatre-going. Otter has likewise drawn attention to the self-reflexivity and reciprocity characteristic of the theatre auditorium, an environment where one might both watch and become aware of one's role as an audience member. For Otter, theatres exemplify the 'oligoptic space', a space of 'mutual oversight', of the Victorian public sphere (libraries are another example), and he draws attention to the way the auditorium provided opportunities for 'personal display' as well as 'for scrutinising the appearance of others'.[93] While in both Armstrong and Otter's books the engagement with the theatre auditorium is fleeting, both examples remind us that self-consciousness and performance were important aspects of looking in the nineteenth century in Drury Lane and beyond.

In the nineteenth century, writers and thinkers repeatedly turned to the auditorium to ask questions about how to look. While professional critics such as G. H. Lewes and William Archer theorized the changing roles of the audience, novelists from Wilkie Collins to H. G. Wells portrayed the trouble caused by the contagious affects and misperceptions which were a distinctive part of theatre-going. In wider debates about the way professionals and the public encountered scientific objects, theatrical audiences came to exemplify the kind of demonstrative, emotional, spectatorial intervention that disrupted the possibility of a sensitive or rational response. However, as this book argues, theatrical looking was also a part of scientific practice, emerging not only when the scientist visited zoos and exhibitions of medical curiosities, but in the comparatively private world of his professional laboratory too. This proximity of scientific observers to theatrical audiences offers a way of thinking about the emotional aspects of scientific practice, but also suggests a resource for thinking about the hard-to-capture embodied experiences of nineteenth-century theatrical audiences too.

The chapters that follow trace the multiple and often contradictory meanings that became attached to recoiling, wincing, and starting between 1872 and 1917, to argue that they became important spectatorial gestures in this period. While we have become accustomed to linking the end of the nineteenth century with the rise of an ideal of the restrained and objective scientific observer, spaces of scientific investigation continued to witness passionate and gestured acts of looking, in which observers flinched from sudden noises, winced at the sight of an animal's pain, and recoiled from

[93] Chris Otter, *The Victorian Eye*, p. 74.

being seen. It was in these moments of embodied and performed looking that the scientific observer's entanglements in the techniques and problems of theatrical audiences came to the foreground. The central claim of this book is that even in a period most closely associated with the ascendency of the modern scientific method, theatrical techniques and problems remained at the heart of experimental life. Opening out this observation to address wider considerations of Victorian visuality, *On Flinching* draws attention to the ways Victorians thought about looking as itself an emotional performance and mode of embodied participation. As a cultural history of flinching and a discussion of the unexpected connections running between science and theatre in the late nineteenth century, the discussions that follow also raise questions about the entwined problems of emotionality, gestures, and spectatorship in an age whose concerns about looking prefigure our own. Like us, those who thought and wrote at the end of the long nineteenth century wondered whether they were merely passive recipients in an image-saturated society or active participants in the creation of visual worlds.

1
Darwin's Flinch

It was called 'one of the greatest attractions of the metropolis'.[1] In 1828, the London Zoological Society moved its menagerie to a newly built complex in the middle of Regent's Park. Originally intended for the expert study of 'specimens', the Zoological Gardens quickly became a place for pleasure and amusement and by the 1840s was attracting almost 170,000 visitors a year.[2] The Reptile House, which opened in 1843, offered close encounters of the more horrifying kind (Figure 3). In the 1850s, the diarist and socialite Eliza Cook wrote with palpable thrill of the 'slimy and creeping things' that 'dart upon their mocking visitors', the snakes and lizards that 'desire to escape', 'writhing upon the earth, or toad-like crouching within some leafy hiding-holes'. 'We dread the bare possibility', she continued 'of encountering the crushing coils of the upbreathing python'.[3] This was a place bristling with imaginary dangers, and the titillating legends of real ones too. The death of the Head Keeper of the Serpent Room in 1852 from a venomous bite after he drunkenly attempted to charm a cobra was a particularly vivid reminder of the horror precariously contained in the looming glass-fronted tanks.[4]

In this unnerving atmosphere, at some point in the early 1870s, the eminent naturalist Charles Darwin (1809–1882) staged a peculiar self-experiment. Tall and thin, and wearing the long, bushy white beard of a Victorian patriarch, the celebrated author of the *Origin of Species* (1859) was by then in his early sixties. He recounted his visit to the Reptile House in the opening pages of his penultimate book *The Expression of the Emotions in Man and Animals* (1872):

> I put my face close to the thick glass-plate in front of a puff-adder in the Zoological Gardens, with the firm determination of not starting back if the

[1] Edward Mogg, *Mogg's New Picture of London and Visitor's Guide to its Sights* (London: Mogg, 1848) p. 196.

[2] Peter Cunningham, *Handbook of London Past and Present* (London: Murray, 1850) p. 562.

[3] Eliza Cook, *Eliza Cook's Journal*, iii, 12 vols. (London: John Owen Clarke, 1850) p. 203.

[4] Anon., 'The Fatal Accident in the Zoological Gardens', *The Times*, 23 October 1852.

> snake struck at me; but as soon as the blow was struck, my resolution went for nothing, and I jumped a yard or two backwards with astonishing rapidity.[5]

The incident, he claimed, 'amused' him. Perhaps, at the time, he let out an embarrassed sort of a giggle, and looked around, wondering if anyone had seen his girlish skitter. As the French philosopher Henri Bergson would remark thirty years later, it is precisely these mechanistic movements, when our limbs involuntary perform one action though 'the circumstances of the case called for something else', that makes our bodies so laughable.[6] Unlike Queen Victoria who gazed unmoved upon the pouncing tiger, the 'firm determination' of the distinguished man of science faltered, leaving him emotionally rearranged in the face of imaginary danger, discombobulated by a flinch he did not mean to perform.

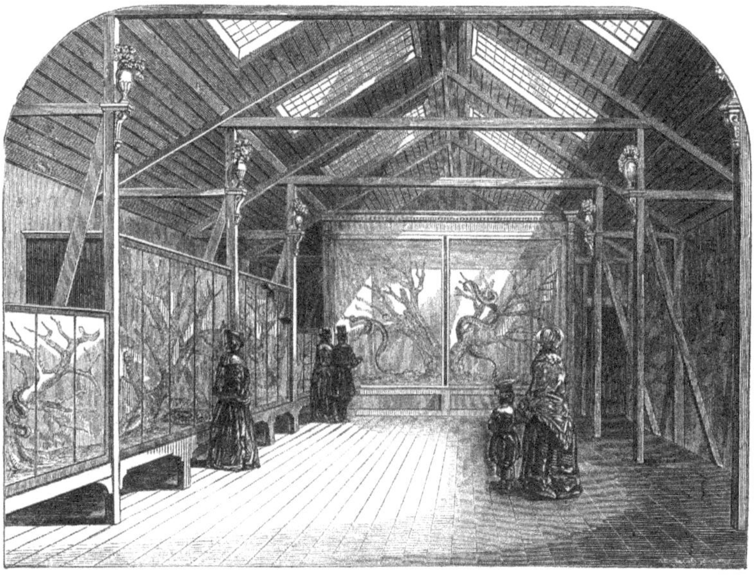

Fig. 3. 'The New Reptile House in the Gardens of the Zoological Society, Regent's Park,' *Illustrated London News*, 14 (2 June 1849), p. 384.

The Bodleian Libraries, University of Oxford. N2288 b. 6

[5] Charles Darwin, *The Expression of the Emotions in Man and Animals* (London: Murray, 1872) p. 38. Hereafter all citations will be to this edition, unless otherwise stated, and will appear as page numbers in parentheses in the text.

[6] Henri Bergson, *Laughter: An Essay on the Meaning of the Comic* (*Le Rire*, 1900) trans. Cloudesley Brereton and Fred Rothwell (London: MacMillan, 1911) p. 9.

The nineteenth century witnessed a transformation in the way the relationship between our inner feelings and their outward expressions were understood. In the seventeenth and eighteenth century, writers including Charles le Brun (1617–1690) and Johann Kaspar Lavater (1741–1801), had spoken of the 'passions' and 'affectations of the soul', arguing that a turmoil of hatred or the delights of love left their imprint on the surface of the body.[7] For these theorists, the body enjoyed a legibility and transparency, part of God's plan to ensure moral behaviour. As Thomas Dixon has shown, in the early decades of the nineteenth century, the emphasis began to shift away from this religious and moral framework, towards an increasingly secular, physiological, and psychological explanation of our feelings, and with it came a new category—the emotions.[8] By the middle of the nineteenth century, talk of the physiological emotions had almost entirely superseded the older theological categories, as men of science began to scrutinize the minute changes that accompanied emotional states, cataloguing the excitations of the body from raised pulses to quickened breathing, an approach which Marshall Hall's account of the simple spinal reflex in 1833 helped to frame in the language of mechanistic, involuntary behaviour. At the forefront of this turn to a physiology of feeling was the Scottish physician Charles Bell's *Essays on the Anatomy and Philosophy of Expression in Painting*, initially published in 1806, but significantly revised in 1844. Bell approached the question of emotional expression in the language of reflex machinery, mapping out the muscular contractions of the lips and cheeks that led to smiles, the circulations of blood that produce blushes, and the convulsions of the viscera in terror. Although Bell followed his eighteenth-century forebears in distinguishing between lower animal appetites and more refined, distinctively human sensibilities, he also reconsidered the relationship between inner feeling and outward expression. It was not simply the case that the body expressed inner feeling; without the body, he argued, the soul could not feel at all. Nevertheless, Bell concluded that his observations proved that God had endowed man with certain muscles—a 'special apparatus'—in order to express, but also experience, passions.[9]

Darwin had read Bell's work in the summer of 1840, and whilst he found many of its anatomical descriptions compelling, he took issue with its broader theistic framework. For Darwin, the fact our pupils dilate when we are surprised or the hairs on the back of our necks rise up when

[7] See, Lucy Hartley, *Physiognomy and the Meaning of Expression in Nineteteenth-Century Culture* (Cambridge: Cambridge University Press, 2001) in particular pp. 44–79.

[8] Dixon, *From Passions to Emotions*.

[9] Charles Bell, *Anatomy and Philosophy of Expression* (London: Longmans, 1806).

we are frightened, was evidence not of intelligent design but of the long processes of our evolution from animals over millennia. Like the fossils half-emerging from the cliffs on the Dorset coast, it was through odd snags in the expected fabric of human emotional behaviour that the evolutionary self declared itself. Why, asked Darwin, did he shut his eyes when thinking of something frightening in the dark? Why did he find soup on a man's beard disgusting, when neither soup nor beards were so? Why flinch from a snake he knew to be securely encased? In such oddities, Darwin's discrete, emotional body revealed itself to be a disobedient bundle of vestiges, gesturing beyond the margins of his own subjectivity to habits and behaviours accumulated by other people, other animals, at other times and in other places. Like Dickens's waterlogged London sinking under 'crust upon crust of mud' where it would not be unexpected to meet a 'Megalosaurus, forty feet long or so, waddling like an elephantine lizard up Holborn Hill', in Darwin's account the emotional body became muddy and mnemonic, and in it worlds collided.[10]

In the last thirty years scholarship on Darwin has been stimulated by numerous interdisciplinary approaches. From the *Origin*'s links with George Eliot's fiction, to the ideas shared between botanical illustrations and Ruskin's ideas about painting, critics such as Gillian Beer, George Levine, and Jonathan Smith have pointed up the ways Darwin's evolutionary ideas were embedded in wider Victorian culture.[11] Underlying their approach is an insistence on the symbiotic relationship between scientific writing and other nineteenth-century cultural forms. Not only were the ideas of evolution assimilated in and challenged by Victorian artistic practices, but also the literary and visual forms through which Darwin articulated his ideas to readers were themselves vital resources for his creative thinking. It is a surprise, therefore, to discover that Darwin's relationship with Victorian theatre has not been more explored.[12] By the time he was preparing the *Expression* for publication, outings to the theatre would have been few and far between for Darwin and his family. Nonetheless, the techniques and problems of actors and audiences remained a distinctive part of Darwin's efforts to study his own emotions and stage those

[10] Dickens, *Bleak House*, 1996, p. 13.

[11] Other works which explore the complex relationship between Darwin's work and wider nineteenth-century culture include: Robert M. Young, *Darwin's Metaphor: Nature's Place in Victorian Culture* (1985); Beer, *Darwin's Plots*; Levine, *Darwin and the Novelists* and *Darwin the Writer* (2011); Jonathan Smith, *Charles Darwin and Victorian Visual Culture*.

[12] Works that specifically address the influence of Darwin's ideas on theatre include: Joseph Roach, *The Player's Passion* and Jane Goodall, *Performance and Evolution in the Age of Darwin*.

of others for observation—from shuddering to himself in the mirror, to persuading strangers to give expressions of grief so he could watch.

As Paul White has pointed out, Darwin's research methodology in the *Expression* is usually approached by historians of science as transitional, combining the 'quaint observations and makeshift experiments' of the nineteenth-century man of science, with the use of indefatigable recording technologies—in the case of the *Expression*, the camera—that were institutionalized in the twentieth-century laboratory with its imperative of objective looking.[13] Yet, Darwin's research into the emotions may also be approached through its sideways relationship to techniques of looking theorized in the 1860s and early 1870s by critics, actors, and philosophers trying to understand theatre's distinctive encounters between spectators and performers. Though he worked in a scientific culture whose demonstrations were already imbued with theatricality, Darwin also made theatrical techniques a part of his private experimental practice. And if theatre played a part in creating the research which would come to shape our modern understanding of the emotions, Darwin's proximity to theatrical audiences may also be regarded as one of the local practices through which this period's culture of scientific objectivity was constituted. In turn, theatre formed an important conceptual resource for Darwin's evolutionary account of emotions, and the picture of a decentred emotional subject it brought into view. Through theatre's unreliable relationships between inner feeling and outward performance, its uncoupling of appearances and realities and its slippages between the here and now and imagined other worlds, cherished notions of autonomous and discrete emotional being were called into question, and Darwin's dynamic and composite conception of the feeling self came to light.

DARWIN'S THEATRE OF EMOTIONS

Charles Darwin was born in 1809 in the small market town of Shrewsbury. The grandson of the philosopher and physician Erasmus Darwin and the son of a wealthy local doctor, it was perhaps inevitable that Darwin should embark on a medical degree. However, his future as a doctor was quickly abandoned when he discovered he was unable to bear the sight of blood and suffering. Instead, Darwin decided to become a country vicar, a career he believed would leave him with plenty of time to indulge his hobby of Natural History. In 1827, Darwin was admitted to Christ's College

[13] Paul White, 'Darwin's Emotions: The Scientific Self and the Sentiment of Objectivity', *Isis* 100 (2010), 811–26 (p. 812).

Oxford, where he proved himself an unremarkable student. However his passion for collecting beetles earned him the friendship of the botanist John Stevens Henslow (1796–1861). It was to be a fortuitous alliance. In 1831, Henslow was invited to travel on the survey ship HMS Beagle as a 'scientific person', but being unable to go suggested Darwin take his place.

The Beagle travelled along the coasts of Africa and South America, and through the Pacific islands, where Darwin collected fossils, plants, and animal specimens. The extensive notes that he took, later transcribed as the *Journal of Researches* (renamed *Voyage of the Beagle*) and published in 1839, are most famous for their observations of the subtle variations in species of tortoises and mockingbirds, now known as 'Darwin's finches', scattered across the Galapagos archipelago. However, Darwin's notes also included reflections on human and animal emotions, observations that would play a vital role in laying the foundations for his theories of common descent and evolution through natural selection. 'It has been said that the love of the chase is an inherent delight in man—a relic of an instinctive passion', he wrote in 1836. 'If so, I am sure the pleasure of living in the open air, with the sky for a roof, and the ground for a table, is part of the same feeling.'[14]

On his return to London, Darwin developed a reputation as a leading naturalist, geologist, and scientific traveller. In 1839, he married his cousin Emma Wedgwood, and in 1842 the couple moved to Downe House in Kent. During this period, Darwin's ideas on evolution through natural selection flourished. Through his reading of the work of the French philosopher Jean-Baptiste Lamarck, as well as that of his grandfather Erasmus, Darwin was already acquainted with the idea that individual species might have evolved along parallel lines into their present forms. Darwin's insight was to blur the boundaries between species, arguing that all living creatures had evolved from a single organism over millennia. Like the tracery of branches that sprout from the trunk of a tree, each successful variation had led to a new species branching off, while no longer serviceable characteristics fell away. It is no coincidence that during this period Darwin was also reading widely on the emotions, and as early as 1838 was speculating about whether the human 'passions', as he still called them, were vestiges of animal ancestors. 'My first child was born on December 27th 1839', he recollected in 1876, 'and I at once commenced to make notes on the first dawn of the various expressions which he exhibited, for I felt convinced, even at this early period, that the most complex and fine shades of expression must all have had gradual and natural origin'. The following summer,

[14] Charles Darwin, *Narrative of the Surveying Voyages of His Majesty's Ships Adventure and Beagle between the years 1826 and 1836*, iii (London: Henry Colburn, 1839) p. 607.

Darwin read Bell's *Essays on the Anatomy and Philosophy of Expression in Painting*, 'and this greatly increased the interest which I felt in the subject, though I could not at all agree with his belief that various muscles had been specially created for the sake of expression'.[15]

The M and N notebooks written between 1838–9 include discussions of three of the core principles through which Darwin would come to understand our emotional expressions. Some evolved as 'serviceable habits', useful movements for defence or preservation, such as the flinch. Others evolved through the principle of 'antithesis': in aggression, a dog's body goes rigid, but when it approaches a friend 'instead of walking upright, the body sinks downwards, lowered and wagged from side and side' (p. 129). The final, but most vague, principle was the 'direct action of the nervous system', through which attention, imagination and so on might influence the expressions we perform. Thus, 'the violence of a start seems to depend partly on the vividness of the imagination and partly on the condition of the nervous system', wrote Darwin, and 'after one violent start' both horses and children are 'very apt to start again' (p. 49). Just as Darwin imagined the living world as malleable and species unlimited in their capacity for change, so emotional expressions were not versions of ideal or essential types with circumscribed boundaries. As they had in the past, so in the future they would continue to be subject to perpetual transformation.

As is well known, though he discussed his ideas on evolution through natural selection with scientific friends, Darwin did not make the theory public until 1858, and only then because he learnt that the naturalist Alfred Russell Wallace was about to publish a similar one. Expanded in 1859 as the bestselling *On The Origin of Species*, Darwin's ideas challenged the prevailing theological orthodoxy and made him a household name. In particular, their implications for the notion of human uniqueness attracted the attention of the Victorian public, intriguing and outraging in equal measures. In the *Origin*, Darwin had been circumspect about the specific applications of his general theory for humans, but in private he continued to gather evidence for the theory of a common ancestor, and it was in part to the emotions that he turned. In 1867, Darwin began his research on the emotions in earnest by distributing a questionnaire to explorers and missionaries across the globe in the hope of gathering evidence for universal expressions of 'natives' in different continents. Inviting potential respondents to document 'any definite description of the countenance under any emotion or frame of mind', but warning them that 'memory

[15] Frances Darwin ed., *The Life and Letters of Charles Darwin*, i (London: Murray, 1887) p. 113.

is so deceptive that I earnestly beg it may not be trusted', Darwin's questionnaire posed seventeen questions, including: 'is astonishment expressed by the eyes and mouth being opened wide, and by the eyebrows being raised?' and 'when a man is indignant or defiant does he frown, hold his body and head erect, square his shoulders and clench his fists?'[16] Darwin had originally intended to gather the answers together, along with his own observations, in the final chapter of his next book the *Descent of Man*, the work that would lay out most unambiguously his conviction that the difference between animals and humans was one of degree rather than kind. However, as soon as he started to collect his notes together, Darwin realized a separate work altogether would be required.

As he confessed in the opening pages of the *Expression of Emotions in Man and Animals*, 'the study of Expression is difficult'. An initial problem arose from the fugitive nature of expressions themselves which were 'often extremely slight, and of a fleeting nature'. Unlike butterflies, smiles and sneers could not be captured and pinned to a board. While Darwin could see the difference between a face crumpled in sadness and one widened in delight, there was never enough time for Darwin to state categorically 'in what the difference consists'. More troublesome, however, was the task of maintaining a dispassionate gaze. As Darwin was quick to realize, watching others in the throes of passion aroused his own feelings, his sympathy so strongly excited that 'close observation' was 'forgotten or rendered almost impossible'. In addition to this, Darwin suspected he tended to 'readily imagine' the presence of certain emotions in his human and animal subjects 'from the nature of the circumstances' (p. 13). From its outset, then, the *Expression* is as much a book about the problems of observing emotion as it is about the emotions themselves.

In the remainder of his introduction to the *Expression*, Darwin laid out the methods and strategies he had employed to circumvent these difficulties. He watched the behaviour of his own and other people's children, who he believed to exhibit more elemental expressions than adults. He collected anecdotes about the insane, believing they 'notoriously give way to all their emotions with little or no restraint' (p. 155). He documented the behaviour of his household pets to which he attributed a perhaps surprising emotional range. Thirty-seven responses to his questionnaire sent from correspondents across the globe arrived at Downe House between 1867 and 1868, and Darwin scoured their diverse descriptions of emotive performances. The anecdotes from his correspondents were supplemented by those gleaned from his extensive reading of previous authors on the

[16] 'Queries About Expression', Darwin's Papers, Cambridge University Library, DAR53.1.B2.

subject of physiology and emotions including the anatomists Charles Bell and Pierre Gratiolet, physicians Thomas Henry Burgess and Duchenne de Boulogne, psychologist Alexander Bain, philosopher Herbert Spencer and artist Charles le Brun. Their examples were marshalled in support of Darwin's conviction that the physiology of our expressions was not designed by God, but had evolved into their present form over millennia.

Darwin also became an avid collector of photographs. From the West Riding Lunatic Asylum in Wakefield, Physician-Superintendent James Crichton-Browne sent images of patients taken in the studio the asylum shared with the local prison. Now gathered together in two fawn-coloured scrapbooks in the Cambridge University Library, these photographs recall playing cards to be swapped and collected, their subjects posing uncomfortably, outlined in pretty red ink: 'Melancholia' is written in looped handwriting under three, 'Imbecile', 'Euphoric Mania', 'The Insane Ears', 'Obstinate Imbecile' are the titles of some of the others.[17] The French physician Duchenne de Boulogne sent a series of photographs he had made of his asylum patients; men and women whose apparently insensible facial muscles were stimulated with a galvanic prod into macabre grins and dreadful expressions of grief. To test whether these artificially produced smiles and gasps were authentic, in the autumn of 1868 Darwin surprised guests staying at Downe for the weekend by asking them to guess the emotions depicted in the Frenchman's photographs. As Jane Gray, wife of the Harvard botanist Asa, confided to her sister, 'it was curious the different meanings given'.[18] Between 1869 and 1870, Darwin travelled frequently from Downe House to the studios around Victoria Station and the Strand. From these greasy commercial enterprises that testified to the bourgeois fashion of having one's portrait taken and the craze for swapping *cartes de visite*, Darwin collected curiosities. One entitled *Der Haarigen Familie von Ambras* depicted a family whose entire bodies were covered in thick hair.[19] Another was a series by the photographer James Landy entitled *Expressive Pets*, in which baleful animals and sorrowful children posed side by side, appearing to mimic each other's expressions.

Such were Darwin's official research strategies, but as the *Expression* reveals, he also made numerous ad hoc experiments and it is in these that

[17] Darwin Papers, Cambridge University Library, DAR59.2 DAR53. Crichton-Browne's photographs are CUL-DAR53.1.A10-A39. The collections can also be accessed through *The Complete Works of Charles Darwin Online 2002–2009*.

[18] Jane Gray's letter to her sister, 28 October 1868. Available: <http://www.darwinproject.ac.uk/jane-gray-on-down.> accessed 12 September 2013. I am grateful to Alison Pearn of the Darwin Correspondence Project for alerting me to this reference.

[19] Darwin Papers, DAR53.1.C7-C10. For a full account of the photographs, see Prodger, *An Annotated Catalogue*.

Darwin's entanglements with the techniques and problems of Victorian theatre come to the fore. From Lavater's *Physiognomy* (1772) to Bell's *Anatomy*, actors and audiences had always formed a significant resource for studies of the passions, and Darwin did not abandon the convention.[20] He cites the example of the actor George Frederick Cooke, who portrayed a 'most determined hate' by drawing up his upper lip and revealing 'a sharp angular tooth' in a snarl not unlike a tiger's (p. 250).[21] Elsewhere in the *Expression* he describes a 'lady belonging to a family famous for having produced an extraordinary number of great actors and actresses', who could contract facial muscles not usually under conscious control to give a remarkably accurate expression of grief (p. 184). Among the photographs found in Darwin's personal library was a folio containing thirty-three albumen prints of the German actor Ernst Schulz in a range of histrionic poses depicting the sentiments pertaining to stock characters, including a wistful star-crossed lover, a prim European lady, and a proud American-Indian chief.

Yet more than a source of curiosities and case studies, theatre—with its slippages between fiction and reality, its over-acting, pretence, and trickery—infiltrated Darwin's work on the expressions in other ways too, becoming a staple, if unacknowledged, part of his research toolkit. Darwin persuaded family members, friends, strangers, and even fellow men of science to act out their emotions so he could watch, noting down the angle of their eyebrows or the action of their zygomatic muscles. On one occasion he observed a young lady who, in the midst of an animated conversation with a friend, would 'hoist the flag of distress…as often as the young lady was beaten, and could not get out her words fast enough, her eyebrows went obliquely upwards, and rectangular furrows were formed on her forehead.' When later Darwin asked the young woman 'to act on her grief muscles,' he found her quite unable to voluntarily produce the expression, though her friend repeatedly performed it 'showing her what was intended' (p. 187). On another occasion, Darwin caught himself 'giving a little involuntary shudder at a painful thought', and during it he 'distinctly perceived' his platysma muscle contracting. 'So it does if I simulate a shudder,' he noted, continuing that when he had 'asked others to act in this manner' he found that sometimes the muscle was engaged and sometimes not. Among those faking it was his son, who 'voluntarily

[20] Lavater complained that he had not been able to study women because his 'opportunities for seeing them at the theatre, at balls, or at the card-table, where they best may be studied, have been exceedingly few'. Johann Kaspar Lavater, *Physiognomy* (London: Cowie, 1776) p. 213.

[21] Darwin cited the example of George Frederick Cooke from Charles Bell, *Anatomy and Philosophy of Expression* (London: Longmans, 1806).

shuddered' at Darwin's request, but whose platysma remained unaffected (p. 320). In his discussion of sneering, Darwin reports that he 'asked four persons to endeavour to act voluntarily' and curl their lips exposing the canine tooth on one side, noting that only one of the four was unable to perform the expression on demand (p. 252). In his discussion of astonishment, Darwin notes that 'a friend asked another man how he would express great astonishment, and he at once threw himself into this attitude' (the attitude in question, with out-flung arms and a gasp, is shown in Plate VII.1, Figure 4) (p. 288).

Perhaps it is not be entirely surprising that such a distinguished Victorian man of science so liberally used theatrical techniques. As I discussed in

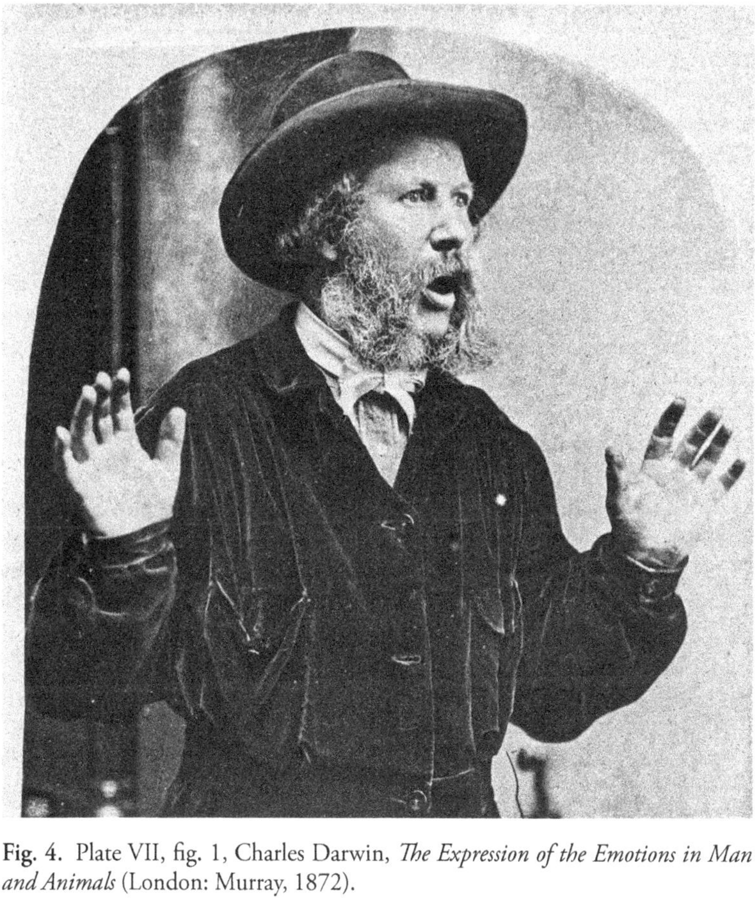

Fig. 4. Plate VII, fig. 1, Charles Darwin, *The Expression of the Emotions in Man and Animals* (London: Murray, 1872).

the introduction to this book (section: 'Theatres of Science'), historians have explored the ways in which Victorian spectacle and science were already epistemologically closer than we might expect to find from our twenty-first century perspective. In the period Darwin was undertaking his work on the expression of emotions, the idea of the professional university scientist, who conducted experiments in a dedicated laboratory, equipped with the latest technologies and adhering to codified methods and techniques, was one still very much in formation. In fact, scientific experiments were conducted in all manner of messily overlapping spaces, including private houses (such as Darwin's home at Downe House), public institutes (such as the Royal Institution, as well as popular exhibition spaces for practical science such as London's Adelaide Gallery and Royal Polytechnic Institution), and indeed at zoos, fairs, and even theatres. As Lightman and Morus, among others, have explored, these spaces were already inflected with the performative, and scientists drew on the showman's techniques and practices—from sleight of hand and misdirection to ratcheted tension and astonishing reveals—to make complex scientific ideas concrete for a general public, 'pulling in crowds and amazing them with nature's secrets'.[22] Such carefully rehearsed scientific spectacles were an important part of Victorian performance culture across the social spectrum. So while audiences at Michael Faraday's lectures, delivered at that preserve of the scientific elite the Royal Institution, were dazzled, shocked, and astonished by scintillating displays of pyrotechnics and electromagnetics, instrument makers and magicians shared the stage at the Polytechnic and the Adelaide with their demonstrations of dissolving views, oxyhydrogen microscopes and electrical induction coils. Not only did scientific demonstrators cast themselves as 'expert showmen', but scientific curiosities themselves wandered between the worlds of entertainment and edification. Pepper's Ghost, a phantagasmoric illusion named after its creator, for example, was first displayed at the Polytechnic in a performance of Edward Bulwer-Lytton's play 'A Strange Story', followed by 'A Strange Lecture' in which the mechanism of the illusion was revealed to a curious public, an event perhaps even more astonishing than the phantom itself.[23] This culture of scientific performance forms an important conceptual and historical backdrop to Darwin's use of actors in his experiments: with theatre already so deeply engrained in scientific practice, the

[22] Morus, '"More the Aspect of Magic than Anything Natural"', p. 337. See also: Secord, 'Extraordinary Experiment', pp. 337–73; Morus, *Frankenstein's Children: Electricity, Exhibition, and Experiment in Early-Nineteenth-Century London* (Princeton: Princeton University Press, 1998); Lightman, *Victorian Popularizers of Science*; Morus, 'Worlds of Wonder'; Martin Willis, *Vision, Science and Literature.*

[23] Lightman, *Victorian Popularizers of Science*, p. 167.

distinguished scientific gentleman would not necessarily have seen the two worlds as epistemologically or socially contradictory.

Yet, while it's important not to overstate the distance between theatre and science in this period, it is equally important not to completely obscure it either. As I discussed in the introduction, historians of science have emphasized the theatricality of spectacular public dissemination of knowledge, but there has been far less attention paid to what Morus has called 'relatively private acts of performing experiments'.[24] Of course, part of Morus's argument is that experimentation and demonstration should not be seen as entirely distinct entities in this period: many conduits of exchange existed between public communication and the framing and creating of knowledge in the nineteenth century—as they continue to today, as Pickering has persuasively argued.[25] All the same, while one might expect theatrical flourishes to emerge at moments when scientists displayed their wares to delight and astonish a paying public, it is more surprising to discover theatrical strategies being deployed in the relative solitude of the ad hoc laboratory, and in particular, as part of the repertoire of techniques used to make experimental observations. Certainly, as I discussed in the Introduction, over the last thirty years historians of science have emphasized the performativity of experiments—by which is broadly meant that the repeated practices and actions of machines and bodies in the laboratory come to produce and constrain a shared reality, in turn making scientific ideas possible. Yet, it is striking that in discussions of 'relatively private acts of performing experiments', the notion of theatrical imposture is less comfortably invoked. This book takes seriously the idea that theatricality, with all its guiltiness, its excess, its pretence, and its slippery relationship between appearances and reality may also be part of 'relatively private' scientific experiments. It argues that attending to the theatricality of experimental encounters—perhaps best seen as a subsection of their general performativity—throws light on particular problems of looking, and in turn highlights distinctive emotional and embodied aspects of scientific practice. In the case of Darwin, theatre both facilitated his study of expressions, and muddled it in surprisingly revealing ways.

While Darwin's research required an array of amateur actors, as a scientific observer he was, more strictly speaking, embroiled in the techniques and problems of theatrical audiences. There are moments in the *Expression* when it becomes clear Darwin strayed beyond the empirically available,

[24] Morus, 'Placing Performance'.

[25] See: Andrew Pickering, 'From Science as Knowledge to Science as Practice', in *Science as Practice and Culture*, ed. Andrew Pickering (Chicago: University of Chicago Press, 1992) pp. 1–28.

inferring inner depths from surface physiological changes. Like a spectator in the theatre, he imagined dramas of inner motivations, desires, and impediments from mere appearances of feeling. For example, sitting opposite a woman in a train carriage, Darwin noticed that 'her *depressors anguli oris* became very slightly, yet decidedly, contracted', a muscular contraction that Darwin knew to usually precede tears. Her expression led him to imagine that 'some painful recollection, perhaps that of a long-lost child, was passing through her mind' (p. 193). Elsewhere in the book, however, Darwin is more troubled by the possibility of a disconnection between emotional expressions and the mental states they are supposed to connote. Negotiating such slippages between seeming and being is a perennial part and parcel of the often unsettling experience of watching theatre and experiencing what Jonas Barish has called its 'ontological queasiness'.[26]

The problems of theatrical emoting come to the foreground in Darwin's discussions of the photographs that illustrate the *Expression*. While some of the photographs in Darwin's collection were of actors, all of them involved acting. With the notoriously slow exposure times of the late Victorian camera, the ability to hold a pose for several seconds or more was crucial if one wanted to 'take well'. In spite of his extensive collection, Darwin decided to commission additional images for his book, choosing the Swedish art photographer Oscar Rejlander for the task.[27] Rejlander had made a name for himself in the 1850s as a tricksy and flamboyant photographer with a penchant for self-dramatization. For example, in his composite work *Two Ways of Life*, a restaging of Raphael's *School of Athens*, the photographer uncannily appears twice.[28] Of the nineteen photographs by Rejlander, six are self-portraits of the photographer posed in sentimental attitudes.[29] In 'Surprise', Rejlander holds his hands up palms facing outwards, his mouth open (Plate VII.1, Figure 4). In 'Defiance', he clenches his fists and pouts (Plate VI.2, Figure 5). To portray 'Helplessness', Rejlander shrugs his shoulders, his head cocked to one side (Plate VI.3–4, Figure 5). For 'Disgust', the photographer positions himself in a kind of flinch or cringe, his hands fending off some invader, his face squashed into a grimace (Plate V.2–3, Figure 6). Today these images look like so much bad acting, but

[26] Jonas A. Barish, *The Antitheatrical Prejudice* (Berkeley and London: University of California Press, 1981) p. 3.

[27] The other photographs were by Crichton-Browne, Duchenne de Boulogne, Adolph Kindermann, and George Charles Wallich. For the provenance of these and the other photographs in the *Expression*, see Prodger, *An Annotated Catalogue*, p. 6.

[28] For Rejlander's self-portraiture beyond the *Expression*, see Lori Pauli, ed., *Acting the Part: Photography as Theatre* (London: Merrell, 2006) p. 20; p. 26; pp. 30–1; p. 69.

[29] There are no less than ten self-portraits of Rejlander in Darwin's collections (not all of them appeared in the finished book), and each reveals a similar combination of flamboyant self-staging and technological chicanery. CUL–DAR53.1.c40-46; 69–73.

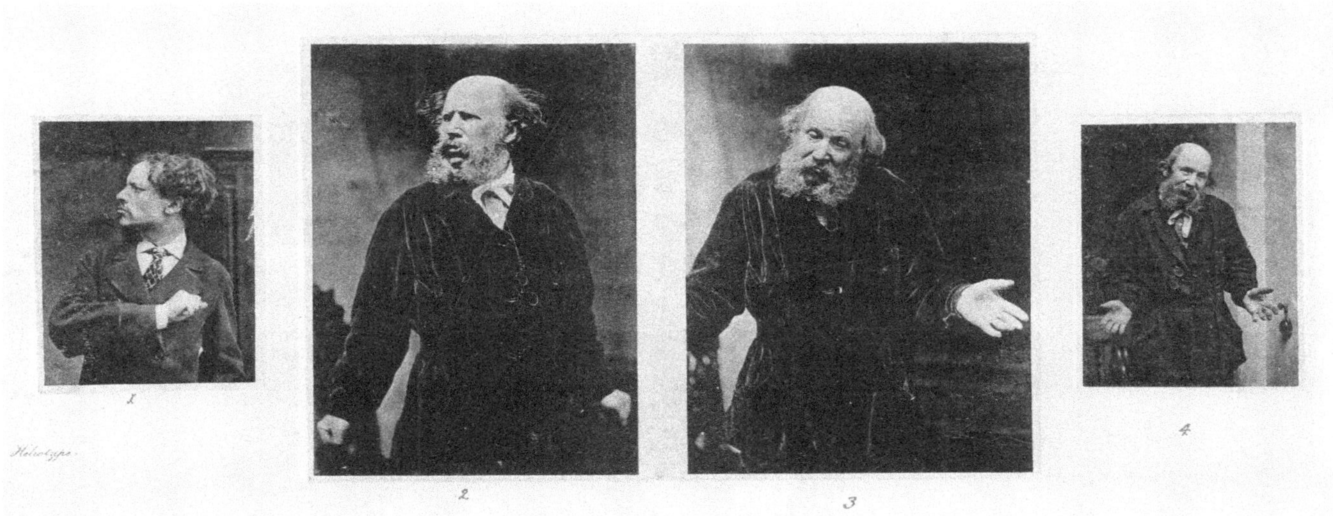

Fig. 5. Plate VI, figs. 1–4, Charles Darwin, *The Expression of the Emotions in Man and Animals* (London: Murray, 1872).

The Bodleian Libraries, University of Oxford (OC) 189 f. 73

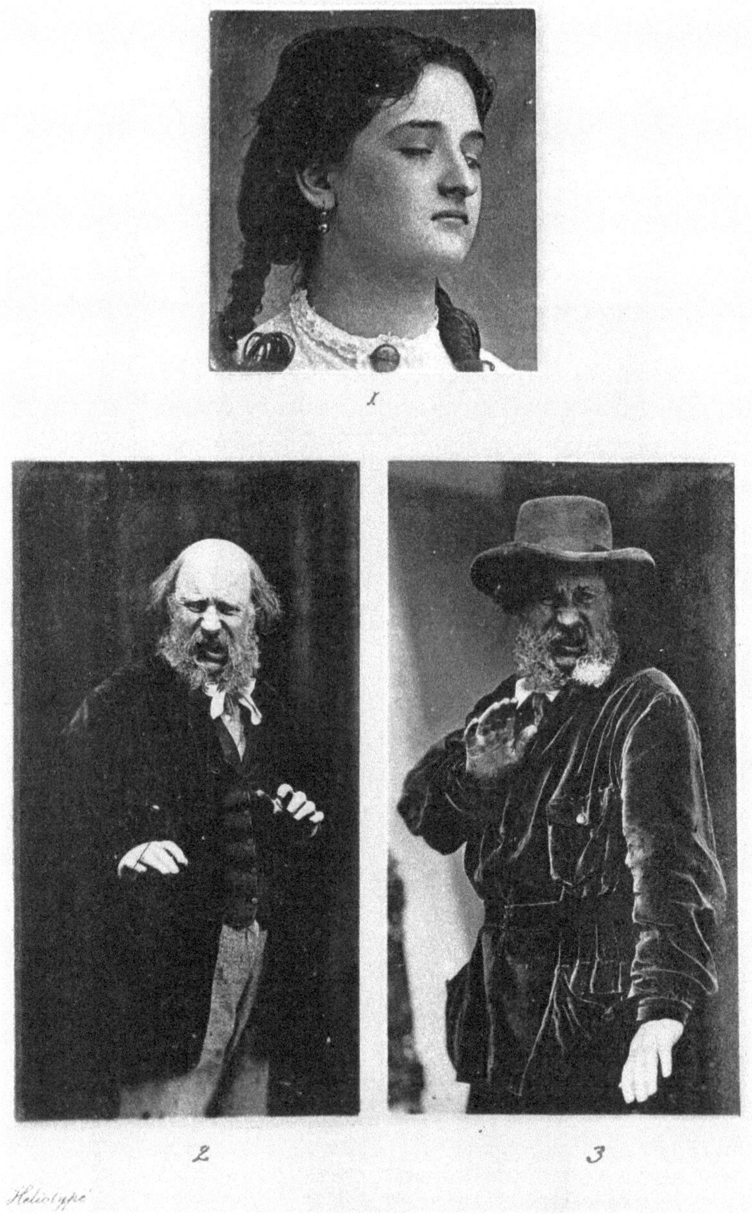

Fig. 6. Plate V, figs. 1–3, Charles Darwin, *The Expression of the Emotions in Man and Animals* (London: Murray, 1872).

The Bodleian Libraries, University of Oxford (OC) 189 f. 73

even in the 1870s, their proximity to theatre would have been apparent. As Jonathan Smith has shown, many of the attitudes in Rejlander's photographs bear a striking resemblance to those depicted in eighteenth and nineteenth-century acting manuals.[30]

In particular, it is Darwin's use of photographs that have led some contemporary critics to argue that Darwin was blind to the Western cultural specificity of his supposedly objective conclusions. Philip Prodger, who characterizes Darwin's search for photographic representations as a hunt for 'specimens', has argued that Darwin became frustrated with the images he collected, that since they were 'produced without proper experimental controls', 'any conclusions that could be drawn from them were tenuous at best'.[31] A similar, if more forceful, claim has been made by Jennifer Green-Lewis, who argues that 'Rejlander's photographs merely substitute for the physiognomist's line drawings, while they appeal to their privileged scientific objectivity as justifications for the author's classifications'.[32] Underlying such an argument seems to be a conviction that Darwin approached the camera as a superior technology of objectivity, as a machine whose self-recording mechanism could simply capture expressions as they passed on a person's face, without any need to rely on the unreliable human eye. In turn, the arguments seem to suggest that Darwin viewed the photographs displayed in the *Expression* as evidence for a stable body, as exemplary physiological types with universal application, not dissimilar from the 'stable body' pedalled by the phrenologists or physiognomists whose theories Darwin sought to undermine.[33] Certainly, if this were true, there would be a profound misalignment between the role of photography in the book, and Darwin's larger project to emphasize transformation through evolution, and life as a process of ongoing negotiation between the body and its environment.

Yet, Darwin was certainly not naïve to the theatricality of the photographs that illustrate the *Expression*, and appeared to have a clear grasp of the contingency of their production. Writing of Rejlander's image of 'Disgust', Darwin draws attention to the gap between spontaneous emotions and representations of them, noting that the photographer had 'simulated the expression . . . with some success' (p. 258). In another photograph, of a moustached man with a downturned mouth and wrinkled forehead, the subject is described as a 'good actor' who 'is shown simulating

[30] Smith, *Charles Darwin*, p. 231; Engel and Siddons, *Practical Illustrations of Rhetorical Gesture and Action*, p. 91.

[31] Prodger, *An Annotated Catalogue*, p. 5.

[32] Green-Lewis, *Framing the Victorians*, p. 159.

[33] John Van Wyhe, *Phrenology and the Origins of Victorian Scientific Naturalism* (Aldershot: Ashgate, 2004) p. 61.

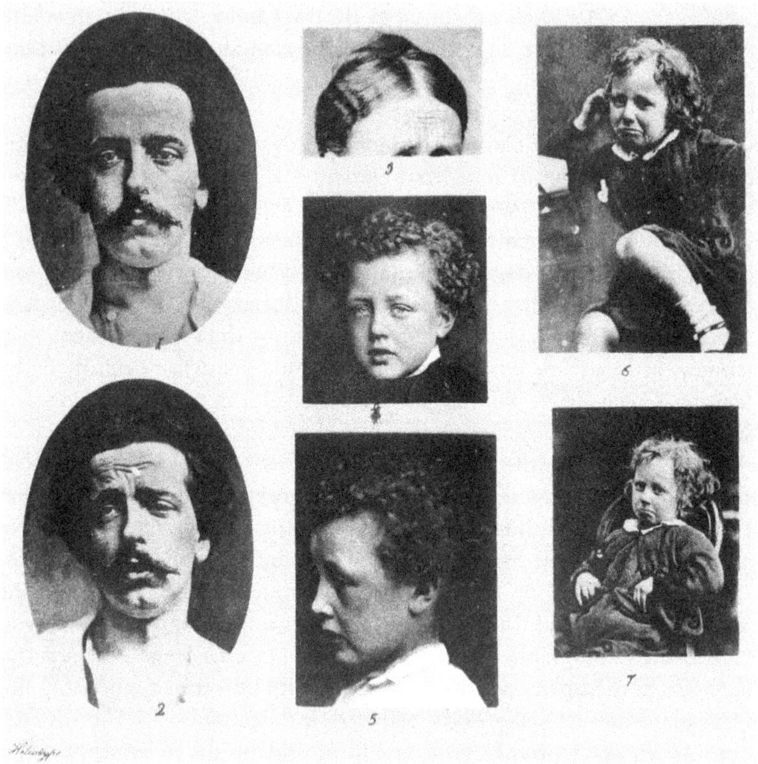

Fig. 7. Plate II, figs. 1–7, Charles Darwin, *The Expression of the Emotions in Man and Animals* (London: Murray, 1872).

The Bodleian Libraries, University of Oxford (OC) 189 f. 73

grief' (Plate II.2, Figure 7) (p. 182). Certainly, Darwin advises his readers to go to the theatre, where the physiology of flinches and cringes as 'common responses' can be 'inferred' from 'the acting of persons who endeavour to express a vividly imagined scene of horror' (p. 307). But at the same time, he reminds us that theatrical representation is one step removed from the thing itself: a prisoner about to be executed, he writes, displayed 'an agony of wildness and despair of which nothing ever exhibited on the stage can give the slightest conception' (p. 294). Framing the photographs as untrustworthy representations, Darwin reminds his readers of theatre's slippery relationship with genuine feeling. Thus, in his description of Plate V.1 (Figure 6), which 'represents a young lady, who is supposed to be tearing up the photograph of a despised lover' (p. 255), the somewhat stingy 'supposed' points up the photograph's inadequacy. Of Plate II.3 (Figure 7), Darwin explains that he has reproduced only the forehead of a frowning woman because as 'she was absorbed in the attempt, whilst being photographed' her expression was 'not at all one of grief' (p. 182). In this case, Darwin's partial reproduction of the photograph reminds us of the compromised relationship between performer and onlooker in the theatre, that Darwin's act of looking was haunted by the incompleteness of theatrical representation and its congenital failures.[34]

As Lorraine Daston and Peter Galison have argued, the concept of objectivity was not a stable one in the second part of the nineteenth century, but rather an idea in formation, constituted through local historical discourses and culturally specific practices. It has been to the apparatuses of the graphic method, such as the sphygmograph for measuring blood pressure or the pneumograph for measuring the breath, as well as stop-action photography and later the X-ray, that cultural historians of scientific looking have turned in order to trace the emergence of an ideal of the 'silent and gestureless' scientific observer of the human body and its fleeting processes. Yet this emphasis on mechanical technologies and graphic representations has obscured other processes deployed in the creation of scientific knowledge about the body in this period. The untrustworthy world of the theatre with its queasy slippages between seeming and being is an unexpected apparatus to hold up as part of the late nineteenth-century's formation of an objective observer, but nonetheless its use does illuminate the embodied and emotional dimensions of experimentation in this period. To invoke a useful distinction made by Peter Galison and Lorraine Daston, scientific observers not only see *that*, but also see *as*, and in the traces of the techniques and practices Darwin used in his research for the *Expression*, it is clear that Darwin was very much '*seeing as*' a theatrical spectator.[35]

Darwin's entanglements with theatre suggest a context for exploring the accidental, emotional, and apparently intangible aspects of his

[34] In his recent edition of the *Expression*, the evolutionary psychologist Paul Ekman reproduced the image of the frowning young woman in its entirety, and then reversed the photographs so that the left-right alignment of the facial muscles was 'correct'. Ekman calls his edition 'the most complete edition ... ever published' (p. xiii), and his work with the photographs reflects his own interest in distinguishing between 'deliberate' and 'spontaneous' facial actions. However, in the case of Darwin's *Expression*, this is a rather redundant strategy, because the photographs were, of course, all staged. It is also misleading, because in doing so Ekman obscures Darwin's own more tentative and sceptical relationship to the photographic representation. See: Charles Darwin, *The Expression of the Emotions in Man and Animals*, ed. by Paul Ekman (Oxford and New York: Oxford University Press, 1998) p. 412.

[35] Daston and Galison, *The Image of Objectivity*, p. 83.

experimental practice. Scientific research is an emotional business: there is the excitement of a new idea, the frustrations of unsatisfactory results, and the thrill of a discovery. In the late 1980s, Christopher Lawrence and Steven Shapin suggested that historians of science might consider a range of other 'embodied human processes' that have characterized laboratory life, asking how one might 'write about the history of scientific (and related) ideas through a history of their embodied form and vicissitudes'.[36] Historians of late nineteenth-century science Otniel Dror and Paul White have separately responded to this call, tracing the presence of emotionality, including that of the experimenters themselves, in the period's scientific practice. Focusing on the turn to human and animal emotion in Anglo-American physiology from the 1870s onwards, Dror has explored the way experimenters attended to the impact of their own affective presence on the moods and responses of their animal subjects, in order to manage the 'emotional ecology' of the laboratory.[37] White, on the other hand, has interrogated the deployment of sentimental rhetoric in the public discourses of science in the second half of the nineteenth century, particularly among vivisectionists eager to represent their humanity to the world (for a further discussion of both White and Dror's work, see Chapter Two).[38] While for Daston and Galison, a moralized and mechanized science coexisted in the development of objectivity, for Dror and White, emotion and scientific observation were similarly constituted together, with the moods, feelings, and affective demonstrations of the experimenter himself playing a key role in the laboratory's delicate ecosystem.

Tracing Darwin's encounters with amateur actors offers an insight into a range of other, perhaps minor, eruptions of emotion that were also part of the experience of the gentleman scientist. For Ridout, going to the theatre to watch actors faking it can swiftly produce a myriad of uncomfortable feelings, from embarrassment and confusion to shame, repulsion, and even illness. 'Theatre being queasy makes me queasy', he writes.[39] Did Darwin catch sight of his friends and family in unseemly self-displays and become embarrassed by their acting? If his involuntary flinch in the Reptile House left him 'amused', did the amateur dramatics of his collaborators also disintegrate into guffawing? Giggling fits (known by actors as 'corpsing'), erupt when cracks appear between the fictional world on stage and the

[36] Lawrence and Shapin, 'Introduction', pp. 2–3.

[37] Otniel E. Dror, 'The Affect of Experiment: The Turn of Emotions in Anglo-American Physiology, 1900–1940,' *Isis* 90 (1999), 205–37 (p. 207).

[38] Paul White, 'Sympathy Under the Knife: Experimentation and Emotion in Late Victorian Britain', in *Medicine, Emotion and Disease, 1700–1950*, ed. Fay Bound Alberti (Basingstoke: Palgrave Macmillan, 2006) pp. 100–24 (p. 101).

[39] Ridout, *Stage Fright*, p. 3.

ludicrous reality, as when an actor notices that his fellow performer, who is delivering a passionate speech about the honour of a Roman gladiator, has a Marks and Spencer underwear label sticking out of his loin cloth. Were there similar breakdowns while Darwin and his 'informants' watched each other mugging surprise or love? Indeed, acting requires playfulness, and can escalate quickly into high spirits and mucking about. A scribbled note on one of the photographs Rejlander sent to Darwin certainly suggests rehearsal room antics. 'Fun only', confided Rejlander under two photographs in which he attempted to mimic his own famous portrait of a child bawling in abject misery, *Jinx's Baby*.

Pretending to experience deep and passionate feelings may well have entertained Darwin and his colleagues, but other, more unnerving affects may have also lingered. Roland Barthes experienced feelings of 'imposture' when he posed for the photomatic, and rather extravagantly suggested that in early photography 'to become an object made one suffer as much as a surgical operation'.[40] Indeed, as a cartoon from *Punch* showed, wincing was a gesture performed in the photography studio by awkwardly posing subjects (Figure 8). Did Rejlander experience the discomfort of sore muscles and self-deception when he arranged himself into an attitude of disgust before his own camera? And while Rejlander was practiced in the art of self-watching, fascinated by the way his image could be doubled, might Darwin's friends, catching sight of their own pretence, have become confounded or momentarily unhinged by the estranged person in the mirror, whose appearance of anger or fear bore so little relation to the actual circumstances of their gesture? Might they too have experienced the *unheimlich* feelings that fifty years later Freud linked to twins, doubles and mirrored images, and to 'the impression of automatic—mechanical—processes that may lie hidden behind the familiar image of a living person'?[41]

It is, then, no coincidence that in a book which opens with anxieties about observing emotional expressions, Darwin signs off the *Expression* with one of Hamlet's most agitated speeches about watching actors: 'Is it not monstrous that this player here / But in a fiction, in a dream of passion / Could force his soul so to his own conceit' demands Hamlet, 'And all for nothing.' Gillian Beer has suggested that the literary allusions in nineteenth-century scientific writing often harbour the theory's wider implications, and this certainly seems the case with Darwin's reference to

[40] Roland Barthes, *Camera Lucida*, trans. Richard Howard (London: Vintage 2000) p. 13.

[41] Sigmund Freud, 'The Uncanny' (1919) trans. James Strachey, in *The Standard Edition of the Complete Psychological Works of Sigmund Freud*, xvii, pp. 217–56 (p. 229).

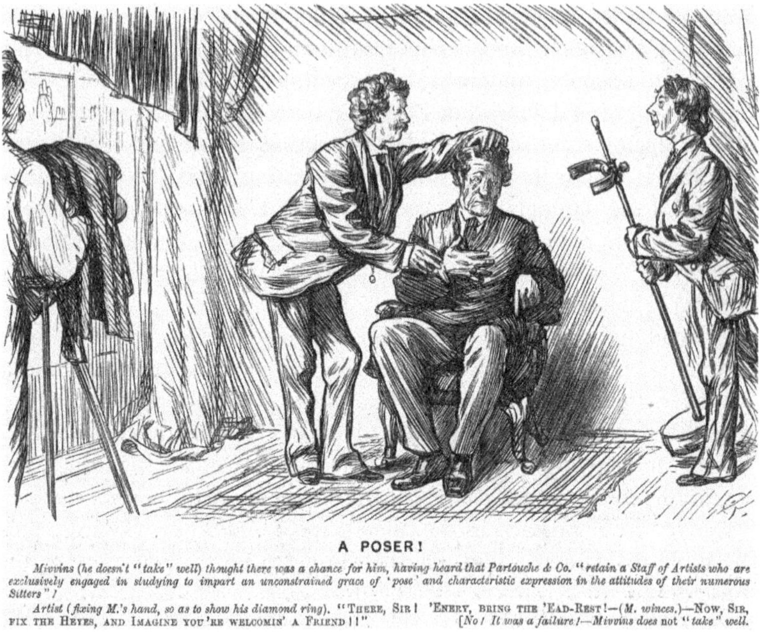

Fig. 8. 'A Poser!' *Punch*, 64 (7 June, Jan/June, 1873), p. 240.

The Bodleian Libraries, University of Oxford, N2706 d. 10

Hamlet.[42] Of all Shakespeare's characters, the Prince of Denmark is the one most disturbed by the fickle relationship between seeming and being, the disjunction between what outward shows and what inward passeth, and the uncoupling of form and content which is the perennial hallmark of theatricality. In both Shakespeare's play and Darwin's scientific tract, theatricality operates as the leading metaphor through which discontinuities and misalignments between the insides and outsides of our emotional selves are explored. As Darwin's evolutionary account of the emotions progresses, so does the creeping realization that in a new age of evolutionary and physiological emotion, our feelings would be not entirely our own.

If the theatrical imagery of the *Expression* served to unsettle cherished notions of a purposeful and reliable emotional body, one that straightforwardly communicated interiority, it also folded the scientist's act of looking into this general condition of instability. It was at the moments when

[42] Gillian Beer, 'Parable, Professionalization and Literary Allusion in Victorian Scientific Writing', in Gillian Beer (ed.) *Open Fields: Science in Cultural Encounter*, pp. 196–215 (p. 215).

the supposedly dispassionate scientific observer studied himself emoting that Darwin's scientific approach became its most theatrical. Darwin's self-experiments were not confined to starting back from lunging snakes in the Reptile House. He also observed himself smiling: 'from my own sensations, I cannot doubt that some of the muscles running to the upper lip are likewise brought into moderate action' (pp. 202–3). At least once he monitored his muscular contractions whilst pretending to shudder, noting that when he shuddered 'at a painful thought', his platysma muscle contracted, and 'so it does if I simulate a shudder' (p. 304). The smell of a dead bird that had not been fully macerated made both Darwin and his servant who were inspecting it 'retch so violently, that we were compelled to desist'. Always alert to his own sensations, Darwin noted that for several days after, any similar skeleton, even ones that barely smelt at all, brought on similar attacks of retching.

In these self-experiments, the discomfort of watching actors was turned on the observer's own body, and the profoundly unnerving feelings of encountering one's theatrical self multiplied. In his self-experiment at the Reptile House, Darwin did not only stage himself flinching so he could observe his response. Even the act of looking ('I put my face up close to the puff-adder's tank') was self-consciously performed in an environment where other spectators, fellow visitors to the Reptile House, might join Darwin in watching himself. Performing his watching—and observing himself turning his face aside, unable to watch any longer—the eminent man of science was both spectator and spectacle, not standing outside the scene he observed but meeting himself on the threshold of his looking. It was precisely in these moments of self-reflexive and emotional spectatorship that the scientific observer of 1872 strayed inconveniently close to the techniques and problems associated with the late Victorian theatrical audience.

TECHNIQUES OF THE SELF-CONSCIOUS OBSERVER

In 1871, the year before Darwin published the *Expression*, Henry Irving made his name playing Mathias in Leopold Lewis's gothic melodrama *The Bells*. The play tells of a local mayor who has been to see a show in a nearby town; 'It was not Punchinello', the mayor admits, 'it was a Parisian who did extraordinary tricks. He sent people to sleep'. The mesmerist provokes in Mathias the memory of a murder he committed twenty years ago, leaving him haunted by hallucinations of the dead man and a sinister cacophony of jangling bells only he can hear. Irving's performance was notorious for its virtuoso flinches. The stage directions describe Mathias '*starting up*' when he hears the bells; he '*starts violently upon seeing the vision before him*'.[43] So spectacular were Irving's flinches and recoils, that each time he staggered backwards he received a round of applause. For the production's publicity photographs, Irving portrayed Mathias at the moment of seeing the ghost, affecting a pose so recognizable it had already become clichéd (Figure 9). As the theatre historian George Taylor notes, by 1871 the start was so firmly embedded as a theatrical gesture that it had become 'universal in pictures of actors, to adopt a "knees-bend" stance, similar to that of a pugilist, swordsman or modern tennis player, so that the actor could start with maximum effect in any direction'.[44]

Throughout the eighteenth and nineteenth centuries starting emerged as a favourite gesture (or 'point') for actors trying to convey moments of sudden perception or crises of recognition. So distinctive was flinching that Henry Morley, an avid chronicler of the theatre, remarked on its various manifestations. One actor, he wrote, 'recoiled with a wild horror' on recognizing her long-lost brother, another 'shuddered and recoiled' when thinking of his daughters.[45] Elsewhere, Morley berated actors for excessive flinching, complaining he was 'quite sure that no Juliet whom Shakespeare in his time had the advising of ever recoiled with such a shriek from the imagined ghost that sought the Romeo', labelling her start a 'claptrap stage-effect'.[46] It was well known that some actors enjoyed flinching a little too much, as one theatre joke made clear: 'Would you not, Sir', said Mr Boswell to Mr Johnson, 'start as Mr. Garrick does, if you saw a ghost?' 'I hope not,' replied Mr Johnson, 'if I did, I should frighten the ghost'.[47] Nonetheless, flinching was supposed to indicate the involuntary expression of depths of feeling. Thus, in one production of *Macbeth*, the Italian actor playing the title role was a particularly prolific flincher, who 'when he shrinks with his mind shrinks with his body also', and when 'he is startled mentally starts bodily, and so, instead of being self-contained is always pouring himself out, even at the very finger tips'. In contrast, this production's Lady Macbeth was, like Hardy's Bathsheba or Dickens's

[43] Leopold Lewis, *The Bells: A Drama in Three Acts* (London: Samuel French, 1871) p. 10; pp. 12–13.

[44] George Taylor, *Players and Performances in Victorian Theatre* (Manchester: Manchester University Press, 1989) p. 31.

[45] Henry Morley, *The Journal of a London Playgoer* (London: Routledge, 1891) p. 306; p. 272.

[46] Morley, *The Journal of a London Playgoer*, p. 337.

[47] William Archer, *Masks or Faces? A Study in the Psychology of Acting* (London: Longmans, 1888) p. 59.

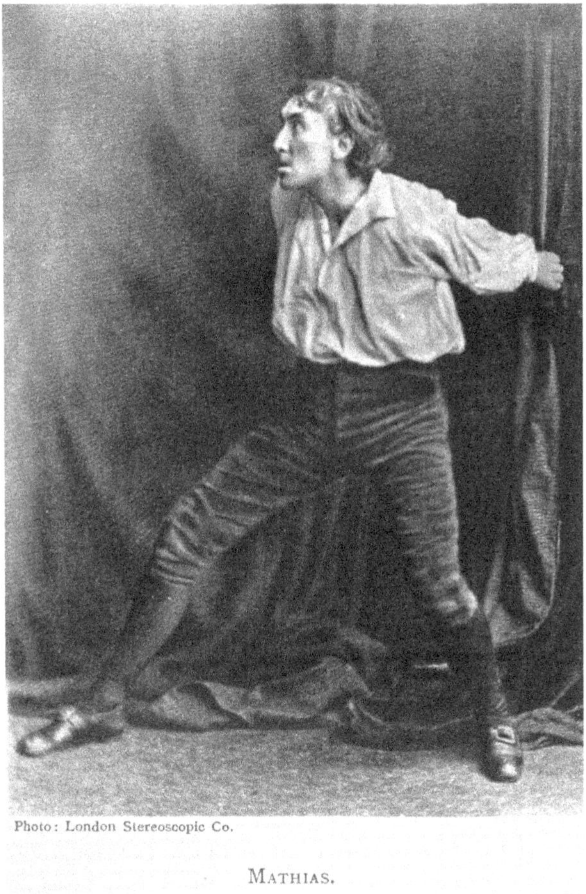

Fig. 9. Henry Irving as Mathias in *The Bells*, 1871, The London Stereoscopic Company.

Plymouth Library Services

Nancy, resolutely unflinching, until she saw Duncan's ghost whereupon she 'flinched bodily' causing her husband to 'recoil' from her 'as from another spectre'.[48]

On the one hand, then, flinching had hardened into a 'stage-effect', a piece of 'business' in which jerking, twitching, and staggering backwards, shielding the face, shrieking, and gasping, were carefully choreographed in order, paradoxically, to suggest a body involuntarily betraying itself. At

[48] Morley, *The Journal of a London Playgoer*, p. 186.

the same time, the gesture, theatrically produced, could also beguile. In his review of *The Bells* the critic William Archer, who later in the century became Britain's chief apologist for theatrical naturalism, was preoccupied by the tantalizing possibility of genuine feeling in the artifice of the stage. He admired Irving's performance, and particularly its flinches which 'seemed not a result of volition, but an involuntary spasm, complicated by extraordinary sidelong and backward skirmishing, reminding one of the moment a napkin-ring shot out from under the forefinger'.[49] In a metaphor that imagines the body's emotions as subject to the forces and pressures of the physical world, Irving's flinch seemed to Archer to be beyond the actor's self-control. Yet, as will always be the case in talk about acting, it only 'seemed' that way. For all its apparent naturalness, Irving's flinch deposited a lingering 'ontological queasiness' in Archer's mind, leaving him wondering whether he had witnessed real fear or a clever simulation of it.

For many of those who thought and wrote about theatre in the second part of the nineteenth century, the problem of emotional authenticity on stage had been resolved through the theories of the eighteenth-century French philosopher and playwright Denis Diderot (1713–1784). Written in 1773, his essay *Le Paradoxe sur le Commédien* ('The Paradox of Acting') remained unpublished until 1830, when its ideas quickly caught on in British theatrical circles well before the book's first full translation into English in 1883.[50] According to Diderot, an actor must be perceptive, adept, and imaginative, a keen observer whose task was to uncover the truths of human relationships and render them in an interesting way. However, for Diderot (and this is the paradox) when on stage the actor should not be emotional. In his nightly forays before an audience, the actor's primary task was to oversee his performance alongside those of the other actors in the scene with him. In this way, he was deemed to have a 'doubled perspective' ('*il est double*'), managing the mirage of the character he had invented through his artistry by maintaining an 'inner distance'.[51] In a similar vein, in 1885 Irving argued that 'the actor never feels', but rather creates for himself a 'double-consciousness in which all the emotions proper to the occasion may have full swing while the actor is all the time on the alert for every detail of his method'.[52] Moreover, actors

[49] William Archer, *Henry Irving, Actor and Manager* (London: Routledge, 1883) p. 63.

[50] Denis Diderot, *The Paradox of Acting* (1773), trans. Walter Herries Pollock (London: Chatto & Windus, 1883).

[51] Denis Diderot, *Oeuvres Esthétiques*, ed. P. Vernière (Paris: Garnier, 1965) p. 195. Quoted in Gunter Gebauer and Christoph Wulf, *Mimesis: Culture, Art, Society* (Berkeley and London: University of California Press, 1995) p. 176.

[52] Henry Irving, 'The Art of Acting' (1885), repr. in *The Drama* (London: Heinemann, 1893) pp. 55–6.

would practice their 'double-consciousness' both on and off the stage. In an anecdote that vividly recalls the way Darwin noticed the muscles engaged whilst shuddering at a 'painful thought', Irving remembered the actor François-Joseph Talma, who 'when deeply moved', found himself 'making a rapid and fugitive observation of the alteration of his voice and on a certain spasmodic vibration which it contracted in tears'.[53] If actors maintained an 'inner distance' that allowed them to uncomplicatedly observe the outward appearances of their emotional expressions, in the case of theatre audiences, the situation was rather less straightforward.

In 1862, *The Times* reported 'the introduction of a new word into the theatrical vocabulary'. The word was 'sensation' and it referred to the 'sensation drama' and its all-important 'sensation scene'. [54] Sensation plays were hybrid forms, combining the basic plots, characters, and situations from melodrama, with one climactic scene of thrilling technological effects. Burning houses, collapsing bridges, and narrow escapes from oncoming express trains featured in scenes of alarming verisimilitude engineered to 'hold the spectator breathless, to harrow up his soul, to excite him' and most of all 'to make the flesh creep'.[55] One such play was *The O'Dowd*, first performed in 1872 at the Gaiety Theatre in London's West End and written by sensation's leading exponent, Dion Boucicault. In its climactic scene, those aboard a capsizing ship are dramatically rescued during a ferocious gale. According to the stage directions, in its extravagant finale *'The stormy sea and a vessel's topsails are seen by the flashes of the lightning—wind—storm—fountains of spray are thrown from time to time over back-pieces on to stage'*—splashing the audience members in the pit where the cheapest seats provided the most thrilling proximity to the action, and almost certainly making them flinch. Accompanying the visual spectacle were startlingly loud noises made by a thunder machine, a wind machine and the continuous onstage firing of guns and flares from the sinking ship, choreographed to make an already tense audience jump out of their skins. In the sensation scene, the rescue coincides with a melodramatic reunion of the estranged Mike with his mad father O'Dowd, a recognition scene punctuated by starts and recoils:

> MIKE: (*staggering back and sinking on the ground*) My God! My father!

A gesture that is echoed and reversed when his father recognizes him:

> O'DOWD: (*staggers forward*) My God! 'tis he—'tis Mike. Oh, it is my son.

[53] Irving, 'The Art of Acting', p. 56.

[54] *The Times*, 13 March 1862, quoted in Michael Diamond, *Victorian Sensation, or, the Spectacular, the Shocking, and the Scandalous in Nineteenth-Century Britain* (London: Anthem Press, 2003) p. 218.

[55] 'Sensational Dramas', *The Era*, 22 January 1881.

At least once, these onstage recoils performed by actors coincided with those elicited from audience members by the sonic choreography:

> Mike: Father! Father! (*two guns fired in succession*).[56]

As a reporter for *The Times* put it, the 'sensation scene' was the moment in which 'the interest of the audience' was 'visibly concentrated'.[57] Michael Diamond has suggested that for Victorians 'a sensation' referred not simply to a particular event or object but to a general 'condition of excited feeling produced in a community by some occurrence'.[58] Already overwrought by the tense drama onstage, gunshots and flashes of light were supposed to produce mass visceral and visible affects in the audience. Like Darwin in his self-experiments, and like the Germans gawping at the human zoos in Berlin, these audiences enjoyed *Schaulust*: both gazing upon and performing alongside the actors. Not least, the excitement of the sensation audience was conspicuous because in 1872, the auditorium was still illuminated, a place where spectators could easily see one another by the soft glow of gas lamps.

Those who regarded themselves to be cultivated theatregoers attacked sensation audiences for their naïve consumption of theatrical excess. Though on the one hand sensation audiences were thought to collude in the explicit artifice of sensation theatre, on the other, the relationship between spectators and actors was characterized as an asymmetrical one, with actors controlling the fiction through their 'inner distance', but spectators naïvely enjoying it. If the 'Adelphi play' (so-called after the London theatre which became most famous for staging sensation dramas) was a box of cheap tricks, it was the 'popular craving for sensation' that paid for it.[59] The great theorist of the sublime Edmund Burke (1729–1797) imagined spectators of shipwrecks and storms who could not 'but shudder' in terror at nature's awesome power.[60] In contrast, the theatre spectator who winced when water splashed over the wooden painted flats and into the pit, or flinched from bangs and crashes produced by the thunder machines backstage, was colluding in a shabby fiction. The audience member was, wrote one reviewer, 'merely thrilled and startled' for 'like Virgil's hero, [he] feeds his eye with an empty picture'.[61]

56 Dion Boucicault, *The O'Dowd* (London and New York: Samuel French, 1908) p. 51; pp. 48–50.

57 *The Times*, 13 March 1862.

58 Diamond, *Victorian Sensation*, p. 1.

59 'Theatre Royal', *Birmingham Daily Post*, 12 November 1867.

60 Edmund Burke, *A Philosophical Enquiry* (1757) (Oxford: Oxford University Press, 1998) p. 63.

61 'Theatres', *The Graphic*, 19 March 1881.

In fact, as the theatre historian Lynne Voskuil has argued, sensation theatre audiences presented their own paradox: 'While its spectators experienced the hair-raising thrills as spontaneous somatic events, they courted such thrills knowingly.'[62] Theatre spectators were self-aware enough to know that they were watching a fiction. There are no reports of sensation audience members rushing up onto the stage to untie the hero from the train tracks. Such percipience distinguished theatrical audiences from other consumers of sensation in the 1860s and 1870s. Those who read sensation fiction, or gossiped about the latest sensational court case, or believed the predictions of 'sensation scientists' who warned of the evolution of gnats into killer mosquitoes and the destruction of London by tiny bottles of explosive liquids, were caught up in a rapid and contagious excitement that quickly obscured the boundaries between what was real and what was theatrical exaggeration.[63] 'Ladies, who had spent their nights and days over captivating novels', warned one instruction manual, 'gave evident proofs that they were of a mind occasionally deranged'.[64] In contrast, theatre audiences were regarded as significantly more sophisticated customers, ones 'practiced at decoding spectacle and awake to its mechanisms and bodily effects', and 'fully at home in the consumerist culture of late-Victorian England.'[65]

Unlike Diderot's actor who 'never feels' but simply observes his emotional performance onstage, theatre spectators simultaneously experienced emotions and monitored them too. In a review of an 1872 production of Boucicault's hit sensation play *The Colleen Bawn* at London's Gaiety Theatre, the audience was described as entranced when the heroine, the hunchbacked villain, and the gallant rescuer all plunged into a deep pool of water. 'The great sensation scene of the water cave exercised its old spell on the house', the reviewer wrote. However, that same night a technical fault interrupted the action bringing the curtain down prematurely, a blunder which the 'highly wrought audience immediately perceived and strongly objected to, and for which Mr Boucicault came forward and apologized'.[66] This audience, in turns spellbound and aware of the terms of the contract they had entered into on purchasing a ticket, had gone to the theatre to consume their own emotions, paying to watch actors present symbolic near-death experiences so that they might enjoy the pleasure of their own flinches, and in turn, the vicarious relief of crises averted. Theirs

[62] Lynn M. Voskuil, *Acting Naturally: Victorian Theatricality and Authenticity* (Charlottesville: University of Virginia Press, 2004) p. 250.

[63] Anon., 'An Gnattempted Sensation', *Judy*, 26 October 1881; Anon., 'Sensation Science', *Funny Folks*, 28 September 1878.

[64] *Health for the Million* (1858) quoted in Gesa Stedman, *Stemming the Torrent: Expression and Control in the Victorian Discourses on Emotion, 1830–1872* (Aldershot: Ashgate, 2002).

[65] Voskuil, 'Feeling Public', p. 250.

[66] 'Drama', *Daily News*, 6 May 1872.

was not a naïve encounter with, or a complete enslavement to, the fictional world on stage. Rather, these audiences consumed their own vivid feelings, in the knowledge that mere simulations of terrors had produced them.

This canny ability of the audience to both be moved and simultaneously consume emotions as visceral objects was brought sharply into focus in literary representations of theatre going in the late nineteenth century. Wilkie Collins's sensation novel *Man and Wife* (1870), for example, features a moment when the spectator's ability to distinguish between fact and fiction fails. An innocent country girl called Blanche finds herself in a shady corner of the metropolis. 'I had never been inside a theatre in my life,' she admits, as she is accidentally swept into the entrance of the pit in a rowdy West End playhouse. Blanche is nervous that she might lose herself in the drama. 'It struck me that I might get taken, as it were, out of myself, if I saw something that was quite strange to me, and heard something which would put new thoughts into my mind.' Yet, as the play reaches its crescendo, she makes a far more alarming discovery. It is not she who has been 'got' but the rest of the working-class audience who stand around her. While the characters on stage had 'murder in their minds', the terrified Blanche realizes that 'all the people about me' were 'laughing and clapping their hands'. She is both confused and enraged by their response. 'The noise they made angered me. I don't know how to describe the state I was in. My eyes wouldn't serve me, and my ears wouldn't serve me, to see and to hear what the rest of them were seeing and hearing.' She tries to warn her fellow spectators of the murderous intentions of the actors ('nobody knew it but me'), but finding her 'tongue was tied' picks up her skirts and scurries out.[67] Blanche makes an error only hopelessly inexperienced theatregoers in stories can do. Confusing fictional representation for the real thing, she also mistakes the audience's enthusiasm for a kind of tragic naïvety, when of course it is she who is credulous, blind to theatre's encoded spectacles.

As Davis and Emeljanow have shown, the pit was habitually characterized as a threatening place by Victorian novelists and social reformers who portrayed working-class audiences as boisterous and disorderly. In these depictions of the audience, a dangerous propensity to over-identification with the fictional situations of the characters was juxtaposed with the cynical opportunism of cut-throats, prostitutes, and thieves (the reality, Davis and Emeljanow argue, was probably merely that such audiences produced 'a certain degree of noise').[68] Collins's novel certainly inscribes two distinct

[67] Wilkie Collins, *Man and Wife* (1870) (Oxford: Oxford University Press, 1995) p. 601.

[68] Jim Davis and Victor Emeljanow, 'Victorian and Edwardian Audiences', in *The Cambridge Companion to Victorian and Edwardian Theatre*, ed., Kerry Powell (Cambridge: Cambridge University Press, 2004) p. 95.

emotional communities in the theatre, contrasting the indifference of the privileged audience who received the play as 'something wearisome', with the overwrought excitements of the poorer spectators in the pit.[69] Yet, as Blanche's traumatic experience makes clear, the same working-class patrons who were seen to noisily express their voluble emotional responses to the scenarios played out on stage before them, were also the ones who most nimbly distinguished between the fictional appearance of the characters, and the reality of the performer's undertaking. If Collins's novel drew attention to a distinctively knowing pattern of emotional theatrical looking, the philosopher, scientific writer, playwright, critic, and erstwhile actor George Henry Lewes expanded the idea to advance a theory of self-reflexive and impassioned spectatorship in the theatre auditorium and beyond it.

INTROSPECTION AND THE 'OPTIQUE DU THÉÂTRE'

In 1875, G. H. Lewes (1817–1878) published a collection of his writings about theatre as *On Actors and the Art of Acting*. The partner of novelist George Eliot, and a close associate of Thomas Carlyle and John Stuart Mill, Lewes was a highly regarded intellectual. Alongside his work as a theatre critic, Lewes established a reputation as a writer on scientific ideas, his work taken so seriously that it was rumoured that Darwin proposed his membership to both the British Medical Association and the Linnaean Society.[70] In *On Actors* Lewes addressed the style and technique of some of the eighteenth and nineteenth century's most important theatrical performers including Edmund Kean and William Charles Macready, and through these studies advanced his own theory of the expression of emotion on stage and in the auditorium.

For Lewes, as it was for Diderot and Irving, acting was less a question of feelings than of skilful representations of them. He adopted the phrase *optique du théâtre* from the French actor Talma to describe theatre's distinctive machinery for representing and generating feeling. Lewes argued that theatrical performance would falter if actors were to attempt to perform 'passion in its real rather than in its symbolic representation'. 'All art is symbolical', he argued, continuing that if an actor 'presented emotion in its real expression it would cease to move us as art; sometimes cease to move us at all, or move us only to laughter'. 'Emotion,' he concluded, 'does

[69] Collins, *Man and Wife*, p. 426.

[70] Hock Guan Tjoa, *George Henry Lewes: A Victorian Mind* (Cambridge, MA and London: Harvard University Press, 1977) p. 24; p. 30.

not utter itself in verse nor in carefully chosen sentences'. Lewes emphasized theatre's separation of form and content, shining a light on the void that lies at the heart of the theatrical encounter where authentic feeling ought to be. 'The look and the tone may come from a man so drunk as to be scarcely able to stand; but the public sees only the look, hears only the tone, and is irresistibly moved by these intelligible symbols.'[71] To describe the actor's task of monitoring his own enactment of these 'symbols', Lewes used the term 'introspection', a term that for Lewes meant turning one's gaze *on* oneself, as well as turning it inwards.

The audience's role in the *optique du théâtre* is less clear in Lewes's discussion. At times, spectators are 'readers' of symbolic emotion, 'irresistibly moved by these intelligible symbols'. Elsewhere he understood their emotional experience to be rather more self-conscious, not unlike the theatricality attributed to audiences of sensation theatre. The audience 'sees at once that as a matter of fact the emotions represented by the actor are not agitating him as they would agitate him in reality; he is representing a fiction which is to move us as a fiction, and not to lacerate our sympathies as they would be lacerated by the agony of a fellow-creature actually suffering in our presence'. In contrast with his earlier more romantic description of spectators being 'irresistibly moved', Lewes advances a more complex idea where, like the actor's own masquerade, spectator's emotions are emptied of depth when they enter the theatre. Unlike real life in which our sympathies are lacerated by genuine suffering, theatre produces an environment of emotional simulacra on both sides of the footlight. 'The tears we shed are tears welling from a sympathetic source', wrote Lewes, 'but their salt bitterness is removed, and their pain is pleasurable'.[72]

It is fairly common to describe Victorian theatre, particularly in the early and middle parts of the century, as a place where people went not only to see, but also to be seen. For example, in his book on Victorian visuality, Chris Otter describes the auditorium as an 'oligoptic space', a space of 'mutual oversight', which provided opportunities for 'personal display' as well as 'for scrutinising the appearance of others'.[73] G. Engelman's painting *Spectacle Gratis* (early to mid nineteenth century), for example, gives some indication of how raucous—and self-absorbed—the auditorium could get: even the spectators hanging over the front of the balcony have turned their heads away from the stage compelled by the fight going on behind them. However, Lewes takes this point further, making

[71] George Henry Lewes, *On Actors and the Art of Acting* (London: Smith, Elder & Co., 1875) pp. 98–9; p. 91.

[72] Lewes, *On Actors*, pp. 94–5; p. 91; p. 100.

[73] Otter, *The Victorian Eye*, p. 74.

self-consciousness pivotal to the creation of meaning in the theatre. Rather than a place for the production of romantic interiorities, through Lewes's account the auditorium becomes a space of interrupted and mediated visuality, in which actors and audience members, in an estranging art of surfaces, knowingly perform emotions alongside each other. 'We are all', he concluded, 'spectators of ourselves'.[74]

Lewes returned to the theme of self-watching two years later when he published the *Problems of Life and Mind* (1875). A testament to Lewes's keen intellectual appetite, its five volumes range from the ethics of animal experimentation to the metaphysics of free will. In the fourth volume, Lewes dedicated a chapter to discussing the validity of introspection as a scientific technique, a subject of fierce debate among those working in the new sciences of mind. In one camp were those who subscribed to the positivist theories of the French philosopher of science Auguste Comte. Following Immanuel Kant and François-Joseph Brousais, Comte had absolutely ('contemptuously' according to Lewes) rejected self-observation as a justifiable method of gathering information about our emotions and sensory experiences, arguing that the conscious mind could not pay attention to itself without being transformed through the process. In the opposing camp were those who followed the German pioneer of scientific psychology Wilhelm Wundt. In his laboratories at Leipzig, Wundt believed he had developed techniques that allowed researchers to report their own experiences whilst eradicating individual bias (Wundt's strategies will be discussed in more detail in Chapter Three).

Lewes's position was poised between the two. He dismissed the notion that we might have privileged access to our interior experiences through the existence of some 'internal eye': 'the physiologist knows of no such organ,' he wrote. Rather, he believed that our attention might just as easily be directed to fluctuations in our sentient affections as to the activities of the physical world. 'We observe changes of Feeling no less than changes in the External', he argued, and when 'an animal moves before us, we observe either its motions, its shape and colour, or the effect (curiosity or fear) produced in us'. In this way, Lewes sidestepped Comte's criticism that the mind is able to directly observe all operations, except its own. Instead, he suggested that the true object of introspection was not a remote, private self, but what he called 'Experience'.[75]

Lewes's concept of experience bears further discussion, not least because it echoes the dynamic model of social interaction evoked in his description

[74] Lewes, *On Actors,* p. 102

[75] George Henry Lewes, *Problems of Life and Mind*, iv, 5 vols. (London: Trübner, 1879) p. 82; p. 84.

of the *optique du théâtre*, as well as Darwin's own account of the emotional self in the *Expression*. According to Lewes, when we look at the ebb and flow of our own experience, we can detect an amalgamation of forces at work. Experience transcends 'the facts of individual feeling' to 'include those of the race'. In other words, it is a mutual process in which other people's emotions and behaviour enter the slipstream of our own consciousness. While Lewes believed that we are not 'conscious of what passes in the mind of another', he nonetheless argued that 'through Observation and Inference, and that sympathetic inward movement which may be called mental contagion' other people's feelings impinge on our inner lives, becoming an 'element in our Experience'. As such, Lewes believed experience could be a valid object of scientific study, as to observe it was to go beyond the idiosyncrasies of the individual 'specimen', and enter the realm of the collective and social, from which 'general laws' may be deduced. 'The experiences of millions of men', he concluded, 'co-operate in the determination of the thoughts and acts of the individual'.[76]

It is an idea strikingly similar to Darwin's account of the emotional mind and body as a bundle of emotional vestiges. Like Lewes's concept of experience, Darwin's emotional body emerges as a composite which harbours the 'thoughts and acts' of men, women, and animals over millennia. Moreover, in both, the observer can never entirely separate himself from the field he observes, but rather is always an active participant in it, the subject and object inseparable from one another. Indeed, for Lewes, it was only through introspection that 'what passes in the mind of another' can be witnessed and understood. While Darwin invoked *Hamlet* to articulate an anxiety that the appearances and reality of other people's feelings might not equate, Lewes turned to *Troilus and Cressida* to capture his belief that to access our own inner terrain we must journey beyond our boundaries and see ourselves reflected in the eyes of others:

> For speculation turns not to itself,
> Til it hath travell'd and is mirror'd there
> Where it may see itself. This is not strange at all.
>
> (*Troilus and Cressida* III.iii.104–6)[77]

For Achilles, 'it is not strange at all' that to discover ourselves we must turn not within but without; in both Shakespeare's and Lewes's description of self-formation, identity is produced through the specular processes of reflection. Just as Darwin repositions the emotional subject in the ebb

[76] Lewes, *Problems of Life and Mind*, p. 92.
[77] Lewes, *Problems of Life and Mind*, p. 93.

and flow of social encounters, concentrating on slippery outward performances rather than the security of inner feelings, Lewes's account of introspection is one in which we do not gaze within so much as upon. To see ourselves, our eyes must roam back and forth.

By the end of the nineteenth century, the concept of a self formed through specular and interactive processes had become well established. Interestingly, it was the new technologies of photography, with their inherent theatrical self-fashioning that provided writers and philosophers with a leading metaphor. Thus, in 1890, the French sociologist Gabriel Tarde described the formation of selves as an 'inter-psychical photography', the action of which consists 'of a quasi-photographic reproduction of a cerebral image upon the sensitive plane of another's brain'.[78] Yet, for Lewes and Darwin, it was the older technology of the theatre that provided the conceptual resources through which to think and write about a self-decentred. In the dynamic *optique du théâtre*, spectators and performers discovered each other and themselves in a hall of mirrors, in which mirage-like surfaces opposed, reflected, refracted, and distorted each other. It is perhaps no coincidence that Darwin's self-experiment in flinching took place in a similarly mirrored and reflective environment. Surrounded by the 'thick glass' tanks housing snakes and lizards, Darwin's experience as a spectator in the Reptile House was one of interrupted visuality, his own reflection appearing on the threshold of his looking. As Isobel Armstrong has argued, nineteenth-century glass acted as 'both *medium* and *barrier*' (original italics), and a repository for anxieties about visibility.[79] Her description of Victorian glass as pock-marked, cloudy, thick with the glass-blower's breath and dim with the exhalations of those who, like Darwin, peer up against it, is strikingly reminiscent of the visuality of sensation theatre with its smoke-filled auditoria and hazily lit stage, its gauzes, projections, and mirrors that permitted the illusions of death-defying leaps and near-drownings. For Darwin, these shifting veils come close to the mutability of the eye itself which is 'slowly changing in form':

> If we must compare the eye to an optical instrument, we ought in imagination to take a thick layer of transparent tissue, with spaces filled with fluid, and with a nerve sensitive to light beneath, and then suppose every part of this layer to be continually changing slowly in density, so as to separate into layers of different densities and thicknesses, placed at different distances from each other, and with the surfaces of each layer slowly changing in form.[80]

[78] Gabriel Tarde, *Laws of Imitation* (1890), trans. Elsie Clews Parsons (New York: Holt, 1903) p. 77.

[79] Armstrong, *Victorian Glassworlds*, p. 7.

[80] Charles Darwin, *On The Origin of Species* (London: John Murray, 1859) p. 188.

Darwin's problem of looking in the *Expression* may be understood as caught up in what Crary has identified as the nineteenth-century's broader disenchantment with the observer. In the eighteenth century, the *camera obscura* provided a primary metaphor for looking, one that insisted on the separation of the observer's body from the world he gazed upon. In contrast, Crary argues, the early decades of the nineteenth century saw the observer increasingly lodged within the 'unstable physiology and temporality' of his own body.[81] While the *camera obscura* prevented the observer from seeing himself as part of the representation, in Darwin's *Expression* even the act of looking becomes part of the instability of the emotional world he sought to study—and it is the live co-presence of theatre, rather than an optical toy, which brings this complicity into focus. Performing his act of watching surrounded by looming glass tanks, Darwin's flinch is a theatrical display of both perception and feeling. Reminiscent of Irving's starts and recoils from imagined terrors on the stage of the Lyceum, Darwin's flinch also serves as a reminder that the onlooker cannot stand outside the *optique du théâtre* and its dynamic affective interactions. In the Reptile House, an environment of excitement and danger, of dispassionate observation and vivid, visceral pleasures, Darwin dramatized precisely this problem of looking. Like a theatrical spectator, he was not only a gesturing emotional onlooker experiencing involuntary nervous responses, but was also a self-conscious performer, alert to his own passionate acts of looking, his gestures multiplied in the glass tanks lining the walls.

DARWIN'S STAGE DIRECTIONS

Darwin wrote the *Expression* at the height of his fame and popularity, and it quickly became a bestseller, with 9,000 copies sold in the first four months alone. 'It is now the rage amongst the people in town', wrote a columnist in the *Globe* newspaper, 'to talk of this wonderful book, and a wonderful book is made of it when its facts and theories are imperfectly recollected and incoherently stated'. 'Mr Darwin', the columnist continued, was bound to become 'a boudoir favourite', his book as much requisite for 'young ladies' as 'the regulation three volumes of romance'.[82] Reviewers also lingered on the *Expression's* 'fascinating' surface, 'enriched by the most diversified illustrations and brightened by all manner of

[81] Crary, *Techniques of the Observer*, p. 70.

[82] Anon., 'Darwin in the Drawing-Room', *The Globe*, 7 November 1872, *Darwin Papers*, CUL—DAR226.2.129.

curious anecdotes', and its photographs, which for the first time in a scientific publication appeared in the body of the text on shiny, slippery paper.[83] Both photographs and anecdotes were deemed capable of producing intriguing emotional effects. One press clipping found among Darwin's private papers compared reading the *Expression* to going to the theatre. There is nothing, the critic wrote:

> Which excites a wider sympathy than the expression of the emotions. The whole charm of art lies in this expression, and no art is so powerful as the dramatic, in which words are interpreted by looks and gestures. Any one who has seen a great play well acted will know that even the most powerful words convey only half their meaning without a visible embodiment.

According to the reviewer, closely watching emotions is stimulating, it 'excites sympathy', and the emotions of others exert an almost magical influence, a 'powerful charm'. Moreover, it is only by producing a 'visible embodiment' of expressions that the fullness of feeling may be communicated. Nonetheless, he also regarded these photographic depictions to be potent, warning women that 'some woodcuts and photographs at the end, descriptive of the feelings of pain, horror, and agony' might 'perhaps occasion a distressing shock under some circumstances. But if these could be kept out of sight, we should recommend to mothers a series of photographs of sulky, screaming, and smiling children.'[84]

For the philosophers Gilles Deleuze and Félix Guattari, 'a book itself is a little machine'.[85] In the case of the *Expression*, the mechanism is theatrical: through it, self-consciously emotional encounters between spectators and performers are repeatedly staged. Much of the *Expression* serves to emotionally rearrange its readers. Not only its illustrations, but also its highly affecting anecdotes of men and women caught in triumphs and tragedies by Darwin's 'informants' (p. 269) entice readers into emotional worlds. A doctor reports being visited by 'a very young Dhangar woman from Nagpore' who was 'nursing her baby who was at the point of death. He distinctly saw the eyebrows raised at the inner corners' (p. 188). Another 'informant', this time a woman, writes of seeing 'a negro towing a boat on the Nile, and as he encountered an obstruction she observed his grief-muscles in strong action' (p. 187). These 'curious scraps of descriptions', more 'curious', no doubt, for their often exotic provenance, could titillate. Thus, in Darwin's discussion of blushing, he reported the

[83] Anon., 'The Expression of the Emotions in Man and Animals', *The Times*, 13 December 1872. *Darwin Papers*, CUL—DAR226.2.142–144.

[84] Anon. 'The Expression of the Emotions in Man and Animals', *The Times*, 13 December 1872.

[85] Deleuze and Guattari, *A Thousand Plateaus*, p. 4.

case of a female asylum patient aged twenty-seven, who was examined by Crichton-Browne 'while she was in bed'. Her doctor noted that 'she blushed deeply over her cheeks and temples; and the blush spread quickly to her ears', and that, when he 'unfastened the collar of her chemise in order to examine the state of her lungs' a 'brilliant blush rushed over her chest, in an arched line over the upper third of each breast and extended downwards between the breasts' (p. 314). In a similar vein, the surgeon Sir James Paget reported a case in which 'a little girl, shocked by what she imagined to be an act of indelicacy, blushed all over her abdomen and the upper parts of her legs' (p. 314). Just as Darwin attributed emotional depths to the tightened muscles around the eyes of a young woman sitting opposite him on the train, such anecdotes invited readers to imagine dramatic scenarios and rich inner lives from descriptions of mere physiological changes.

In other cases, Darwin's stories seem intended to emotionally arouse his readers through their deployment of sentimental conventions. The tales of Darwin's pets are a particularly vivid example of his 'romantic materialism'.[86] Darwin 'formerly possessed a large dog,' he informs us, 'who was much pleased to go out walking' and who 'showed his pleasure by trotting gravely' before the naturalist 'with high steps' (p. 57). However, when Darwin interrupted his walk to visit his experimental plants in his hot house, the dog was overcome by a 'great disappointment', displaying a 'look of dejection' which was 'piteous and hopeless', 'the head drooping', 'the whole body sinking', 'the ears and tail falling', 'the tail was by no means wagged' (p. 60). In this drama of dashed hopes, Darwin's dog performs as coercively as the travelling circus animals described by Dickens, who tug insistently at the reader's heart-strings:

> 'That dog' said Jerry, pointing out the old leader of the troop, and speaking in a terrible voice, 'lost a halfpenny to-day. He goes without his supper.' The unfortunate creature dropped upon his fore-legs directly, wagged his tail, and looked imploringly at his master. 'You must be more careful, sir' said Jerry, walking coolly to the chair where he had placed the organ, and setting the stop. 'Come here. Now, sir, you play away at that, while we have supper, and leave off if you dare.' The dog immediately began to grind most mournful music. [87]

In his emotive descriptions of animals and children, Darwin seems to deliberately instil in his readers the experience that he himself hoped to overcome at the beginning of the *Expression*: one of the things that makes

[86] Beer, *Darwin's Plots*, p. 37.
[87] Charles Dickens, *The Old Curiosity Shop* (1841) (Harmondsworth: Penguin, 1972) p. 202.

the study of emotional expression 'difficult' is that observing and understanding emotions often goes hand in hand with sympathetically feeling them too.

The *Expression* works as a theatrical machine in more explicit ways too. From its pages, Darwin issues stage directions, tantalizing and explicit requests that his readers artificially reproduce emotions. To observe the expression of a screaming baby, Darwin advises his readers to 'make a person first raise his eyebrows' and then 'contract all the muscles round the eyes with as much force as possible' (p. 148). To observe surprise, he hints that 'any one who will try to open his eyes as quickly as possible before a mirror' will find that their eyebrows are automatically raised (p. 281). Encouraged to stage each other and themselves, the readers' performances are meant to corroborate Darwin's descriptions, as well as authenticate the *Expression*'s photographic representations. But the mode of address also recalls discussions of the art of gestures already familiar from acting manuals of the period: to produce the appearance of 'joy', for example, Johann Jacob Engel advises the actor to 'sink the arms lower on each side; give less force to the muscles so that the figure may insensibly elevate itself; place the two feet lightly upon the earth, and make the edge of the teeth visible by a feeble and fugitive motion of the mouth'.[88] In a similar manner, Darwin coaxes his readers to compare themselves with two 'fairly good representations of men simulating indignation', Plate VI.1 and 2 (Figure 5), through a carefully guided acting lesson:

> Any one may see in a mirror, if he will vividly imagine that he has been insulted and demands an explanation in an angry tone of voice, that he suddenly and unconsciously throws himself into some such attitude (p. 247).

It is perhaps no coincidence that the gesture they arrive at bears a striking resemblance to that of 'Anger' in Engel's *Practical Illustrations of Rhetorical Gestures*.[89]

Responding to these stage directions, those who pick up the *Expression* are encouraged to experience the text both theatrically and somatically, observing their own emotional performances as they study the emotional expressions of others. Acting along with the *Expression*'s descriptions, comparing their own performances of 'indignation' with those appearing on the photographic plates, the book's readers echo Darwin and Rejlander's self-experiments, Irving's careful gestures, and the 'double-consciousness' of the audiences of sensation theatre. As a theatrical experience, the *Expression* brought together a range of Victorian domestic practices,

[88] Engel and Siddons, *Practical Illustrations of Rhetorical Gesture*, p. 280.
[89] Engel and Siddons, *Practical Illustrations of Rhetorical* Gesture, fig. 41 'Anger'.

from reading aloud and in groups to the craze for *tableaux vivant* and the increasingly popular use of home science kits. It is not too far-fetched to imagine groups of the Victorian middle classes in drawing rooms up and down the country pretending to be insulted with each other, and making all kinds of frightening grimaces in the lustre on the mantelpiece. As Jane Gray admitted, after the experiment at Downe House with Duchenne de Boulogne's photographs, 'it came out at dinner, that several of us had been trying to move certain muscles before the glass!'[90]

Comparing one's own facial expressions to those portrayed on the *Expression*'s heliotype plates and engravings created plenty of opportunities to be 'struck with admiration at the truthfulness of all' (p. 14).[91] The device is artful, and might well be construed as manipulative, a way of producing and reinforcing a taxonomy of normative emotions that Green-Lewis or Stedman have found in the *Expression*. Certainly, it is in these stage directions that Darwin's book comes closest to the acting manuals with which it shares so much of its visual style. Yet, in mobilizing an *optique du théâtre* in which readers observe themselves and one another emoting, the *Expression* also blurs the boundaries of the discrete emotional subject. Haunted by the slippages of theatrical mimesis, its mismatched relations and laughable failures, the encounter between the *Expression*'s readers and its pages emphasizes malleability rather than fixity. The *Expression* argues for continuity and similarity between species, at the same time as it insists on the principles of transformation and mutation at the heart of evolutionary theory. In her study of the *Origin*, Gillian Beer emphasizes Darwin's use of 'expressive rather than rigorous' language, his deployment of multi-vocal metaphors that have a 'tendency to dilate and contract across related senses, to oscillate between significations'. The *Origin*'s final sentence contains Darwin's bold and poetic assertion that 'endless forms most beautiful and most wonderful have been and are being evolved'. As Beer has put it, in this moment the author of evolution 'alternates in the sentence the principles of stasis and motion, of completion and continuity', setting in motion an 'imaginative release into a continuing and undescribed future' which she regards as 'remarkable when it is set alongside the positivistic emphasis on *finality* which we find in Comte' (original italics). For Beer, Darwin's 'language practice and his scientific theory coincide'.[92]

[90] Jane Gray's letter to her sister, 28 October 1868.

[91] When Darwin examined Duchenne de Boulogne's photographs of galvanized facial muscles without their captions, he was left feeling 'perplexed', but with the descriptions attached, he was 'struck with admiration at the truthfulness of all' (p. 14).

[92] Beer, *Darwin's Plots*, p. 38; p. 64; p. 33.

Theatre performs a similarly unsettling role in the *Expression*. Darwin's aim was not to demarcate a series of ideal emotional types. Rather, by producing mirages of bodies reflecting one another, the *Expression* performs a rhetorical gesture of its own, echoing the lengthy processes through which expressions evolve. It is no coincidence that for Darwin, mimicry was a vital mechanism for the evolution of emotional expression. Musing on the tendency of butterflies and moths to transform their appearance to those of their predators, Darwin demanded to know 'why, to the perplexity of naturalists, has Nature condescended to the tricks of the stage?'[93] Ten years later in the *Expression*, he wrote of man's 'strong tendency to imitation', citing Charcot's work on the 'echo sign' (pp. 356–7) as an example. In copying others, and becoming aware of the way others echoed them, Darwin's readers were invited to experience the disconcerting feelings of such an imposture. Just as Darwin encountered his body to be composite and out of control at the moment of his flinch, in reading the *Expression* his readers discovered that their feelings were not entirely their own.

INSIDES, OUTSIDES, AND ASIDES

One of the things that can be frustrating to today's readers of the *Expression* is the fact that it offers no consistent, or even coherent, theory of emotion. Although Darwin describes how individual expressions evolved, he offers no overarching philosophical or physiological account that explains how the subjective, felt aspects of emotions and their outward expressions are connected. Nonetheless, the larger philosophical problem is never far from his writing, emerging in asides and fleeting comments that overlap and contradict one another. In some places, Darwin's rhetoric invokes a reliable and predictable causal relationship between feelings and their outward performance. Emotions such as terror and joy, he writes, 'naturally lead to certain lines of actions and produce certain effects on the body' (p. 288). Elsewhere, however, this unidirectional relationship is provocatively muddled. Darwin notes that 'most of our emotions are so closely connected with their expression, that they hardly exist if the body remains passive' (p. 239), later acknowledging that 'even the simulation of an emotion can arouse it in our minds' (p. 366). His stage directions go further in highlighting the reciprocity between emotional mind and body, pointing up the way physical movements and the imagination cooperate to produce spontaneous visceral affects: by vividly imagining one has been

[93] Charles Darwin, 'Review of Contributions to an Insect Fauna of the Amazon Valley. By Henry Walter Bates, Esq.', *Natural History Review*, 3 (April), 219–24 (p. 220–1).

insulted, and demanding 'an explanation in an angry tone of voice', the actor 'throws himself' into an attitude of defiance (p. 247).

Today, when psychologists specializing in the emotions such as Paul Ekman and Daniel Goleman turn to the history of their discipline, it is with Darwin that their story begins. While they draw attention to Darwin's reliance on unsubstantiated anecdotes, they also emphasize his use of modern scientific research methods, most of all photographs. It is unsurprising, perhaps, that such histories overlook the role of theatre in Darwin's experiment. After all, theatre, with its shabby pretence, has long been regarded the antithesis of scientific enquiry: in contrast to the empirical exactitude of the experimental method, theatre deals, as Francis Bacon put it, merely in 'worlds of illusion'.[94] Yet, the techniques and problems of theatre were deep within Darwin's experimental work on the emotions. Acting and watching actors were vital, if problematic, tools in his research kit, allowing him to stage emotions—whether in person or through the medium of photography—in order that he might observe and study their physiological changes. If Darwin came close to the condition of the self-conscious audiences of sensation theatre, so his readers too became performers when they responded to the stage directions in the *Expression*, their own assumption of emotional attitudes bringing Darwin's ideas home in very concrete ways. Finally, as was the case with Lewes, in Darwin's writing theatricality became an important metaphor for his proposition of a decentred emotional self, one formed through the specular and interactive processes of mimicry in an ongoing negotiation between bodies and their environments.

By endlessly deferring the subjective dimension of the emotions in order to concentrate on their performance, Darwin's writing undoes the clasp that formerly held inner feeling and outward expression together. His flinch before the puff adder's tank in the London Zoological Gardens encapsulates a broader historical moment in which our bodies were taken out of our sole possession, becoming theatrical even to ourselves. Although Darwin does not explicitly theorize the relationship between emotional expressions and their mental states, his lack of clarity reflects a wider ambivalence in the second part of the nineteenth century around the causal link between body and mind. In this period of transition, a new physiological account of the body's relationship to the outside world was being charted, one which called into question cherished notions of a purposefully feeling and perceiving subject, and suggested new ways of thinking about the relationship between self and other, observer and subject,

[94] Francis Bacon, *Novum Organum* (1620).

and inside and outside. This broader moment of uncertainty found, albeit only momentarily, a radical resolution in the definitive writing of William James, in his proposal of what has become known as the James-Lange theory of emotion. In *What Is An Emotion?* published twelve years after the *Expression* in 1884, James argued that while 'common sense says' that 'we meet a bear, are frightened and run', the 'most rational statement' is that we 'feel afraid because we tremble', and that 'without the bodily states following on the perception, the latter would be purely cognitive in form, pale, colourless, destitute of emotional warmth'. James's essay offered a radical resolution to the question Darwin had raised but deferred. However, like Darwin's, James's account emphasized the dynamic, interactive nature of emotions and the anxieties that tenaciously shadow our passions. Like Darwin, James draws on a theatrical metaphor to pinpoint the sociality of looking and feeling: for James, 'stage fright' epitomizes the continuous awareness that when we look, we know we are looked at too.[95]

[95] William James, 'What is an Emotion?' p. 190; p. 195.

2

Monkey F Startled

At 3pm on the 4 August 1881, a group of a hundred eminent physicians, among them the surgeon Joseph Lister, biologist Rudolph Virchow, and neurologist Jean-Martin Charcot, walked from London's Royal Institute of Physicians on Albemarle Street to the physiology department of King's College on the Strand. They were ushered into a large laboratory by a thirty-eight-year-old Scottish neurologist, a 'slight and erect, genial and alert' man by the name of David Ferrier. Earlier that morning, the distinguished physicians had heard Professor Ferrier deliver a paper to the International Medical Congress as part of a heated debate entitled 'Discussion of the Localization of Function in the Cortex Cerebri'.[1] His adversary was the Professor of Physiology at Strasburg University, Friedrich Goltz (1834–1902), a large and imposing figure with a walrus moustache. Defending the prevailing medical view, Goltz, following the French pioneer of experimental brain science Jean Pierre Flourens (1794–1867), argued that the brain worked as an indivisible network of perceptions, sensations, and volitions, in which 'one stimulated point in the nervous system stimulates all others, one weakened point weakens all'.[2] In a radical departure from this established theory, Ferrier argued that discrete areas of the brain were the control 'centres' for distinct operations of the body such as hearing, taste, smell, and the movement of limbs. Ferrier's audacious claim was that he could map the functions of the brain, an idea which Goltz, along with most of Europe's scientific elite, found dangerously regressive. Dividing the labour of the brain and identifying physical locations for each

[1] For full transcripts of the debate, see William MacCormac, *Transactions of the International Medical Congress, Seventh Session*, i, 4 vols. (London: J. W. Kolckmann, 1881) pp. 218–28.

[2] This theory was derived from the work of the French pioneer of experimental brain science, Jean Pierre Marie Flourens (1794–1867). See: Jean Pierre Marie Flourens, 'Experimental Researches on the Properties and Functions of the Nervous System in Vertebrates', in Edwin Clarke and Charles Donald O'Malley, *The Human Brain and Spinal Cord: A Historical Study Illustrated by Writings from Antiquity to the Twentieth Century* (Berkeley and Los Angeles: University of California Press, 1996) p. 487.

task seemed a return to the outlandish claims of the quack phrenologists who had been so roundly discredited earlier in the century.[3]

In their respective papers Ferrier and Goltz had described the results of experiments performed on animals. It was to adjudicate their evidence that the hundred eminent scientific witnesses found themselves jostling for space among the benches of the King's physiological laboratory. First, Goltz led in a dog. The creature had undergone five operations, by the end of which all the areas Ferrier hypothesized to be the somatosensory and motor centres of the cerebral cortex had been destroyed, the grey matter flushed away with a compressor and rubber hose. Nonetheless, the dog was still able to walk and run, accept food, see, smell, and flinch when its flesh was pinched. The only change in the dog's behaviour was that it now displayed limited intelligence and attention: it acted 'idiotic', as Goltz put it. Because of this, Goltz believed the dog proved conclusively that discrete areas of the brain could not control particular functions, but rather that if the brain was injured 'the degree of dementia is proportionate to the spatial extent of the lesion'.[4]

Next Ferrier was invited to exhibit his evidence and from the animal enclosure in the basement two monkeys were led in. Like Goltz's dog, both monkeys had undergone operations in which specific areas of their brains were destroyed (a procedure known as 'cortical ablation'), but in Ferrier's experiment a more precise area of tissue was burnt away with a wire cautery. The first exhibit named only by the letter C, ambled lopsidedly into the laboratory. Though she was able to smell, taste, hear, and see, the primate was entirely paralysed on the right-hand side of her body, and when Ferrier approached her holding out a biscuit she was only able to accept it with her left hand. The area the neurologist hypothesized to be the motor cortex on the right hand side of her brain had been completely destroyed, whilst all other areas were left undisturbed. She presented, the doctors agreed, the 'typical features (viz. the semiflexed arm, and rigidly clenched fingers) of hemiplegia with late rigidity as seen in man'.[5] '*C'est un malade!*' ('it is a patient!') cried the French neurologist Jean-Martin Charcot excitedly, for if medical research could identify the root of such

[3] See: John van Wyhe, *Phrenology and the Origins of Victorian Scientific Naturalism* (Aldershot: Ashgate, 2004).

[4] Friedrich Goltz, 'Uber die Verrichtungen des Grosshirns', *Archiv fur die gesamte Neurologic und Psychiatric*, 26, 1–49, translated in Stanley Finger, *Origins of Neuroscience: A History of Explorations into Brain Function* (Oxford and New York: Oxford University Press, 2001) p. 54.

[5] David Ferrier, 'Cerebral Localisation. The Marshall Hall Prize Oration', *Medico-Chirurgical Transactions*, 67, 3 (1884), 33–49 (p. 37).

maladies in monkeys then the possibility of a cure for humans might not be far behind.[6]

The keeper then led in a second primate, called by Ferrier Monkey F. This small female seemed, unlike her predecessor, to be in good physical health. Alert and spirited, Monkey F 'bounded about and climbed hand over hand with the greatest agility and vivacity'.[7] To demonstrate Monkey F's affliction, however, Ferrier had decided upon an altogether more spectacular staging. Instructing the hundred eminent men of science to stand together at one end of the laboratory, he cajoled Monkey F and Monkey C to sit together on the floor facing the audience. The laboratory servant then passed Ferrier a pistol. While the monkeys sat distracted by the audience, Ferrier crept upstage behind them. Undoubtedly he moved stealthily, perhaps on tiptoes. It was imperative that the monkeys should be oblivious to the sudden movement he was about to make. When he was as close as possible to the monkeys, 'in their immediate proximity' as the official transcripts of the demonstration recorded, Ferrier squeezed the trigger. The cap exploded into the air. The hundred eminent men of science jumped out of their skins. The laboratory servant ducked. Ferrier flinched. Monkey C 'started very emphatically', but Monkey F seemed completely unmoved.[8] Two years later, Ferrier joked that Monkey F 'was the only animal in the room that was not startled by the explosion which I made'.[9]

The experiment was repeated several times, each with the same peculiar result. Ferrier then turned to his audience to explain that the region he had hypothesized to be the auditory cortex, the *temporo sphenoidal convolution*, had been destroyed (Figure 10). Far from stoically controlling her emotions, achieving the dizzying heights of Queen Victoria's own self-mastery, Monkey F had not flinched because she had not heard the pistol's unexpected blast. With such compelling evidence for two competing theories, the hundred scientific gentlemen called for the animals to be 'sacrificed', as was the official terminology at the time, and their brains removed for post-mortem inspection. Goltz's 'idiotic' dog and Ferrier's hemiplegic Monkey C were taken away to be etherized, and the unflinching Monkey F returned to the animal enclosure where she would continue to be the subject of experiments and observations for a further year. On closer examination, the lesions made by Goltz were found by a committee of experts to be less extensive than he had believed. The use of a water

[6] MacCormac, *Transactions*, p. 237.
[7] Ferrier, 'Cerebral Localisation', p. 38.
[8] David Ferrier, 'Schäfer on the Temporal and Occipital Lobes', *Brain*, 11, 1 (April 1888), 7–30 (p. 16).
[9] Ferrier, 'Cerebral Localisation', p. 38.

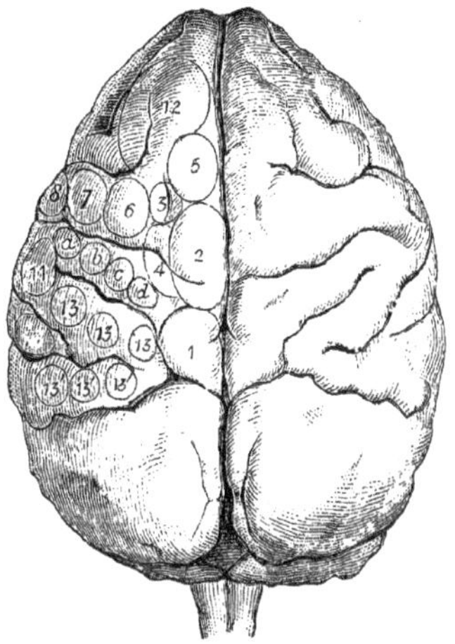

FIG. 69.—Upper Surface of the Hemispheres of the Monkey. (Royal Soc.)
The circles and included numerals are explained in the text.

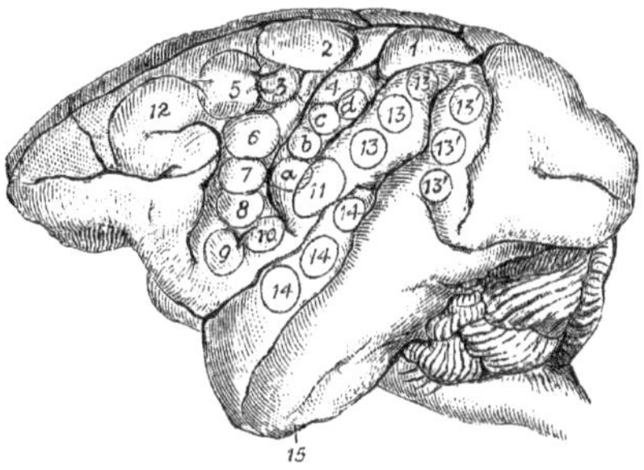

FIG. 70.—The Left Hemisphere of the Monkey. (Royal Soc.)
The circles and numerals have the same signification as in last figure.

Fig. 10. Cortical Maps of the Brains of Macaque Monkeys, figs. 69–70, David Ferrier, *The Functions of the Brain*, 2nd edn. (London: Smith, Elder and Co., 1886) p. 240. The region of the superior tempero-sphenoidal convolution is marked number 14.

jet had meant the injuries on the dog's brain were superficial, and that very little damage to either the motor or the visual areas had been sustained. In contrast, the committee agreed that the use of a wire cautery had enabled a more precise and thorough injury to the tissue, so that Monkey C's injuries were accurately localized to the predicted areas. It was clear to the scientific experts that the primate's injuries and subsequent behaviour provided incontrovertible evidence of the surprising theory of cortical localization. Ferrier had won the day, and his experiments would usher in a new era in the science of the brain.

Ferrier's demonstration took place as part of the seventh session of the 1881 International Medical Congress, an annual meeting of physicians, physiologists, and neurologists that year held in London between the 2nd and 9th of August. With 3,000 delegates attending, including such luminaries of the age of science as Louis Pasteur and James Paget, and representatives from at least seventy countries, the Congress was something of a sensation—*The Times* for example devoted thirty-five separate columns to it. Alongside lectures and demonstrations on subjects as diverse as obstetric medicine, surgery, diseases of children, and experimental physiology, there was a museum collection filled with specimens, photographs, illustrations, and machines, and a series of morning exhibitions of living patients that were so popular that 'every morning, at the hour announced, the room filled', producing great 'confusion and crowding'.[10] There were also lavish social events: a garden party thrown by Baroness Burdett-Coutts (Figure 11), a reception for 12,000 people in the concert room at the Crystal Palace,

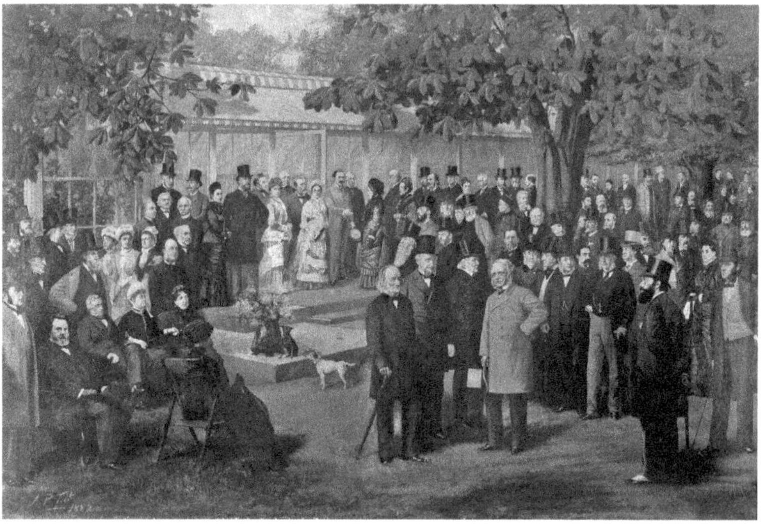

Fig. 11. Baroness Burdett-Coutts's garden party at Holly Lodge, Highgate, for members of the International Medical Congress, 8th August 1881, A. P. Tilt, (1881–2).

Wellcome Library, London

[10] MacCormac, *Transactions*, pp. 118–19.

and an ostentatious display of pyrotechnics which 'consisted in the fire portraits of Sir James Paget, M. Charcot, and Professor Langenbeck'.[11] In his rousing opening speech James Paget acknowledged the excitement and drama of the Congress, speaking of the 'multitude and diversity of minds' in attendance, of the 'novelty' of their discoveries, of the 'stir and controversy' he anticipated and, with a rhetoric shot through with appropriately Darwinian themes, urged those in attendance to be 'pliant and quick to adjust themselves' to new ideas. The Congress was certainly exhilarating, no less spectacular than Michael Faraday's infamously theatrical Christmas Lectures at the Royal Institution. With a fanfare the Congress alerted the general public that medicine had followed in the footsteps of chemistry and physics, and that the understanding of bodies and their maladies was rapidly improving because medicine had become 'more scientific'.[12]

In 1865, the French physiologist Claude Bernard argued that understanding illness and its treatment had moved away from that 'blind faith in theories which is only scientific superstition' and towards a genuinely 'experimental medicine'.[13] The pursuit of a fully materialist account of the body was facilitated by the invention of new machines such as the cardiograph (which measured the heart's contractions), the pneumograph (which traced respiration), the photograph and the X-ray that gave graphic representation to phenomena previously too minute or fleeting to be seen by the human eye. With these new and often costly technologies came an increasingly professionalized university scientific culture, and by the 1880s, the amateur tradition of the gentleman of science with his privately funded laboratory—a tradition to which Darwin had belonged—was on the wane (although, as the following chapter makes clear, it did not disappear altogether). Most importantly, the 'experimental medicine' heralded a new injunction, or as Lorraine Daston and Peter Gallison have characterized it, an 'ethical imperative', for objectivity. The scientist was compelled to remain aloof, detached from that which he witnessed. Modelling his gaze on that of his self-recording machines, he withdrew from the scene of looking, protecting his results from any interference that might arise as a result of his own presence as an observer.

Ferrier's contribution to the International Medical Congress has been depicted as a 'dramatic' turning point in the emergence of a modern scientific study of the brain, and in turn some historians have been quick to characterize Ferrier as an embodiment of the new experimental spirit

[11] MacCormac, *Transactions*, p. 107.

[12] James Paget, 'President's Address', *British Medical Journal*, 2, 1075 (6 August 1881), 195–8 (p. 195).

[13] Claude Bernard, *An Introduction to the Study of Experimental Medicine* (1865) trans. H. Copley Greene (London: Macmillan, 1927) p. 37.

of self-restraint. While Goltz has been described as an 'engaging speaker with a flair for the dramatic', Ferrier emerges as a 'short, thin, and dapper Scot', who 'looked more like a military officer'.[14] Certainly, a 'flair for the dramatic', though it might have been vital for the popular exhibitions of the period, might seem to be at odds with the empirical objectives of the new scientific medicine. Yet, it is clear from his demonstration on 4 August 1881, that Ferrier was not immune from the lure of the spotlight. Creeping up undetected behind the monkeys, with his finger hovering over the trigger, the neurologist bore more than a passing resemblance to a murderous stage villain. The great chronicler of Parisian theatre Honoré Daumier had depicted an almost identical *tableau* in a painting finished around 1860, entitled *At the Theatre (The Melodrama)* (Figure 12): the gun-wielding miscreant, standing upstage of his unsuspecting female victim but in full view of the audience, pulls the trigger. The parallels between Ferrier's demonstration and the late nineteenth-century theatre do not end with the performances on stage. In their choreography of passionate gestures, Daumier's wincing and gasping working-class spectators anticipate the eminent flinching audience at Ferrier's demonstration. Moreover, if Daumier's main focus was the theatrical reactions of the Parisian audiences, so eliciting extravagant spectatorial responses was also Ferrier's aim. It was vital for the success of Ferrier's demonstration that his audience should perform spectacular flinches, and that they should become aware of their own involuntary affective responses as well as those of their colleagues. Only by staging a comparison between the startled spectators and the oblivious primate could Ferrier bring Monkey F's deafness starkly into view.

To produce this theatrical audience in the laboratory Ferrier utilized a well-known bit of stage business. It was a technique that would be used to great effect the following year when a young Russian doctor turned playwright named Anton Chekhov (1860–1904) began work on his first naturalistic drama *Ivanov* (1882). In Chekhov's play, the curtains part to reveal an elderly gentleman quietly sitting facing the audience, absorbed in his newspaper. A second character, Mischa, appears upstage, holding a shotgun. The tension mounts as Mischa, who it transpires has been drinking and is also wearing large boots, tiptoes tipsily across the length of the stage, his gun aimed directly at Ivanov. The longer the actor playing Mischa takes to cross the stage, the more twigs he breaks and near-stumbles he recovers from without disturbing Ivanov, the closer the audience gets to the edge of their seats. Finally, the barrel of the gun comes level with the unsuspecting reader's nose:

[14] Stanley Finger, *Minds Behind the Brain: A History of the Pioneers and their Discoveries* (Oxford: Oxford University Press, 2000) p. 155.

IVANOV: (*seeing Mischa, starts and jumps up*) Mischa, God knows what... you frightened me... And as it is I'm in a state, your silly jokes.[15]

Both Mischa and Ferrier's performances enlist the same convention of a melodramatic finale to get their audience 'in a state'. In Chekhov's opening scene, of course, the convention is subverted in its final moments: only Ivanov 'starts and jumps up', leaving the rest of the audience with the lingering sense of unease that would come to characterize

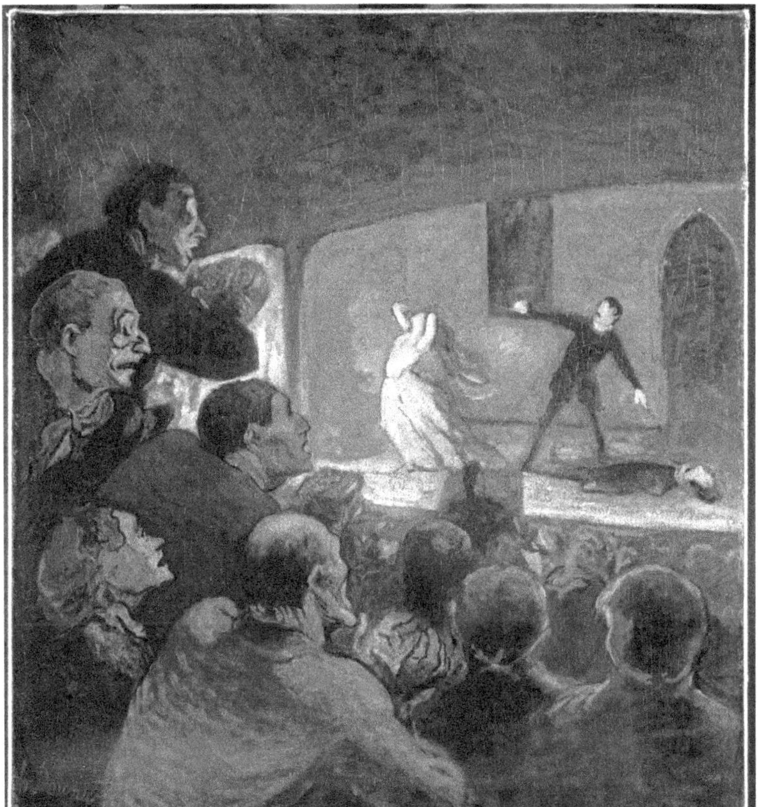

Fig. 12. *At The Theatre (The Melodrama)*, Honoré Daumier, *c.*1860.

bpk / Bayerische Staatsgemädesammlungen, Munich

[15] Anton Chekhov, *Ivanov* in Peter Carson (ed. and trans.) *Anton Chekhov, Plays* (London and New York: Penguin, 2002) pp. 1–79 (p. 3).

the playwright's future work in the naturalistic style. In contrast, Ferrier's theatre had the scientist tiptoeing around behind the monkey to ratchet up the nervous anticipation and guarantee a generous display of flinches at the pistol's discharge. While the invention of the light microscope brought cells into view, and tools such as the cardiograph gave graphic representation to the heart's beats, Ferrier's demonstration used the tricks of the stage to make the remote terrain of subjective experience visible for the distinguished scientific gentlemen. While the audience subjected Monkey F to a scrutinizing gaze, reading the legible signs of her body, they also found themselves participating in the experiment, turned into jumpy, nervy audience members in a laboratory theatre, their own bodies appearing in the foreground of the scene they had come to observe.

Ferrier's experiments with Monkey F and her fellow primates provided the first sustained evidence of localized function in the brain. In doing so, they helped pave the way for brain surgery on humans and provided the conceptual framework for present-day neuroscience. However, it is not what Ferrier discovered as much as how he discovered it that is the focus of this chapter. Perhaps the use of theatre in Darwin's ad hoc emotional experiments is not altogether surprising; but even a decade or more later in the increasingly professionalized environment of the physiological laboratory, theatrical practices and problems lingered. Ferrier's year and a half long observation of Monkey F reveals that questions about dissimulation and representation haunted the encounter between the observing vivisectionist and his performing animal subjects. Moreover, the neurologist himself became a theatrical performer, flinching over and over again in his laboratory. The startled audience at Ferrier's demonstration recalled sensation theatre's spectators who consumed their own visceral responses as part of the pleasures of theatre's live encounter. However in his day-to-day laboratory work the neurologist's recoils resembled performances associated with audiences of the naturalistic drama emerging across Europe in the 1880s. The architects of theatrical naturalism revolted against the excesses of the Romantic stage. They sought instead to turn a scientific gaze on its characters and portray physiological and psychological 'truth'. In this naturalist aesthetic, theatre audiences, like scientific observers, were under a growing imperative to disappear from view, to be outside looking in. Nonetheless, their choreography of hiding, emerged as a type of self-conscious theatricality, through which they remained aware of the social dimensions of their looking. Tracing the connections running between these spectatorial performances in both laboratories and theatres in the 1880s, a distinctive pattern of embodied and gesturing spectatorship comes into view.

'GALVANIC SPARKS'

David Ferrier was born in Aberdeen on 13 January 1843.[16] Whilst studying classics and philosophy at Aberdeen as a pupil of one of the early proponents of scientific psychology Alexander Bain (1818–1903), Ferrier found himself drawn to the new physiological methods in the study of the mind. On finishing his degree in 1863, Ferrier travelled to the University of Heidelberg in Germany, where he enrolled as a student at the physiological institute under the direction of the physicist Hermann Helmholtz (1821–1894). Unlike the empiricist Bain, whose seminal works *The Senses and the Intellect* (1855) and *The Emotions and the Will* (1859) relied mainly on inference and anecdotal evidence, Helmholtz approached the core problems of psychology with reference to the laws of physics and chemistry. In particular, it was by pioneering the use of ophthalmoscopes to understand the workings of the eye, and phonautographs to trace and record sound waves, that Helmholtz was able to develop a fully materialistic account of perception. In 1864, equipped with the experimental psychological techniques that would underpin his future research, Ferrier left Heidelberg and returned to Scotland, where he enrolled as a student of medicine at Edinburgh University. Upon qualifying, Ferrier was appointed as a lecturer in physiology at the Middlesex Hospital, and two years later, as a professor in Forensic Medicine at King's College Hospital. It was whilst at King's in the early 1870s, that Ferrier met John Hughlings Jackson.

Hughlings Jackson (1835–1911) was a highly influential figure in late nineteenth-century neurology. From 1862 he worked as a physician at London's National Hospital for Paralysis and Epilepsy (founded in 1859), where he recorded in painstaking detail his clinical observations of patients suffering diseases of the brain and nervous system. Hughlings Jackson's interests were wide-ranging, and included work on aphasia, or the loss of language, which in 1871 Paul Broca had argued originated in damage to a specific 'language' area of the brain. Hughlings Jackson also explored the relationship between 'higher' and 'lower' operations of the nervous system, work which earned him the admiration of Henry Head. However, it was Hughlings Jackson's work on epilepsy that proved most influential to the young David Ferrier. Hughlings Jackson had observed among his epileptic patients a distinctive type of fit that began with local spasmodic movements, for example, the repeated raising and lowering of the left arm,

[16] For further biographical details see: G. H. Brown (ed.) *Lives of the Fellows of the Royal College of Physicians of London*, iv, 1826–1925 (London: Royal College of Physicians, 1955) pp. 246–7; 'Obituary—Sir David Ferrier', *The Lancet*, 211, 5456 (1928), 627–9; 'Obituary—Sir David Ferrier', *British Medical Journal*, 1, 3407 (1928), 525–6.

the trembling of an index finger or the twitching of the right eyebrow, before developing into a full chronic convulsion (this type of fit, 'in which parts of the body are affected one after another' later became known as Jacksonian Epilepsy). Observing that the areas in which the convulsions began reliably corresponded to diseased parts of the cortex found later during patient autopsies, Hughlings Jackson hypothesized that specific regions of the brain controlled particular parts of the body. In a pivotal 45-page pamphlet *A Study of Convulsions* (1870), he outlined his theory, one developed, as he put it, by observing the 'experiment performed by disease' upon the body.[17]

Hughlings Jackson was not alone in hypothesizing that specific 'centres' of the brain controlled discrete bodily movements. In 1870, the same year that Ferrier was appointed to his chair at King's, two German physiologists Gustav Fritsch and Eduard Hitzig published the first tentative experimental evidence for Jackson's ideas. It had been whilst working as a medical officer during the Prusso-Danish war that Fritsch first stumbled across the idea of cortical localization. Asked to clean the head-wounds of an injured soldier, he noticed that when he accidentally touched the exposed cerebral cortex on one side, the opposite side of the soldier's body twitched. On returning home, Fritsch joined forces with a physiologist Hitzig, who offered his Berlin apartment as an ad hoc laboratory for a very gruesome series of experiments. Working with dogs, who received no anaesthetic, the pair first exposed the brain and then set to work stimulating different areas of the cerebrum with blunted electrodes, noticing that irritating different parts of the left side would evoke distinct spasmodic jerks of the forepaw or hind leg on the right. The application of an electric current to living animals was hardly a new phenomenon—at the beginning of the nineteenth century, Marshall Hall had used 'galvanic sparks' to make decerebrated frogs withdraw their hind legs—but what was unique to Fritsch and Hitzig's experiment was the direct stimulation of the brain itself to produce marionette-like movements of the body.[18]

Ferrier was familiar with Fritsch and Hitzig's findings, but was angry that the Germans had overlooked the debt they owed to Hughlings Jackson's clinical insights. In 1872, Ferrier, by now twenty-nine years old, accepted an invitation from Darwin's friend and correspondent the alienist James Crichton-Browne to direct a laboratory of experimental neurology at the West Riding Lunatic Asylum. In Yorkshire Ferrier had a fully supported

[17] John Hughlings Jackson, 'A Study of Convulsions', *Transactions of the Saint Andrews Medical Graduate Association*, 3 (1870), 162–204 (p. 204).

[18] Hall, 'On The Reflex Function of the Medulla Oblongata and Medulla Spinalis', p. 656.

laboratory at his disposal, and access to a supply of experimental animals with which to develop Fritsch and Hitzig's work on cerebral localization. By controlling the intensity of the electric current, and also by working with primates 'sufficiently narcotised to abolish all sense of pain', he was able to discover a far greater range of excitable areas in the cerebrum and map the cortical centres in far greater detail. Moreover, where the Germans had only been able to observe spasmodic jerks, Ferrier elicited distinct bodily movements, from the swish of a monkey's tail to the closing of its eyes: when the *superior* or *postero-parietal lobe* was stimulated on one side, the 'opposite hind limb advanced, as if walking', and if Ferrier stimulated the area of the *ascending parietal convolution*, the monkey clenched its fist. In one instance, Ferrier produced if not a start, then at least a poise of attentiveness when, on stimulating the *superior tempero-sphenoidal convolution*, he observed 'pricking of the opposite ear, head and eyes turn to the opposite side, pupils dilate widely'.[19] In 1805 the Italian physicist Giovanni Aldini had produced ghastly demonstrations before a crowd of bystanders at Newgate by applying a galvanic pile to the bodies of freshly executed criminals: by electrically exciting the 'remaining vital forces', 'the jaws of the deceased criminal began to quiver, and the adjoining muscles were horribly contorted, and one eye actually opened'.[20] Seventy-five years later, Ferrier was able to make an etherized primate perform similar tricks by the direct stimulation of the cortex itself.

Ferrier's experiments in Yorkshire confirmed his view that the bodily movements habitually understood to spring from emotional feelings were, in fact, mere 'responses to various forms of sensory stimulation'. Even animals deprived of their cerebral hemispheres, he argued, 'start at sounds, flinch at light thrown in their eyes, respond by movements expressive of disgust or discomfort at unpleasant nasal or gustatory stimuli', but this 'outward manifestation of feeling is a purely instinctive or reflex act, one over which we have little or no control'.[21] If stimulating the *superior tempero-sphenoidal convolution* elicited a pricked ear, a turned head, and dilated pupils, it was not because the monkey was experiencing fear or shock, but because it had evolved to respond physiologically to acoustical stimulation. Similarly, 'intense and definite' movements of the eyes, ears, tongue, and nostrils elicited by cortical stimulation were indexed to subjective sensations of seeing, hearing, tasting, and smelling. From these conclusions, Ferrier published a series of cortical maps in the Asylum's own

[19] David Ferrier, *The Functions of the Brain*, 2nd edn. (London: Smith, Elder and Co., 1886) p. 243.

[20] *The Times*, 22 January 1803.

[21] Ferrier, *The Functions of the Brain*, p. 146.

journal, later gathering them together in the first edition *The Functions of the Brain*, which he dedicated to Hughlings Jackson. These maps recalled the phrenologist's diagrams, but rather than finding in the lumps and bumps of the skull affection, arrogance, or an aptitude for being educated, Ferrier located the centres of movement, taste, hearing, smell, and sight in the brain. For this pioneering albeit highly contentious work, Ferrier was elected a fellow of the Royal Society in 1876.

In 1880, Ferrier returned to London to take up a post as physician in charge of outpatients at King's College Hospital, where alongside clinical work, he intended to develop the research begun in Yorkshire. One of the criticisms levelled against Ferrier's earlier experiments was that he had only been able to study the effects of stimulating specific regions of the brain for very short periods of time. What he had been so far unable to observe conclusively was that damage to specific regions of the cerebrum could lead to a permanent paralysis or loss of sensation of the kind witnessed in human patients. At King's a solution presented itself in the figure of the Professor of Physiology Gerald Yeo (1845–1909). He would prove a wary but generous accomplice, who would later admit that he commenced the experiments with Ferrier 'with distinct misgivings', believing that the existence of discrete centres of the brain was 'highly unlikely'.[22] Born in Ireland and raised in a military family, Yeo was a well-known advocate of experimental physiology who had eschewed clinical work in favour of a life of laboratory research and teaching.[23] In 1880, the same year that Ferrier arrived at Kings, Yeo delivered the College of Surgeons' Arris and Gale Lectures on Anatomy and Physiology, which he used to demonstrate the many advances gained as a result of experiments on animals. British physiologists, unlike their counterparts on the Continent, had found themselves increasingly under attack by a highly vocal animal rights lobby that had been gathering momentum since the early 1870s. In response to charges that vivisectionists were heartless, callous, and consumed by a lust for knowledge that blinded them to the suffering before them, Yeo emphasized that all experiments in his laboratory were conducted on anaesthetized animals and in full co-operation with the new Cruelty to Animals Act (1876) which distinguished experiments of life-saving purpose from those undertaken 'merely out of curiosity'.[24] A skilled and licensed vivisectionist, Yeo was also familiar with the principles of aseptic surgery, which had been developed in Glasgow by Joseph Lister (1827–1912). Until this point any surgery on

22 MacCormac, *Transactions*, p. 238.

23 For biographical details of Gerald Yeo, see: Anon., 'Obituary, Gerald Yeo', *Nature* 80, 2063 (1909), 314–15.

24 Anon., 'The Charge Against a Vivisectionist', *Daily News*, 18 November 1881.

the brain was almost certain to be fatal, however, the use of carbolic acid to prevent post-operative infection meant that Yeo and Ferrier were able to devise their series of experiments. Working under the direction of Ferrier and with the cortical maps drawn in Yorkshire at his side, Yeo would use a galvanic cautery to make a lesion on an agreed region of the primate's brain. The animal would then be kept under observation for a year or more in his laboratory for Ferrier to periodically visit and inspect. Once Ferrier had determined whether any motor or sensory ability had been lost, the animal would be 'sacrificed' and its brain removed for inspection.

Meddling in the brains of monkeys, producing surprise and excitement with the dull thud of an electric shock, reducing feelings to a series of automatic physiological responses, and fixing them in the flat representational schema of a map, Ferrier's work on cortical localization certainly suggests an attempt to master the body. In rendering the monkey's nervous system transparent and legible, Ferrier's 'loquacious gaze' emerges as powerful and controlling.[25] Jeremy Bentham's panopticon, which allowed a guard to watch all the inmates of a prison, school, or asylum from a hidden 'inspection house' without their knowing whether or not they were being observed, created, as Bentham put it, 'a new mode of obtaining power of mind over mind'.[26] Foucault adopted panopticism as an archetype of 'disciplinary' power in modern societies, but it is a model which many have applied to late nineteenth-century scientific practice. With its urge to taxonomize and regulate the body, and its pursuit of fixity and stasis, Victorian physiology has been linked to what Deleuze and Guattari, and the post-human theorists after them, have called 'the signifying totality of the organism'—as opposed to the anarchical indeterminacy of the 'body without organs'.[27] Yet, while Ferrier's conclusions certainly suggest a totalizing perspective, the relationship which emerges in his laboratory practice suggests a more nuanced and complex interchange. As Martin Willis has recently argued, visual experience in late nineteenth-century scientific practice did not always fit neatly into Foucauldian structures, not least because 'acts of seeing were performances of extraordinary variation'. Visual technologies just as frequently 'undermined visual authority, or came to stand as metaphors for vision's fragility' than shored up a mastering perspective: as Willis puts it, 'scientific observation (even without the use of instrumental aid) was rarely able to proclaim itself as an ultimate authority, and never for very long'.[28] Indeed, in practice, where Ferrier

[25] Foucault, *The Birth of the Clinic*, p. xi.

[26] Jeremy Bentham, *Panopticon; or The Inspection House* (1787), repr. Jeremy Bentham, *The Panopticon Writings*, ed. Miran Bozovic (London: Verso, 1995) pp. 29–95 (p. 29).

[27] Deleuze and Guattari, *A Thousand Plateaus*, p. 4.

[28] Martin Willis, *Vision, Science and Literature*, pp. 2–4.

observed the emotional life of Monkey F, he came closer to the condition of the theatre audience than the prison guard. His looking was often troubled by the unstable relations between visible surfaces and hidden interiors in the monkey's laboratory performance. And while the primate's performance became theatrical, when Ferrier hid from his experimental subject, he also became a show. In a twist on the conventionals of the panopticon, the observer and observed found themselves embroiled in a play of hide-and-seek, their theatrical interaction one of the emotional practices through which the regime of late nineteenth-century scientific objectivity was shaped and articulated.

A GLIMPSE OF A MONKEY'S FEELINGS

A faded, cracked leather notebook, one of a series kept at the Royal Institute of Physicians, reveals that on 22 June, 1881 Ferrier and Yeo commenced work on Experiment F.[29] A young female macaque, 'an unusually active and intelligent monkey' with a good sense of hearing was selected.[30] She was 'thoroughly narcotized with chloroform', and the *temporo-sphenoidal convolution* on both hemispheres of her cerebral cortex—the part Ferrier believed to be the auditory centre (Figure 10)—was exposed and the tissue in the area cauterized using an electric current.[31] The wound was sutured and bandaged, and Monkey F was left alone in her cage to come round. Later that day Ferrier went down to the animal enclosure in the basement of King's physiology department to observe the effects of the operation, recording his observations in a scientific language shot through with unexpected dashes of tenderness. It was to be an intimate and intriguing encounter between scientific observer and his subject, between the spectacle of a performing monkey and a watching audience, and between a scientist-performer and his audience of animals.

> 3.35pm
>
> Placed in cage alone, it dozed for some minutes then suddenly lurched up wide awake. Came to bars of cage and climbed up hand on hand, clinging

[29] David Ferrier's unpublished notebooks from 1873–1883 are kept at the Royal College of Physicians Heritage Centre, GB 0113 MS-FERRD. A transcript of the notes relating to Experiment F are included as Appendix A. Hereafter all references to Ferrier's laboratory notebooks are to Appendix A, and dates appear in parentheses in the text.

[30] Ferrier, 'Schäfer on the Temporal and Occipital Lobes', p. 13.

[31] David Ferrier and Gerald F. Yeo, 'A Record of Experiments on the Effects of Lesion of Different Regions of the Cerebral Hemispheres', *Philosophical Transactions of the Royal Society of London*, 175 (1884) 479–564 (p. 480).

properly with hands ... now hanging on to the bars.... Its companion in next cage is making plaintive howls but not the slightest sign of reaction is given by F who does not turn its head.

3.45pm

Touching its hands or feet with the point of a pencil causes the animal to withdraw its hands sharply as if from pain. It lurches about and places its hands on the bars of cage.

5.30pm

Animal well—moves about.... Companion allowed in cage with it, went to it when it saw it. Not the slightest indication of hearing it. Various sounds made, whistle, tapping the bars... No attention to whistling... the companion always started. So other monkeys with same sounds. (22 June)

Between 22 June 1881 and 27 July 1882, Ferrier returned repeatedly to the animal enclosure to observe Monkey F, initially several times a month. On 23 June she was 'very dull and drowsy-looking', her right eye partially closed, but while she ate greedily, seemed able to smell when oil of bergamot was wafted under her nose, and went about easily, climbing 'from one cage to the other through small door', she paid 'no attention whatsoever to whistling in its ear'. By 25 June, three days after the operation she was 'quite bright and active' running about and seizing pieces of bread and eating cold boiled potato 'apparently with relish', but nonetheless was always very quiet, and a 'scratching sound which caused F's neighbours to be always very frightened caused not the slightest semblance of hearing on the part of F'. A fortnight later, Yeo and Ferrier removed F's dressings and found that the wound on her scalp was 'perfectly healed'. On this day, Ferrier performed his first test with the explosive sound of the 'percussive cap', noting that she 'occasionally seems to start, but other times pays no attention'. By 25 July, Monkey F had settled into life with her blind cage-mate 'companion' Monkey G, and seemed 'perfectly well'. Ferrier praised F's hunting abilities ('is very expert in catching flies, which it watches carefully and pursues skilfully'), noting that while she occasionally grunted upon seeing food or water, she made no noises in response to those of her companion. On 26 July, Monkey G was 'sacrificed', an experience which left F bereft. 'Owing to the death of G., F., which has been disconsolate and occasionally uttering plaintive cries' was transferred to the cage of another primate, the hemiplegic Monkey C. Two days later, Ferrier attached an electric bell to the side of their cage, noting that 'ringing it suddenly caused C. to be very much disturbed and annoyed, whereas F. paid no attention whatever'. By the end of July, Ferrier felt confident enough in F's deafness to demonstrate the pistol test to the psychologist and friend of

Darwin's, J. G. Romanes (1848–94), perhaps rehearsing for the upcoming Congress: the unexpected crack of the pistol caused 'no reaction or starting' in F, 'while its companion was invariably much startled and annoyed' (29 July 1881). The entry for 4 August, the date of the demonstration at the International Medical Congress states 'a percussion-cap was exploded close to it several times before the audience, and it gave no sign whatever of starting; whereas C. started very emphatically'.

In Ferrier's published accounts of his experiment with Monkey F, any animal who flinched or jumped in the proximity of a loud noise was judged to have heard it. Recoiling, scampering away, crying out, and other movements of 'excited attention' were, in Ferrier's articles and in both editions of *The Functions of the Brain*, described as involuntary responses, part of the 'animal economy' of muscular contractions that characterized the mechanistic simple reflex arc first described by Marshall Hall in 1833. Flinches and starts, wrote Ferrier in 1876, are 'movements either of defence or preservation, and are in general adapted to withdraw the part from the source or irritation or to repel the irritant itself'.[32] The gesture was not an expression of emotion, but purely an 'instinctive or reflex act' that necessarily followed from the perception of an unexpected sound. Thus, he characterized a flinch as a 'landmark' on the topography of the nervous system, a stable and straightforward signifier of the monkey's interior experience. Visible protrusions on the body's surface, winces and starts rendered the primate transparent and made her invisible subjective auditory sensations (or lack of them) manifest.[33] As far as the rhetoric of Ferrier's published account of the experiment was concerned, the difference between a monkey who heard and flinched, and one who was deaf and remained unmoved, was a clear and distinct one: F 'was the only animal in the room not startled by the explosion which I made', he proclaimed. Yet, it is striking that on closer inspection of his private notebooks, observing a monkey's emotional responses—or more precisely, the more troublesome task of observing the lack of them—was not as straightforward as Ferrier wanted it to seem.

The language with which Ferrier recorded Monkey F's behaviour in his notebooks is unstable, moving back and forth between the emotive and empirical. At one extreme, Ferrier's notes brim with imaginative flights of fancy, recording amusing or poignant details that suggest a full investment in the psychodrama of the creature's day-to-day experience. Delighted by the taste of cold mashed potato, grieving at the death of her companion, F is also prone to tantrums. She 'squabbles' with her new cage mate, who

[32] Ferrier, *The Functions of the Brain*, p. 73.
[33] Ferrier, *The Functions of the Brain*, p. 114.

in turn is 'very indignant' at having to share the food (27 July 1881), yet when left alone, Monkey F 'utters a short cry of loneliness' (12 December 1881). If F is 'most totally unconcerned' with the sound of the pistol, her companion is often 'annoyed' by the sounds Ferrier makes, and at worst is left 'in abject terror, shrinking, winking, and twitching its ears' (30 June 1882). At the other end of the spectrum, Ferrier records his observations in language that resolutely clings to the observable facts alone, deliberately, even suspiciously, drawing attention to the possibility of a disconnect between surface appearances and the interior experiences to which they are habitually linked. On 22 June 1881, Ferrier wrote that touching the animal's palms with the point of a pencil caused her to withdraw her hand 'sharply *as if* from pain'. The following day, he noted that wafting oil of bergamot under her nose caused her to '*apparently* smell', and that acetic acid placed on her tongue caused her to make 'movements of tongue and mouth *of tasting*'. Four days later, when noises were made in her vicinity, Monkey F gave no '*indication*' of hearing them (my italics).

Certainly the conflicting rhetorical styles of Ferrier's notebooks reflect a wider transition occurring in the late nineteenth century in written accounts of animal behaviour. On the one hand, Ferrier's anthropomorphism recalls the multispecies ethologies that had become so popular earlier in the century, a genre made most famous by Darwin in his accounts of affectionate beetles, possessive crustaceans, submissive monkeys, and loving dogs who experience 'the feeling of religious devotion' towards their masters.[34] On the other hand, the sceptical detachment that sits alongside the emotional descriptions in Ferrier's notebooks reflects the emergence of a new style of record-keeping to accompany the 'experimental method'. Though experiments on animals emphasized a physiological continuity across species and vivisectionists paid great attention to the physiological changes that accompanied emotion, scientists were also obliged to separate observable physiological phenomena from apparent motivations and feelings. As G. H. Lewes had cautioned in 1858, observers should discard 'all anthropomorphic interpretations' when looking at animals in 'scientific seriousness', warning against construing animal behaviour 'according to the analogues of our own structures'.[35] Whilst emotions were physiological responses described in terms of surface phenomena such as raised heartbeats, flushing skin, quivering muscles, and retracted limbs, the scientist was nonetheless compelled to defer subjective correlates of these observable facts in his explanations. Yet, wavering between over- and under-identification in his written accounts of observing Monkey F,

[34] Charles Darwin, *The Descent of Man*, p. 68.

[35] George Henry Lewes, *Sea-Side Studies* (London: Blackwood and Sons, 1858) p. 365.

Ferrier's notebooks also point up the deeper problem of looking haunting his experiment.

As the theatre historian Jackie Bratton has pointed out, in the music halls of the 1880s monkeys appeared alongside sideshow 'freaks', dancing frogs, and blackface performers, as 'speciality acts'.[36] Even whilst staging their unnerving proximity to the 'civilized' men and women of Western Europe through amusing charades of drawing room manners and marching soldiers, monkey mimics were also uncanny curiosities and resolutely othered. The task of witnessing Monkey F's emotional performances in the laboratory was similarly troubled by a doubled perspective which slid back and forth between identification and distance. Observing the responses of an animal unable to give voice to its own feelings, Ferrier's problem of looking came close to the queasy experience of watching actors in theatre's less-than-transparent optic, where signifiers and the feelings they were supposed to denote were easily uncoupled. It is a problem particularly evident in Ferrier's descriptions of his attempts to observe F's flinches, and the lack of them, moments when the scientist's gaze foundered.

Monkey F was, after the operation, 'excessively on the alert, and it follows every movement, and is with difficulty surprised' (27 July 1881). Her compromised hearing making her particularly watchful and distinctly jumpy, it appears that F did flinch, and these movements left Ferrier circumspect about his conclusions. 'Occasionally seems to start, but other times pays no attention' he wrote 7 July, 1881; 'Sometimes it appears to start when a pistol cap is exploded, so that occasionally it is judged to hear', he confided on 12 December 1881. While by 27 July 1881, 'the signs of reaction (*which have caused so much doubt*) to sound are less evident' (my italics), nonetheless, the neurologist's uncertainty lingered in question marks and obscure double negatives: 'ears are now mobile and seem to twitch at sounds?' he wrote 7 July 1881, and while other monkeys flinched upon hearing a pistol, Ferrier 'failed to detect any unequivocal indication of this on the part of F' (27 July 1881). On 27 July 1882, well over a year after beginning the experiment, Ferrier was still recording these odd manifestations, what he termed *appearances* of flinching. 'Occasionally, as before, there was an *appearance* of a start, or a look round, *apparently* conditioned by the noise', but these were later deemed to be 'mere coincidences' (my italics).

[36] Jackie Bratton, 'The Music Hall', in *The Cambridge Companion to Victorian and Edwardian Theatre*, ed. Kerry Powell (Cambridge: Cambridge University Press, 2004) pp. 164–182 (p. 178). See also: Goodall, *Performance and Evolution in the Age of Darwin*.

These moments of failure, moments when the neurologist's cartography of the body seemed blurred and indistinct, draw attention to the indeterminacy of the primate's emotional performance. Watching flinches that were merely 'appearing' and 'seeming', but not unambiguously *being* one thing or another, found Ferrier beset by the 'ontological queasiness' of watching actors. Indeed, such language alerts us to the possibility that studying the emotional behaviour of monkeys in the animal enclosure at King's was less like *reading* a map than it was like watching a live theatrical performance. Ferrier's descriptions of the monkey's apparent flinches recall William Archer's description of watching the actor Irving in *The Bells*: the actor's flinches were so lifelike that they almost 'seemed' to be the result of an 'involuntary spasm'.[37] For scientific observers, as for theatre audience members, the relationship between surface appearance of behaviour and the interiorities they supposedly described became an unstable liaison, one that swung moodily between the excesses of passionate sympathy (she 'utters a short cry of loneliness'; it 'recoils in abject terror') and a landscape in which there are merely the impressions, facades, even illusions of feelings (the bergamot causes her to 'apparently smell'; the primate 'apparently' flinches). Indeed, it is quite possible that for Ferrier the monkey was herself *acting* flinching. As Romanes who was himself at the time busy studying the primates in London Zoological Gardens observed, monkeys are 'animals that imitate for the mere sake of imitating'.[38] If the keeper going down to the animal enclosure set 'all the others on the *qui vive*' (25 June 1881), would not F, who was watchful, nervous, and always on the alert, have mimicked them in mere 'appearances' of excitement, perhaps indistinguishable from the real thing? Such enigmatic performances left the scientific observer beguiled, his gaze unable to penetrate the interior of the monkey's brain. Instead, it ricocheted off the hard surface spectacle of her emotions, leaving the watchful scientist uncertain of their provenance or authenticity.

THE 'ILLUSION OF THE STAGE'

To read the theatre into Ferrier's experiment and tease out his doubt and 'ontological queasiness' may offer a new way to think about the emotionality of the vivisectionist's laboratory, a topic which over the past ten years has been of interest to a number of historians of science charting the

[37] William Archer, *Henry Irving, Actor and Manager*, p. 63.

[38] George Romanes, *Mental Evolution in Animals* (New York: Appleton, 1884) p. 477.

affective dimensions of late nineteenth-century laboratory life.[39] As Paul White and Otniel Dror have both explored, objectivity and emotionality were not mutually exclusive categories in late nineteenth-century scientific discourse, not least because so many emotional states—from 'steely nerves' to a mastery of empathetic instincts were attributed to scientists, and particularly vivisectionists, by their defenders.[40] Within the laboratory itself, emotions were an object of enquiry in their own right, and as Dror points out, this led to an increased sensitivity to the laboratory's 'emotional ecology', and the introduction of the 'qualitative emotional descriptors into the quantitative language of their experimental science'. The scientist who wanted to observe the physiological changes of emotion in his animal subject, had to do so against a neutral backdrop, and thus scientists and laboratory servants paid attention to their own emotional presence, conscious of the need to create an atmosphere of relaxed calm: 'animals were literally petted and stroked while awaiting their planned—imminent—death'.[41] The collision between emotionality and objectivity in Ferrier's looking emerges in the moments when the neurologist's own passionate performance of looking took centre stage. An ethical imperative associated with limiting the possibility of the observer's own participation, Ferrier's virtuoso attempts to hide from his experimental monkey also became a surprisingly theatrical display. In its performance of hiding, Ferrier's looking not only intersects with the new regime of objectivity, but also with techniques increasingly associated with theatre audiences in the 1880s.

By the 1880s, the vogue for the excesses and excitements of sensation theatre was rapidly on the wane: 'we are all up to all the secrets of the style', wrote one critic; 'the "illusion of the stage" is a thing so much more talked about than felt', wrote another. In 1881, a critic in *The Times* perceived a shift in the style of acting towards the unforced, the 'refined and cultivated': 'English acting', he wrote 'has risen much beyond its old standard. It is possible to be present at an English performance now without indignation at the contempt which managers must have entertained for their patrons to impose upon them mere burlesques of human emotions.'[42] In place of these emotional burlesques, writers on the continent began to formulate a new style of acting that they hoped would have all the precision of an anatomy lesson.

[39] See: Dror, 'The Affect of Experiment'; Jed Mayer, 'The Expression of the Emotions in Man and Laboratory Animals', *Victorian Studies*, 50, 3 (2008), 339–417; Paul White, 'The Experimental Animal in Victorian Britain', in *Thinking with Animals: New Perspectives on Anthropomorphism*, eds. Lorraine Daston and Gregg Mitman (New York: Columbia University Press, 2005) pp. 59–82 and 'Darwin's Emotions'.

[40] White, 'Sympathy Under the Knife', p. 101.

[41] Dror, 'The Affect of Experiment', p. 207; p. 227.

[42] Anon., 'Sensational Dramas', *The Era*, 22 January 1881; Anon., 'The Court Theatre', *The Times*, 9 November 1881; Anon., 'The Decay of Drama', *The Times*, 17 June 1881.

In 1888, seven years after Ferrier began his experiments with Monkey F, the Swedish dramatist August Strindberg (1849–1912) wrote *Miss Julie* (*Fröken Julie*), a play he subtitled 'A Naturalistic Tragedy'. Set on Midsummer's Eve in the kitchen of a large country house, it tells the story of a young aristocratic woman, Julie, who becomes infatuated with her family's servant Jean. While the guests at a garden party dance and chatter excitedly offstage, inside the kitchen Julie tests, provokes, and spars with Jean's affections, finally seducing him. As the evening wears on, the couple make a daring plan to elope, all the while acutely aware of the transgression they are committing. Mounted on the wall of the kitchen is an electric bell, which the master of the house uses to summon Jean to his duties, not dissimilar to the contraption attached to the cage of Monkey F. The bell looms over the action, threatening to startle the couple from their illicit conversations, and reminding the audience of the imbalance of power onstage. For Jean, the condition of servitude is stubbornly ingrained in the operations of his nervous system, made manifest through his reaction when his master rings for him: 'I only have to hear that bell up there', he confides to Julie, 'and I start like a frightened horse'. In the closing moments of the play, Jean's resolve crumbles, and while Julie hesitates on the threshold of the door, Jean informs her that he must stay behind. As if to reinforce the inevitability of their tragedy, the sound of the bell pierces the auditorium, his recoil from their agreement echoed in an involuntary physiological response:

(*The bell rings twice loudly. Jean flinches, then straightens up.*)
JEAN: It's horrible! But there's no other way!—Go!
(*Miss Julie walks firmly out through the door. Curtain.*)[43]

In 1881, the year that Ferrier began his work on Monkey F, the French critic, playwright and novelist Émile Zola wrote a manifesto he called 'Naturalism in the Theatre', in which he proclaimed 'we are an age of method, of experimental science. Our primary need is for precise analysis'. Pitting a modern science that verifies 'what is' against the distorting excesses of melodrama and sensation theatre, 'the big spectacle with big words, the play of lies that shows off in front of the crowd', Zola argued that theatre should reproduce a doctor's or a scientist's gaze, replacing the 'abstract characters' of 'metaphysical man' with the 'thorough analysis of an organism' and characters 'whose muscles and brain function as in

[43] August Strindberg, *Miss Julie* (1888), trans. Michael Robinson (Oxford: Oxford University Press, 2008) pp. 56–110 (p. 87; p. 110).

nature'.[44] Strindberg had read Zola's swaggering manifesto, and like his Russian counterpart Chekhov, combined writing plays, short stories, and essays with a passion for natural sciences and in particular, the emerging field of scientific psychology. Keeping abreast of pioneering research in the field, from Charcot's work on hysteria to Henry Maudsley's *The Pathology of Mind* (1867), Strindberg also performed his own experiments, publishing his observations on topics as diverse as the life cycle of the Death's Head moth to the nervous systems of plants in two collections of essays. Published in 1887, and then again in 1894, Strindberg called these collections *Vivisections: A Retired Doctor's Observations*, explicitly invoking an ideal of a living dissection in his relationship with the intellectual culture at the time. Like Zola, Strindberg abhorred the excesses of the 'degenerate' Romantic stage, which he regarded to be merely 'a place of amusement' where 'inexplicable events unfold in castle halls'. Instead, with science key to his self-legitimization, he wanted to apply his understanding of physiology to the pursuit of an experimental 'naturalistic' style, a theatre that dissected the psychologies of its characters and scrutinized their behaviour and motivations. He described Molière's comedy *Tartuffe or the Imposter* (1664) as exemplary, calling one scene in particular a 'wonderful vivisection' of the main protagonist.[45] If the dissection of corpses in the anatomy theatres of the seventeenth century had proved a popular spectacle for the curious public, the late nineteenth-century naturalistic drama turned the older medical shows on their head, staging an ersatz living anatomy—or vivisection—before an audience.

At first glance, Jean's flinch at the end of *Miss Julie* encapsulates a desire to stage a living 'organism' with its emphasis on a malleable nervous system and reflex emotions. Jean is repeatedly presented throughout the play as an animal whose automatic responses can be trained and manipulated. Not only does Jean start like a 'frightened horse' upon hearing the bell, but Julie treats him as a kind of pet, training him to leap over her riding crop 'the way you'd teach a dog to jump'.[46] It was not unusual for the emotions of women, children, and members of the working classes to be described as 'brutish' in the nineteenth century. However, the flinch that secures the play's tragic conclusion has a very specific physiological context too. It reflects a growing interest in this period in the possibility of re-educating

[44] Émile Zola, 'Naturalism in the Theatre' (1881), repr. and trans. in *The Theory of the Modern Stage: An Introduction to Modern Theatre and Drama*, ed. Eric Bentley (Harmondsworth: Penguin, 1976) pp. 351–73 (pp. 356–63).

[45] August Strindberg, 'On Modern Drama and Modern Theatre' (1889), repr. and trans. in *Selected Essays by August Strindberg*, ed. and trans. Michael Robinson (Cambridge: Cambridge University Press, 1996) pp. 73–86 (pp. 74–5).

[46] Strindberg, *Miss Julie*, p. 77.

the reflexes, most famously demonstrated in the stimulus-response experiments of the Russian physiologist Ivan Petrovich Pavlov (1849–1936) in the 1890s which showed how the 'psychic secretions' of dogs could be deliberately manipulated.[47] This collision of the physiological and theatrical in Jean's flinch points up a broader entanglement of the scientific and dramatic in Strindberg's work. The theatre historian Amy Strahler Holzapfel, for example, has suggested that Strindberg did not only draw on discoveries of scientific psychology but also replicated its techniques: Strindberg's work is bent on 'investigating and penetrating the interior of a live human or animal body', she argues, revealing 'the interior physiological and pathological mechanisms of his characters, exploring beyond the boundaries of everyday perception'. Her conclusion is that, in his deployment of vivisection as both metaphor and dramaturgical technique, Strindberg reaches towards a theatre that interrogates the idea of looking, and in doing so destabilizes 'the very foundation of theatrical representation: mimesis'.[48] Holzapfel's argument recalls Stanton Garner's contention that in the late nineteenth century 'medicine proceeded in less performative directions'; in both arguments an uncomplicated rhetoric of the anti-theatricality of the scientific gaze predominates. Such language of breaches and display certainly echoes the scientific metaphors deployed by the early practitioners of naturalism to legitimize their theatrical project. Yet, we should be wary of adopting this wholesale, or imagining that it operated as a stable metaphor in their writing. Just as theatricality crept into Ferrier's observations of Monkey F, so those who theorized theatrical naturalism also betrayed an acute awareness of the dislocating, doubling effects of the theatre machine in their work.

The naturalist theatre remained, of course, a place of faking, pretence, and make-believe, in which the portrayal of 'truth' was always unstable, and the 'real' remained as tantalizing but inaccessible as ever. Even Zola, who claimed scientific rigour for drama with such panache, knew that talking of 'truth' on stage would always create confusion. In the opening paragraph of 'Naturalism in the Theatre' he insisted that the 'truth does not need clothing; it can walk naked'. But in a later section on the thorny questions of sets and costumes, Zola sent designers to the main marketplace of *Les Halles* in Paris for inspiration. 'It would be enough to go to *Les Halles* and look about,' he advised. 'Nothing is gaudier or more interesting. All of Paris would enjoy seeing this set if it were realized with the necessary accuracy and amplitude.'[49] The paradox of theatrical naturalism

[47] Pavlov, *Conditioned Reflexes*.

[48] Amy Strahler Holzapfel, 'Strindberg as Vivisector: Physiology, Pathology, and Anti-Mimesis in *The Father* and *Miss Julie*', *Modern Drama*, 51, 3 (2008), 329–52 (p. 334).

[49] Zola, 'Naturalism in the Theatre', p. 368.

is implicit in Zola's own advice: were it possible to recreate the market-place with 'the necessary accuracy and amplitude', ('*le degré d'exactitude et de largeur nécessaire*') the set would be a theatrical sensation, yet such a full and detailed copy would be, of course, an impossibility. According to Holzapfel, Strindberg's naturalist dramaturgy works as a penetration into, and revelation of, the 'interior physiological and pathological mechanisms of his characters'. Yet for Strindberg himself, in an illustration of his ability to master and manipulate the apparatus within which he worked, it was through theatrical devices of *concealment* that nature could be simulated most persuasively. Naturalism, in which the gap between the representation and reality aims to become virtually indistinguishable, operates most effectively not through what is shown, but what is hidden. As Strindberg put it:

> As for the scenery, I have borrowed the asymmetry and cropped framing of impressionist painting, and believe I have thereby succeeded in strengthening the illusion; for not being able to see the whole room or all the furniture leaves us free to conjecture, that is, our imagination is set in motion and we complete the picture ourselves.[50]

Allowing the audience to generate a complete image through the work of imaginative inference is what, for Strindberg, creates the theatrical mirage of reality. It was a technique he deployed quite self-consciously in *Miss Julie*. Just before the end of the first act, Jean is instructed by his exhilarated young mistress to change out of his uniform and into his Sunday best:

> (*[He] goes to the right; his arm is visible as he changes his coat.*)[51]

Half hidden and half in view, Jean's tantalizing striptease highlights the lack of transparency that theatre creates. The careful instruction reminds us that as much as the theatre is an apparatus for *appearing*, it is also one which works through concealment and opacity. In Strindberg's theatre, 'reality' is not revealed or penetrated so much as it is simulated through meanings deferred and feelings tantalizingly out of a reach. Just as in Ferrier's laboratory, in Strindberg's theatre the 'real' lies beneath the shimmering surfaces, or extends beyond the frame of the set, to be evoked through imaginative labour alone.

Capturing this play of the visible and invisible, the director and scholar Herbert Blau has suggested that the 'resistance to being seen is what not only teases us into theatre but teases the theatre out'.[52] Just as the 'resistance' of

[50] Strindberg, *Miss Julie* (Preface) pp. 65–6.
[51] Strindberg, *Miss Julie*, p. 76.
[52] Herbert Blau, *The Audience* (Baltimore and London: Johns Hopkins University Press, 1990) p. 40.

Monkey F's emotional gestures to being uncomplicatedly 'seen' brings the theatre of Ferrier's laboratory to the foreground, so the strategies of hiding and concealment deployed quite consciously by Strindberg reminds us of the playwright's ongoing negotiation with, rather than disavowal of, the theatrical frame in which he worked. What was hidden from view highlighted the enduring theatricality of the vivisectionist's experiment and naturalistic drama. And when we discover the same teasing games of hide and seek being played in the auditorium, it is clear that the audience of naturalistic drama remained deeply committed to their own theatrical performances too.

'PLAYING THE SPY'

It was not only the portrayal of fictional characters that underwent a transformation in the naturalistic theatre. Audiences also found themselves the subject of experimental techniques, designed to command their attention, and focus it exclusively on the stage. In his preface to *Miss Julie*, Strindberg called for his plays to be performed in small rooms, with 'complete darkness in the auditorium'. Unlike the direct-addresses, the winks, asides, and imploring of the audience that were part of the stock in trade of melodramas, Strindberg wanted actors who would never exchange looks with the audience, never entering 'into direct contact outside the frame of the set'. Turning 'the stage into a room with the fourth wall removed' enabled both performers and spectators to collude in the pretence that actors did not act *for* an audience at all, but rather went about their business unselfconsciously.[53] For their part, the audience was being asked to perform the curious task of pretending, whilst sitting in the dark, that they were not really *there* at all.

Lynn M. Voskuil has drawn attention to the way audiences of late nineteenth-century naturalism have been rather overlooked by theatre historians.[54] Audiences from earlier in the century have proved attractive for the public roles they played. The Old Price Riots of 1809, in which audiences vigorously protested the rising costs of tickets at the new Theatre Covent Garden, the call-and-response form of melodrama and pantomime, as well as the tendency for actors to eye-ball the audience—and spectators to shout abuse and throw oranges when dissatisfied—have all contributed to the view that early to mid nineteenth-century audiences were vocal and oppositional, powerful and participatory.[55] By the

[53] Strindberg, *Miss Julie* (Preface), p. 67.

[54] Voskuil, 'Feeling Public', p. 249.

[55] See: Marc Baer, *Theatre and Disorder in Late Georgian London* (Oxford and New York: Oxford University Press, 1992); Hadley, *Melodramatic Tactics*.

end of the nineteenth century, this interactivity of the auditorium has been broadly understood to be on the wane. The naturalist aesthetic, with its 'fourth wall' dividing spectators and performers was only one part of this broader shift. In 1880, the Theatre Royal Haymarket became the first theatre to have the pit, where working class audiences previously stood to watch the show, covered over and replaced with an extension of the stalls. Though this generated additional income for the Bancrofts, and other theatre managements quickly followed suit, the decision banished the demonstrative and audible working-class audiences to the Gods and left the middle-class patrons who 'often came late and were generally unresponsive' in the most direct contact with the stage. Thus, the 'old sense of engagement and interactivity between stage and auditorium was inevitably lost'.[56] A further change was the invention of the incandescent carbon-filament electric lamp, introduced first in 1881 in London's Savoy Theatre. While gas lighting had meant that audiences, as well as the actors, were illuminated for much of the nineteenth century, electric circuits enabled the lights in the auditorium to be dimmed on command, whilst those on stage shone even brighter. It was not unheard of for audiences to sit together in the dark before 1881 (for example, in shows that included phantasmagoric effects) but nonetheless, to routinely 'extinguish the house lights was to cut off almost completely contact between all but the most immediate neighbours in the audience and to substitute a different relationship to the actors on stage'. Where once the stage seemed 'practically an extension of the auditorium', the drama now took place in a great pool of light from which the audience sat separated in shadow: they were outside looking in.[57]

It is striking that this 'fall' of the theatre spectator's predicament—from a condition of interactivity and participation to one in which they were mere outsiders 'looking in'—could equally well describe the way scientific looking has been understood to have changed in the same period. While theatre audiences were increasingly required to demonstrate a 'restraint and due deference for the performer's efforts', in an emerging culture of scientific objectivity the laboratory observer was also compelled to practice 'self-restraint', to withdraw from the scene of looking in order to ensure that their judgement, personality, or even emotions could not interfere with the observation of facts. Yet, as the flinching audience at Ferrier's demonstration showed, it was not always the case that scientific attention

[56] Davis and Emeljanow, 'Victorian and Edwardian Audiences', p. 103.

[57] Terence Rees, *Theatre Lighting in the Age of Gas* (London: Society for Theatre Research, 1978) pp. 187–8.

was turned outwards. Nor was it the case for the spectators in the new naturalistic theatre who sat together in the dark, that interactivity and intervention were entirely lost or superseded.

In their quest for objective, reliable, replicable results in the latter part of the nineteenth century, physiologists became increasingly preoccupied with the affective dimensions of laboratory life, and in particular the animal's experiences of terror, pain, and excitement. As Dror has emphasized, this was driven less by a concern for animal welfare than by what the French vivisectionist Claude Bernard described as the need to 'remove causes for error brought about by suffering'.[58] In the laboratory of the Italian Angelo Mosso, who spent much of the 1880s provoking, recording, and quantifying the physiological changes in fear, even the awareness of being watched could produce a distinctive change in an animal's emotional physiology, akin to shyness or embarrassment. During a series of experiments with rabbits, Mosso noted that the blood vessels in their ears pulsated vigorously. Earlier experimenters had labelled this artery an 'accessory heart', but Mosso discovered that these contractions only appeared when the rabbit knew it was under scrutiny. 'I used certain precautions which others would perhaps have thought superfluous', reported Mosso. 'Instead of watching the rabbit while holding it in my hand I thought to spare it all emotion, by enabling myself to observe the ears without its becoming aware of the fact.'[59] In a specially designed cage which allowed the physiologist to 'watch quite easily, without being seen', Mosso was able to observe a truly 'tranquil rabbit', one whose ears did not pulsate, leading him to call the contractions of the blood vessels a rabbit's 'blush'. Mosso's cage, a kind of panopticon, brought the strategies of objective looking to their logical conclusion: like the theatre audience hiding from the view of the actors, pretending not to be there at all, so the scientist reassured himself that by spying unseen upon his subjects, his mere presence would not impinge upon the natural processes unfolding before him.

If rabbits got performance anxiety, 'blushing' when they knew they were being observed, so could spectators in the naturalistic theatre when their act of watching was exposed. Audiences of the Victorian sensation theatre were alert to their own visceral responses, yet spectators imagined by the architects of naturalism could also be made alert to their bodies and surroundings. Chekhov deliberately pulled such a trick in the final moments of *The Seagull* (1895). From the wings, quite unexpectedly, a shot is fired, marking the suicide of Konstantin. '[*Everybody starts*]' is

[58] Dror, 'The Affect of Experiment', p. 207; p. 227.

[59] Angelo Mosso, *Fear* (1884), trans. E. Lough and Frederich Kiesow (London and New York: Longmans, 1896) p. 11.

Chekhov's stage direction—it can be taken playfully, to refer to those both on- and offstage.[60] Perhaps like Darwin, the first audiences at *The Seagull* became embarrassed by their girlish flinches; at the very least, like the scientific observers at Ferrier's demonstration, the gunshot would have left them with heightened nerves and a feeling of itchy, self-conscious discomfort as they became aware of their own response. Such moments ruptured the skein of naturalistic representation, incurring a kind of spectatorial 'stage fright,' in which audience members became suddenly aware of their own presence in the theatrical encounter.[61] The stage direction '*[Everybody starts]*', then, reminds us that in the naturalistic theatre, the sociality of the auditorium did not simply disappear, but emerged reconstituted, erupting in deliberate moments of audience manipulation, or, as the following chapter will explore, failures of concentration.

If flinching made Chekhov's audience acutely aware of their own bodies, then starts and recoils can also be part of a self-conscious choreography of looking. In Ferrier's observation of Monkey F, hiding itself became a kind of performance, a show of concealment which emphasized the lengths he was willing to go for objective results. Thirty years after Ferrier began his experiment on Monkey F, the playwright and philosopher Bertolt Brecht in the *Messingkauf Dialogues* (1942) invoked the idea of a hidden spectator to complain of the limitations of naturalism. Brecht argued that the naturalist aesthetic turned audiences into voyeurs, stripping them of their potential for political change. Instead, he favoured a style that used direct address among other 'alienation' techniques to remind his audiences of their participation in the encounter. In particular, he believed naturalism's fourth wall and darkened auditorium left audiences forgetful:

> Ah yes, then the audience is tacitly assuming that it's not in a theatre at all, since nobody seems to take any notice of it. It has an illusion of sitting in front of a keyhole.[62]

Brecht's equation between naturalism and disengagement has been very influential among today's theorists of theatre; Susan Bennett, for example, has argued that Ibsen's *A Doll's House* 'excludes audience intervention', with its 'neatly packaged fixed reality', that forces the audience to take a 'voyeuristic role', that demands 'passivity'.[63] For Brecht, the 'illusion of

[60] Anton Chekhov, *The Seagull, Anton Chekhov, Plays*, ed. and trans. Peter Carson (London and New York: Penguin, 2002) pp. 82–141 (p. 141).

[61] Ridout, *Stage Fright*, pp. 1–2.

[62] Bertolt Brecht, *The Messingkauf Dialogues* (1942) trans. John Willett (London: Methuen, 1977) p. 51.

[63] Susan Bennett, *Theatre Audiences: A Theory of Production and Reception* (London: Routledge, 1990), p. 3; p. 24; p. 157.

sitting in front of a keyhole' produced a passive and acquiescent audience. But for the playwright and philosopher Jean-Paul Sartre, in his discussion of shame in *Being and Nothingness* (1943) written the following year, spying was an activity that left him acutely alert to the dangers of being caught looking:

> Here I am bent over the keyhole; suddenly I hear a footstep. I shudder as a wave of shame sweeps over me. Somebody has seen me. I straighten up. My eyes run over the deserted corridor. It was a false alarm. I breathe a sigh of relief.[64]

In this scene of looking Sartre is a voyeur but is also acutely self-conscious. Not only does his body assert itself with a raised pulse and an involuntary start ('I straighten up)', but he also momentarily plunged into the dislocating out-of-body experience of watching himself watching. For Sartre, hiding leaves the observer feeling active, and very much exposed.

In Ferrier's laboratory a similar choreography of illicit spying became part of the official gaze of the scientific observer. Just as Darwin had confessed to the challenges of studying emotions, so Ferrier admitted in 1888 in an article for the new journal *Brain*, seven years after beginning his experiment, that observing the fear, surprise, or irritation of monkeys in the laboratory could be an exasperating affair. 'It was difficult to devise a test to determine whether or not the animal could hear', he wrote, as 'it was not easy to make a sound without in any way attracting its attention by sight'.[65] In an attempt to avoid the gaze of the ever-watchful Monkey F, the neurologist devised extravagant attempts to spy on her. On 12 December 1881, he secreted himself on the top of the staircase that led down to the animal enclosure and, keeping an eye on Monkey F's cage, called out as if coming to visit the creatures: 'the other monkeys are both on the alert, looking eagerly and making sounds of expectation; but F. pays no attention whatever and goes on with its own occupation quite unheeding'. On another occasion he enlisted the help of the laboratory servant, with 'one person going to a distance out of sight, while another watched, and the one in the distance called the Monkeys as if coming with food'.[66] The electric bell on the side of F's cage would undoubtedly have been an ideal contraption for creating noise with the minimum of movement on the part of the experimenter. Nonetheless, when called upon to recount his experiment in 1888, Professor Ferrier, by now a highly regarded member

[64] Jean-Paul Sartre, *Being and Nothingness* (1943) trans. Hazel E. Barnes (London: Routledge, 2000) p. 277.

[65] Darwin, *Expression*, p. 19.

[66] Ferrier and Yeo, 'A Record of Experiments on the Effects of Lesion of Different Regions of the Cerebral Hemispheres', p. 480.

of the scientific establishment, decided to demonstrate his experimental method by describing not the staircase or electric bell experiments, but instead by conjuring a rather theatrical scene.

> While the animal was sitting quietly by the fire, I retired to the other room, and while watching through a chink of the half-shut door, called loudly, whistled, knocked on the door, tinkled glass &c., without ever causing it look round, or give any sign of having heard. I then cautiously approached the animal, and not till it saw me did it give any sign of consciousness of my presence.
>
> When the same experiment was repeated, while the monkey and its companion were quietly seated by the fire enjoying the heat, it gave no sign of hearing; while its companion started with alarm, and came with curiosity to ascertain the cause of the sound.[67]

At first glance, Ferrier's description of concealing himself behind a door to observe Monkey F is reminiscent of Mosso's contraption for hiding from rabbits. However, the two scenes differ in one important respect. Unlike Mosso, Ferrier is not securely hidden, but rather is hiding, skulking around, dodging behind doors, recoiling from being seen, he is almost a caricature of a voyeuristic scientist. It is intriguing that Ferrier, whose work exemplified the gains made through the 'experimental method' and its new imperative for non-intervention, should choose to present his 'self-restraint' in such a dramatic, even theatrical, scenario. Far from being 'silent and gestureless', in Ferrier's scene of looking, the scientist steals the show. This is even more surprising when we consider the probability that Ferrier made the scene up for effect: though Ferrier claimed he undertook this experiment on 8 April at 10am, there is no corresponding entry for it in his laboratory notebooks. Ferrier's description is marked by stealth and trepidation but most of all by a self-consciousness about his own performance as a spectator. Like Quilp, Charles Dickens's nefarious hero in *The Old Curiosity Shop* who plants himself behind a door unable to resist 'the prospect of playing the spy', Ferrier's description hints at the experimenter's heightened alertness of his own physical presence: 'not a sound, not so much as a creaking board, or a stumble against a cobweb', warns Quilp.[68]

The Belgian playwright Maurice Maeterlinck's symbolic drama *Interior* (*Intérieur*), first translated into English by William Archer in 1894, presents the theatre audience as individuals caught up in a similar predicament of 'playing the spy'.[69] It is a short play, set at night, in a garden, in

[67] Ferrier, 'Schäfer on the Temporal and Occipital Lobes', p. 13.

[68] Charles Dickens, *The Old Curiosity Shop* (1841) (London: Penguin, 1972) p. 457.

[69] Maurice Maeterlinck, *Interior* (1895) in *Three Plays By Maurice Maeterlinck*, ed. and trans. William Archer (London and Glasgow: Gowans & Gray, 1911) pp. 57–84. The play

which a group of strangers stand downstage in the dark amid trees, peering up at an illuminated window in which a family 'gathered for the evening round the lamp' are vividly on display. The strangers, who 'enter the garden cautiously' have come to impart the tragic news that the daughter of the house has been found drowned, but they hesitate, hidden in the gloom outside, uncertain how to make their awful interruption. While the family sit sewing and reading unaware they are watched, the strangers peer up from their hiding places, poised, hesitant, ready at any moment to shrink back behind the trees. 'She's looking at us' one stranger whispers urgently. 'No, she's looking at nothing', another, an old man, replies before warning, 'do not go any nearer'. 'If we were to attract the father's attention…' the stranger tentatively suggests.[70] The strangers gathered together in the dark, watching a family enact their domestic rituals around a lamp oblivious to the fact that they are being watched, comments on the condition of Maeterlinck's audience—a group of strangers gathered in the dark to watch an artificially illuminated domestic interior scene. Yet, these strangers also recall the neurologist in his laboratory hiding behind the door watching, preparing to interrupt the monkey and her companion, who are themselves enjoying domestic tranquillity 'quietly seated by the fire enjoying the heat'. Making a show of looking and a show of hiding, Maeterlink's 'strangers', like Ferrier himself, simultaneously watch and put themselves on display. In Charlotte Brontë's *Villette* (1853), Madame Beck, the proprietor of a ladies boarding school, glides 'ghost-like through the house, watching and spying everywhere, peering through every keyhole, listening behind every door'.[71] In contrast, Ferrier's clandestine surveillance of Monkey F was not so much of a disembodied spectral 'gaze' as a fully emotional and corporeal experience, a persistent reminder that at the heart of the act of observation in Ferrier's laboratory was a two-way relationship in which the monkey could glance back.

As Daston and Gallison have emphasized, the scientific observer's responsibility to withdraw from the scene of looking was increasingly rendered in the language of a moral imperative. Yet, so deliberately portraying himself as someone 'playing the spy' so many years after completing his experiment, Ferrier drew attention to the fact that the pursuit of objectivity could also be an affective and theatrical undertaking. Objectivity, which raised the scientist's pulse and led him to be acutely nervous of being caught watching, was also enacted in a choreography of spectatorial

received its premiere at the *Théâtre de l'Oeuvre* in Paris in 1895. Archer's English translation was first published earlier, in *The New Review* in 1894.

70 Maeterlinck, *Interior*, pp. 59–60; p. 59; p. 26.

71 Charlotte Brontë, *Villette* (1853) (Oxford: Oxford University Press, 2008) p. 73.

flinches as part of increasingly heroic attempts to avoid making an appearance. While we are accustomed to thinking of machines such as the sphygmograph as the apparatus through which the imperative of objective looking was framed, the new techniques of theatrical spectatorship linked to naturalist drama also offer an insight into the strategies of scientific looking in late Victorian Britain. Ferrier used the tricks of the stage to demonstrate his experiments, encountered theatrical problems in his attempts to observe the emotional behaviour of Monkey F, and characterized himself in a way that replicated emerging spectatorial practices of avoiding being seen to look. In each case, these entanglements with theatrical spectatorship draw attention to the emotional, social, and bodily dimensions of his role as an experimenter. However, the entwined practices of theatricality and scientific objectivity did not only surface in Ferrier's laboratory, but became the subject of wider debate when, in the 1880s, the 'vivisection question' once more struck at the heart of Victorian society.

'THE SPECTACLE OF DYING CATS'

The summer of 1881 with its International Medical Congress had proved triumphant for Ferrier and secured his reputation in the medical establishment and beyond. So it must have felt like a particularly brutal reversal of fortunes when, on 3 November 1881, three months after the fêted demonstration, Ferrier received a summons to appear at Bow Street Magistrates Court. A Mr Waddy QC, acting on behalf of the Victoria Street Society for the Protection of Animals from Vivisection, had lodged a case against the renowned professor, claiming that his much publicized experiments on monkeys had contravened the new Cruelty to Animals Act (1876). The passions and problems of observing monkeys, previously only the subject of Ferrier's private notebooks, were about to become the focus of intense public speculation.

While cruelty to domestic animals had been outlawed in 1822, the rapid expansion of physiology in British universities in the 1870s had brought with it a surge in unregulated experiments on cats, dogs, mice, and monkeys that attracted the condemnation of animal rights campaigners. The 'vivisection question' as the ensuing debate was popularly known, garnered powerful voices on both sides. Prominent anti-vivisectionists included writers and critics such as John Ruskin, Vernon Lee, and Lewis Carroll, as well as feminists and educationalists most prominently Frances Power Cobbe and her Victoria Street Society. They described barbaric conditions and agonizing procedures in their letters, lectures, and pamphlets, attacking the medical establishment for its arrogant 'indifference to suffering', its 'recklessness and pitilessness' and its 'moral depravation'.[72] In turn, members of the scientific elite including Darwin, Louis Pasteur, and Thomas Huxley accused the animal rights lobby of sentimentalism and sensationalism, arguing that British vivisectionists were careful to minimize the suffering of animals, but that their work was far from an indulgence. Since physiology had the ultimate goal of saving human lives, they argued, and 'can not possibly progress except by means of experiments on living animals', 'he who retards the progress of physiology commits a crime against mankind'.[73] So volatile was the situation that the organizers of the Congress forbade delegates from performing 'anything like a distinct vivisection experiment', not wanting the event to become marred by the vivisection question.[74] Moreover, despite a complaint registered by forty-three qualified female practitioners, the organizers barred women from attending, fearing that anti-vivisectionists, who were predominantly female and closely linked with the suffragettes, would disrupt proceedings with protests.[75]

Passed in response to these fierce and emotive debates, the Cruelty to Animals Act imposed a series of limitations on vivisectionists, requiring them to hold a license and stipulating that all experiments 'calculated to give pain' were to be performed under anaesthetic and that the animal should be killed before the anaesthetic wore off. If, after a painful operation, an animal was to be kept alive for observation and further experimentation, an additional license was required, granted on a case-by-case basis by the Secretary of State. The Act also outlawed public demonstrations of animal experiments: 'the experiment shall not be performed as an illustration of lectures in medical schools, hospitals, colleges, or elsewhere.'[76] The Victoria Street Society had it on the authority of the Home Office that Ferrier had never applied for a license to conduct animal experiments. In a further apparent snub to the legislation, the neurologist had not only kept the monkeys alive after painful procedures, but had also demonstrated his

[72] Frances Power Cobbe, 'The Moral Aspects of Vivisection', *New Quarterly* 4 (1875) 222–37 repr. in Susan Hamilton (ed.) *Animal Welfare and Anti-Vivisection 1870–1910: Nineteenth-Century Woman's Mission* (New York: Routledge, 2004) pp. 99–114 (p. 102).

[73] Charles Darwin 'On Vivisection', *The Times*, 22 April 1881.

[74] Anon., 'The Charge against Professor Ferrier under the Vivisection Act: Dismissal of the Summons', *The British Medical Journal*, 2, 836 (1881), p. 840.

[75] W. F. Bynum, *Science and the Practice of Medicine in the Nineteenth Century* (Cambridge: Cambridge University Press, 1994) p. 144.

[76] 'An Act to Amend the Law relating to Cruelty to Animals', *Public General Statutes Passed in the Thirty-Ninth and Fortieth Years of the Reign of Her Majesty Queen Victoria, 1876* (London: Queen's Printing Office, 1876) pp. 459–64. See also: Andrew H. Ryan, 'History of the British Act of 1876: An Act to Amend the Law Relating to Cruelty to Animals', *Journal of Medical Education*, 38 (1963), 182–94.

experiments before an audience at the International Medical Congress. 'That frightful and shocking injuries had been inflicted upon two monkeys, and that the Act had been undoubtedly infringed' were recorded as the grounds for the complaint.[77] The date for Ferrier's hearing was set for thirteen days later.

It is a surprise to find in the reams of print dedicated to the vivisection question in the 1870s and 1880s almost as much attention paid to the feelings of those who inflicted pain on animals as to the suffering of the animals themselves. Multiple and competing emotional discourses sprang up around the vivisectionist's laboratory, which was portrayed both as a place of cold detachment, where a cat's yelps of pain would be ignored so that the size of its pupils could be observed, and of morbid fascinations and sinister infatuations, where 'ruthless passions' were 'unleashed'.[78] The 'notorious vivisector' of H. G. Wells's *The Island of Dr Moreau*, who, in a nod to Ferrier, honed his skills in the Gower Street laboratories in the early 1880s, was described as falling 'under the overmastering spell of research', his eyes gleaming and his limbs itching when each new stock of animals arrives.[79] While in his opening speech at the International Medical Congress, William MacCormac had given the pleasures of scientific research an almost transcendent twist speaking of 'the delight—the really elemental happiness—of watching the unveiling of a mystery', continental physiologists gained notoriety in the anti-vivisectionist lobby for characterizing vivisection as quasi-aesthetic undertaking.[80] As the Russian-born physiologist Elie de Cyon advised students, 'the true vivisector', should approach a difficult vivisection with 'joyful excitement': 'the sensation of the physiologist when, from a gruesome wound, full of blood and mangled tissue, draws forth some delicate nerve thread has much in common with that of a sculptor. He who shrinks from the section of a living animal, he who approaches a vivisection as an unpleasant necessity, may perhaps be able to repeat one or two particular vivisections, but will never become an artist in vivisection.'[81]

De Cyon's treatise on vivisection was often quoted by advocates for animal rights as evidence for the fact that physiologists were brutalized by an ongoing exposure to the sights, smells, and sounds of mutilated creatures. As the mathematician and author Lewis Carroll argued, no one

[77] Anon., 'Charge Against A Vivisectionist', *London Daily News*, 4 November 1881.

[78] White, 'Sympathy Under the Knife' p. 101.

[79] H. G. Wells, *The Island of Dr Moreau* (1896) (London: Penguin, 2005) p. 34.

[80] MacCormac, *Transactions*, p. 346.

[81] Elie de Cyon, 'Atlas zur Methodik der physiologischen Experimente und Vivisectionen (1876)', quoted in Frances Power Cobbe, 'Vivisection and its Two-Faced Advocates', *Contemporary Review*, 41 (1882) 610–26 (p. 611).

was immune from the degrading effects of inflicting and witnessing horrific pain. Carroll described how the scientist's 'first instincts of horror', his urge to cringe or recoil from his subject's anguish, became 'deadened by familiarity', and the spectacle of suffering animals turned 'first a matter of indifference, then a subject of morbid interest, then a positive pleasure, then a ghastly and ferocious delight'. Medical students were seen to be particularly vulnerable to these degrading effects, and one anonymous physiologist confided to Carroll that 'when the unfortunate creatures cried and moaned under the operations, many of the students actually mimicked their cries in derision!' causing the informant to abandon the lecture 'the writhing animals and the fiendish behaviour of the audience' so sickening him.[82] Fear about the audience's moral health underpinned the Act's prohibition on performing experiments as demonstrations 'in medical schools, hospitals, colleges, or elsewhere'. But it also reflected a far wider anxiety about spectatorship and theatricality in the late nineteenth century. The Victorian sensation theatre had come under attack for deranging its audiences, provoking such intense visceral responses that spectators seemed almost shaken off their own emotional axes. In the 1880s, witnessing animal experiments might likewise decentre the watching subject, sweeping him up in the emotions of others and rendering him unfamiliar even to himself.

For the feminist and social campaigner Frances Power Cobbe (1822–1904) the audiences of vivisection experiments were being exposed to explicitly theatrical dangers. Cobbe was a prolific writer who between 1855 and 1898 produced forty-nine books and pamphlets and numerous collected articles, many on the subject of vivisection. Even the most principled student in the laboratory auditorium, she argued, could not resist absorbing the lascivious excitement of his peers, just as those among crowds at Jubilee celebrations would find themselves aroused by an intense patriotic feeling, or audience members in a theatre could be 'infected' by their neighbour's laughter. While contagions of patriotism and giggling were, to Cobbe's mind 'an altogether wholesome and beneficial thing', elsewhere she argued that the feelings produced were shallow imitations, 'mere contagions of sentiment'.[83] Recalling the furor over sensation audiences, and anticipating the concerns of the crowd psychologists of the 1890s, Cobbe argued that spectators caught up in 'contagions of sentiment' were

[82] Lewis Carroll, 'Some Popular Fallacies about Vivisection', repr. in Wilkie Collins, *Heart and Science* (1883), ed. Steve Farmer (Peterborough: Broadview, 1997) p. 346.

[83] Frances Power Cobbe, 'The Education of the Emotions', *Fortnightly Review*, 43 (1888) 223–36 repr. in Hamilton (ed.) *Animal Welfare and Anti-Vivisection 1870–1910,* pp. 231–44 (p. 232).

a species of actor. According to Cobbe, actors had a 'superficial sensibility and exaggerated mode of expressing the same' because they were always mimicking the feelings of others.[84] It was a similar feverish and sensationalist emotional appetite that characterized the unusually 'mournful' spectacle of the medical students' 'passion for vivisection'.[85] Cobbe offered an incident from St Augustine's *Confessions* as an example of the contagious power of bloodlust. The law student Alypius was forced to attend a gladiator fight, but detesting the idea, he vowed not to look. Yet upon taking his seat he was overcome by the excitement surging about him, and seeing 'the blood, he therewith drank down savageness; nor turned away, but fixed his eye, drinking in pleasure unawares', no longer 'the man he came, but one of the throng he came into'.[86] So potent was the bloodlust Cobbe imagined coursing through the audience's veins, that she wondered if the teaching of physiology in universities was not a slippery slope that would inevitably culminate with young ladies in boarding schools up and down the land being 'entertained by the spectacle of dying cats'.[87]

The scientific establishment defended their work, energetically insisting on a separation of the worlds of the laboratory and the theatre. As James Paget explained, experimental animals experienced no more suffering than those creatures trained to appear in the music hall, but while performing monkeys endured harsh punishments for the purpose of profit and entertainment, laboratory creatures suffered in the service of nobler ends. Moreover, far from enjoying the spectacle of suffering animals, scientific observers portrayed themselves as heroically mastering their natural sympathies. 'There can be little doubt that to most civilized people the mere sight of suffering is painful', wrote the Scottish physician Thomas Lauder Brunton in 1882, but 'instead of yielding to the natural tendency to shun the sight of suffering', vivisectors, like surgeons, taught themselves to 'overcome this impulse'.[88] Suppressing an instinct to turn aside, recoil, and 'shun the sight' required fortitude but also skill, training, and a strict adherence to laboratory regimes. Burdon-Sanderson's highly influential *Handbook for the Psychological Laboratory*, for example, set out the instructions for a series of vivisection experiments through a 'purely

[84] Cobbe here quotes a remark by 'one of the most gifted of the profession', but does not name her source. Cobbe, 'The Education of the Emotions', p. 232.

[85] Cobbe, 'The Moral Aspects of Vivisection', pp. 104–5.

[86] St Augustine, *Confessions* Bk vi. C.8, quoted in Cobbe, 'The Education of the Emotions', p. 238.

[87] Cobbe, 'The Moral Aspects of Vivisection', p. 112.

[88] Thomas Lauder Brunton, 'Vivisection and the Use of Remedies' (1882), in Hamilton (ed.) *Animal Welfare and Anti-Vivisection 1870–1910*, iii: pp. 215–23 (p. 216).

objective description of anatomical facts and methods'.[89] By cultivating an 'objective' stance vivisectionists like the surgeons before them, learnt what Brunton called the 'power of controlling one's own emotions, of disregarding one's own feelings at the sight of suffering'. Nonetheless, it was far from easy, as the maleficent vivisector of Wilkie Collins's novel *Heart and Science*, which was serialized in 1881–2 and written as a direct response to the vivisection question, argues:

> Have I no feeling, as you call it? My last experiments on a monkey horrified me. His cries of suffering, his gestures of entreaty, were like the cries and gestures of a child. I would have given the world to put him out of his misery. But I went on. In the glorious cause I went on. My hands turned cold—my heart ached—I thought of a child I sometimes play with—I suffered—I resisted—I went on. All for Knowledge! All for Knowledge![90]

In the vivisectionist's laboratory it is those whose guard is down, whose training has been forgotten or whose capacity for self-mastery has weakened through exhaustion or addiction, that find themselves turning aside and shrinking away. Thus, the over-worked and fatigued narrator of *Heart and Science*, himself a physiologist, 'recoiled from' the very idea that animal experiments were taking place in Benjulia's laboratory, a place that had become 'an object of horror to him'. Similarly, Montgomery, Dr Moreau's doctor companion on the island, has succumbed to alcoholism as he finds he is unable to bear the horrific experiments any longer:

> A sharp horse cry of animal pain came from the enclosure behind us. Its depth and volume testified to the puma. I saw Montgomery wince.[91]

As Paul White has pointed out, the ability to master one's sentiments 'and perform like well-tuned instruments' was key to the 'self-legitimization' of the vivisectionists. It was the anti-vivisectionists who were accused of being 'slaves to their sentimental affections', and of inciting the emotions of others through exaggerated, sensationalized tales of suffering.[92] Ferrier's collaborator Yeo, who published a defence of vivisection in the periodical the *Fortnightly Review* in March 1882 accused Cobbe and her comrades of being simultaneously 'weak-minded' and cleverly manipulative in broadcasting 'oft–told tale of horrors' from Claude Bernard's laboratory

[89] J. Burdon Sanderson, *A Handbook for the Physiological Laboratory* (Philadelphia: Blackiston, 1884) p. vii. See also: Mayer, 'The Expression of the Emotions in Man and Laboratory Animals', *Victorian Studies*, p. 405.

[90] Wilkie Collins, *Heart and Science*, pp. 190–1.

[91] Wells, *The Island of Dr Moreau*, p. 37.

[92] White, 'The Experimental Animal in Victorian Britain', p. 74.

in France or Paolo Mantegazza's in Italy. These European physiologists, he argued, had little to do with British experimentation and Yeo himself regarded their practices 'with pain and loathing'.[93] Yet for Cobbe, anti-vivisectionists were far from undisciplined. While at times she had tempered her descriptions to avoid 'harrowing the reader', in other pieces she hoped to challenge her readers to look unflinchingly upon the suffering of animals, laying out the details of the experiments so as to dispel any illusion from the mind of those 'persons who shrink from the miserable subject'.[94]

On 17 November 1881, Ferrier presented himself at Bow Street Magistrates Court, before the Yorkshire-born Chief Police Magistrate Sir James Ingham (1805–1890). The courtroom was tense with anticipation. Inside, 'ladies and gentlemen interested in the case occupied seats on the bench'. Outside, a crowd of almost 500 medical students showed their support for Ferrier by 'howling and cheering' and 'frequent jeering and groaning, the sounds of which were distinctly audible in court'.[95] Mr Waddy QC, prosecuting on behalf of the Society for the Protection of Animals opened the proceedings by stating the facts of the case, namely that Ferrier had 'offered to exhibit two monkeys' to the Congress, and that these monkeys had sustained deliberate injuries inflicted on their cerebral cortex that resulted in permanent disabilities. He concluded his summary with a rhetorical flourish, designed, not unlike Ferrier's pistol shot, to make his audience cringe. Appearing as though he were only halfway through describing the grisly details of the operations themselves, Waddy closed the published account of the demonstration, saying he refused to read out any more. He 'did not want to make a sensational business of the case', he claimed, 'it was too serious for that'.[96] It was a feint, a cynical ploy: in fact the published account contained no further details, upsetting or otherwise. Just as Ibsen knew that withholding information allowed the audience's imaginations to conjure a far more vivid reality than he could ever present, so Waddy, by hinting at the existence of details too gruesome to be heard, undoubtedly intended to stir the imaginations of all those sitting in the gallery, causing them to wince in horror.

Waddy's feint draws attention to the drama of the nineteenth-century courthouse, a place where sordid entanglements with scandalous conclusions were played out and regaled to newspaper customers as 'keenly

[93] Gerald Yeo, 'The Practice of Vivisection in England', *Fortnightly Review*, 37 (1882) 352–68 (p. 358).

[94] Frances Power Cobbe, 'Light in Dark Places', (London: The Victoria Street Society, 1883), repr. in *Animal Welfare and Anti-Vivisection 1870–1910*, pp. 99–114, p. 294.

[95] Anon., 'The Vivisection Case', *Glasgow Herald*, 18 November 1881; Anon., 'The Charge Against Professor Ferrier', *The Times*, 18 November 1881.

[96] Anon., 'The Charge against Professor Ferrier', *The Times*, 18 November 1881.

interested over the details of a deed of crime, horror, and bloodshed as the most ignorant occupant of the fourpenny gallery in a suburban Theatre'.[97] Yet the courtroom was also a live theatrical environment, where as one might expect, barristers gave emotional performances, but so did the spectators, the jury, and even the judge.[98] In *Forbidden Fruit*, one of Dion Bouccicault's last sensation dramas, which premiered at the Adelphi in the summer of 1880, the messy overlap between justice and showbiz was parodied. The curtains part to reveal Zulu, a glamorous young circus 'artiste' who proudly claims to be 'the first person that ever submitted to serve as a Cartridge in a Cannon', standing in a lawyer's fusty chambers in Lincoln's Inn. She has come to persuade the Barrister Cato to let her star as a witness in the Great Brighton Scandal Case:

> ZULU: For three years I've worked hard to get well displayed before the public, and never obtained more than three lines in the daily press, but here, sir, everybody is talking about the business and witnesses in this case, perfectly unknown people until you called them in the witness-box, once there they get columns of notice—I want to be a witness!

Swept up in the fantasy, Zulu helps her leading man imagine the scene: 'I shall be covered with charming confusion here', she says, standing in an imaginary witness box, 'and you', she says, pointing to a make-believe courtroom floor 'will make the most of it for the amusement of the jury'. To which the rotund and aging barrister lasciviously replies, 'I would prefer to enjoy your charming confusion here'.[99] Thus, the barrister's chambers is transformed into an imaginary courtroom, which in turn is revealed to be mere theatre where those who watch and witness are also acting.

Having recounted the details of the experiments, Waddy laid out his claim that Ferrier had openly violated the Act. Not only was the neurologist 'without a licence, but he did not even administer an anaesthetic, and further, the experiments were performed as an illustration to a lecture, which again was contrary to the Act'. Ingham immediately dismissed the idea that Ferrier had committed an offence by showing the monkeys to an audience, pointing out that 'the professor did not experiment there and then'. 'No sir,' Waddy conceded, 'but the case does not rest upon that'.

[97] Anon., 'Sensational Dramas' *The Era*, 22 January 1881.

[98] Sir James Shaw Willes (1814–1872) was known for weeping when commuting the death sentence. See: Thomas Dixon, 'The Tears of Mr Justice Willes', *Journal of Victorian Culture*, 17, 1 (2012), 1–23.

[99] Dion Boucicault, *Forbidden Fruit*, in *Forbidden Fruit and Other Plays*, ed. Allardyce Nicoll and F. Theodore Cloak (Bloomington: Indiana University Press, 1964) pp. 7–48 (pp. 10–11).

Waddy continued 'by the provisions of the Act, no experiments can be performed except by persons who are licensed', and as the initial summons stated, Ferrier was known to have never applied for the certificate. Again, the magistrate dismissed the line of questioning, reminding the prosecution that Yeo, the fully licensed professor of experimental physiology at Kings, had conducted the operation, not Ferrier himself. However, Waddy had a further allegation prepared, namely that 'the victims—or as that may be an offensive term, I will say the subjects—of the initial part of the experiment were kept alive by Dr Ferrier for the purpose of experiments'. Keeping animals alive after a serious injury after the effects of the anaesthetic had worn off violated section three of the Act. As Ingham conceded, the problem of whether Ferrier was accountable for keeping the animals alive would depend on the precise definition of the word 'experiment': was the experiment only the 'cruel act of cutting', or could the year-and-a-half long process of testing and watching also be termed an experiment which Ferrier, rather than Yeo, had plainly conducted.[100] The question of whether to *observe* the results of a painful experiment was also to intervene in it, or in short whether to watch was also to act, was one on which Ferrier's future reputation would depend.

Historians have explored the ways that the debates over vivisection of the 1860s and 1870s brought to the foreground changing attitudes to the relationship between humans and animals, challenged received notions about pain and who experienced it, and raised questions about the relationship between gender, emotion, and scientific knowledge by pitting feminine sensibility against a masculinist gaze. However, Ferrier's trial also drew attention to the status of the scientific witness in late nineteenth-century Britain, and in particular the relationship between observation and participation. Despite Waddy's best efforts to argue the opposite, according to Judge Ingham, observing a painful experiment was not the same as taking part in it. To Ingham, Ferrier was 'only' a spectator, who had performed 'observation alone'. If watching the behaviour of post-operative monkeys was tantamount to an experiment, he continued, then anyone observing Monkey F would be culpable: 'you mean to say that the hundred scientific gentlemen who attended the laboratory were partakers of the cruelty?' he scoffed.[101] Ingham concluded that while 'there is no doubt that some facilities were afforded to Dr. Ferrier to inspect those animals from time to time, and that he did inspect them, and took very great interest in the physiological results of the experiments made by Dr. Yeo', nonetheless, 'it

[100] Transcript of the court case printed in Anon, 'The Charge Against a Vivisectionist', *Daily News*, 18 November 1881.

[101] Anon., 'The Vivisection Case', *The Leeds Mercury*, 18 November 1881.

does not seem that there was anything more than he took great interest in the results of a cruel operation performed for the purposes of science no doubt by another person'.[102] With these words, the case against Ferrier was dismissed, and in the midst of the public uproar over the 'vivisection question,' the exemplary figure of the scientific observer, remote and invisible, one who merely looks on but does not intervene, hardened into a legal category of unaccountability.

In the autumn of 1884 at the National Hospital for Epilepsy and Paralysis Dr Rickman Godlee (1849–1925) carried out the first modern brain surgery.[103] His patient was a twenty-five-year-old man who had presented himself with a complete paralysis of the left hand and arm. The consultant Dr Hughes Bennett, who was familiar with Ferrier's cortical maps, was able to correctly diagnose the presence of an 'encephalic growth, probably of limited size, involving the cortex of the brain and situated at the middle part of the fissure of Rolando'. The patient urged his physicians to remove the growth, and on 25 November 1884, the operation was performed with Ferrier himself in attendance. The initial diagnosis had proved correct and Godlee was able to excise the tumour. The patient initially recovered well, but despite the use of carbolic acid for antisepsis eventually succumbed to a post-operative infection and died. Following the patient's death there was a public outcry, with many accusing the physicians of taking unnecessary risks. Nonetheless, the operation was deemed a success for its correct identification of the site of the growth, and paved the way for further attempts throughout the 1880s to locate and remove brain tumours using Ferrier's cortical maps. As the distinguished brain surgeon Sir Charles Balance later claimed, 'it was Ferrier, not any surgeon who was the originator and founder of modern cerebral surgery'.[104]

The recoiling body was central to the development of Ferrier's work on the brain. Viewed by him as involuntary reflexes and part of a fully mechanistic account of human emotion, flinches performed as Ferrier's clues to the secrets of interior sensation. But they were also a surprising part of his laboratory life in other ways, a source of consternation and

[102] Anon., 'The Charge Against A Vivisectionist', *Daily News*, 18 November 1881.

[103] Hughes Bennett, Rickman J. Godlee, 'Hospital for Epilepsy and Paralysis, Regent's Park: Excision of a Tumour from the Brain', *The Lancet*, 2, 3199 (1884) 1090–1. The claims for Bennett and Godlee's priority have been contested: the Scottish surgeon William Macewen carried out surgery for intercranial disease at the Glasgow Royal Infirmary in 1883, however contemporary historians have disagreed over the extent to which he used knowledge of localization in his work. See: M. Macmillan, 'Localization and William Macewen's Early Brain Surgery', *Journal of the History of Neuroscience*, 14, 1 (2005), 24–56.

[104] Charles Balance, 'The Thomas Vicary Lecture: Being a Glimpse into the History of the Surgery of the Brain', *The Lancet*, 1 (1922), 111–16.

frustration as well as an opportunity to stage himself and his colleagues as simultaneously passionate and objective. As Victoria's reign drew to a close, the shrinking subject came under scrutiny again when physiologists and psychologists grew increasingly interested in the malleability of the sensorium. It was in an attempt to chart the body's unpredictable and changeable responses to tactile stimuli—from the tickle of cotton wool to the stab of a needle—that in 1903, a young neurologist called Henry Head embarked on a peculiar self-experiment.

3

Henry Head's Wince

In April 1903, in a book-lined study in St John's College, Cambridge, the psychologist W. H. R. Rivers (1864–1922) and the neurologist and psychologist Henry Head (1861–1940) posed for a photograph (Figure 13). Rivers, on the right, somewhat younger looking, and smart in his suit, industriously held a scientific instrument, a notebook beside him. Head, on the left, bearded, older, and wearing a light-coloured smock, sat with his eyes closed, his chin cupped in his palm of his right hand and his face tilted away from the camera. It was a carefully choreographed pose to suggest one lost in reverie—although Head must have been bracingly self-aware not to jump when the camera bulb popped. On the table, stretched out between the two men, lay Head's left arm. Scattered around it, a number of scientific instruments: the pressure-aesthesiometer (for measuring sensitivity to pressure), the spring algesimeter (for measuring thresholds of pain), a pitcher of iced water, a box brimming with the softest jeweller's cotton wool and a series of fine wire 'hairs'.[1] For this photograph, the two men fashioned themselves into a *tableau vivant*, to represent an arduous and daring experiment. On 3 April 1903, Head underwent an operation to sever the radial nerve of his left arm. Over the four-and-a-half years that followed, once a week, Head and his colleague Rivers tested the gradual and faltering return of sensitivity to the limb. Their aim: to understand the physiology of sensation, at the time considered to be 'one of the most obscure regions of neurology'.[2]

The experiment required a distinctive and rather peculiar technique of introspection. By entering a trance-like state he called a 'negative attitude of attention', Head believed himself able to gain unmediated access to his own sensory experience.[3] Once Head achieved this state of reverie, Rivers applied various stimuli to the affected hand, from pricking

[1] Henry Head, 'Methods of Examining Sensation', *Studies in Neurology*, i, 2 vols. (London: Hodder & Stoughton, 1920) pp. 12–34.

[2] Gordon Holmes, 'Henry Head, 1861–1940,' *Obituary Notices of Fellows of the Royal Society*, *3*, 10 (1941), 665–89 (p. 669).

[3] W. H. R. Rivers and Henry Head, 'A Human Experiment in Nerve Division', *Brain*, 31 (1908), 323–450 (p. 345).

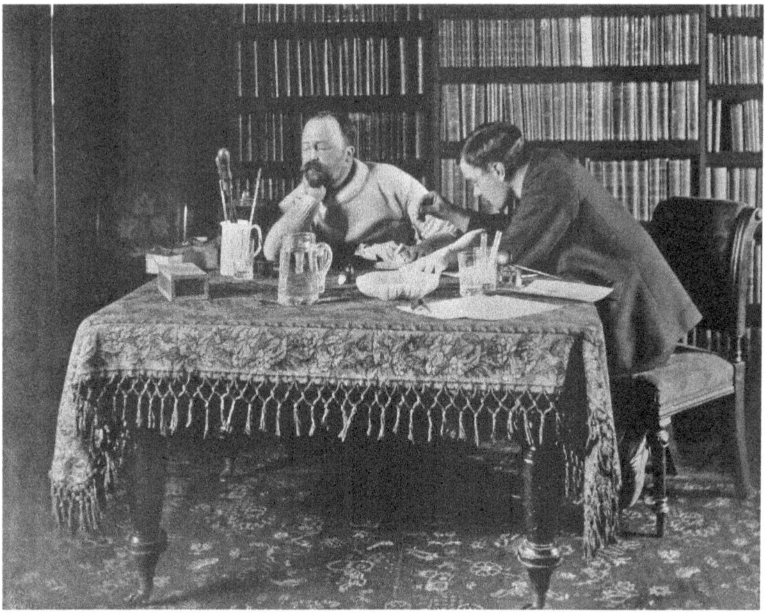

Fig. 13. Henry Head and W. H. Rivers working in Rivers's 'writer's room' at St John's College, Cambridge. Reproduced in Ronald A. Henson, 'Henry Head's Work on Sensation', *Brain: A Journal of Neurology* vol. 84, part IV (1961) 535–50, (p. 537).

Wellcome Library London

it with a pin to brushing it softly with cotton wool, and Head reported the minute changes in his responses. Although today such an approach would be dismissed as unscientific, between 1870 and 1920 introspection was a codified practice routinely used in laboratories dedicated to experimental psychology in Europe and America, and Head's 'negative attitude of attention' sits squarely within this tradition. The trance-like state, Head believed, minimized the chances of the participant-subject becoming embarrassed and self-conscious whilst performing in the experiment, emotional interferences which might distort the accuracy of the self-reports. In contrast to Darwin who deliberately created opportunities to watch himself feeling, Head sought to forget the theatrical conditions of his experiment altogether, by pretending he was not being monitored, or observing himself. In this way, Head believed he was able to directly and objectively access information about the human sensory landscape, a method he argued which bypassed inference or guesswork of the kind that had shadowed Ferrier's work with Monkey F. However, it will probably be no surprise to discover that accessing this condition of reverie was not always straightforward for Head. From being startled by noises drifting into the room from outside, to moments when the pain of the stimuli became unbearable causing Head to shriek, withdraw his hand, and jerk his body away from Rivers in a violent flinch, Head's quiet absorption was easily interrupted.

Head's attempt to achieve a 'negative attitude of attention' was not only part of an established method of introspection at the end of the nineteenth century. It also echoes ideas about sought-after contemplative aesthetic states that were gaining currency in literary and theatrical circles at the *fin de siècle*. Walter Pater, Oscar Wilde, Marcel Proust, the theatre critic A. B. Walkley, and actress Eleanora Duse, among others, each explored and questioned the idea of becoming fully immersed in one's own sensory experience. In the avant-garde theatre of the early twentieth century, actors and audiences took the logic of late nineteenth-century naturalism—and its attempts to ignore the live interaction between stage and auditorium—to its most extreme conclusion. Colluding instead in a deliberate attempt to forget the shared experience of the theatrical encounter altogether, both audience members and actors entered transcendent states of reverie. In a book which explores a pattern of emotional and performative spectatorship in this period, a chapter exploring trance-like states of contemplation may appear out of place. But in fact, in both the theatrical and scientific contexts explored in this chapter, reverie itself became a kind of performance, one which brought the theatricality of the spaces and contexts in which it was enacted to the foreground when it failed—through lost concentration, distraction, shock, or surprise. Head himself, who was an avid theatregoer, frequently described his efforts to achieve this revered condition of aesthetic transcendence in letters and scrapbooks documenting his artistic pursuits. During his trips to art galleries and churches, his reading and writing of poetry, and most of all his visits to the opera and theatre, Head sought out reverie, hoping for an unmediated connection with his own emotional and sensory experience. As in the laboratory, however, Head was often disappointed. The co-presence of the theatre audience proved particularly troublesome, as when irksome fellow spectators rustling their programmes startled Head out of his reverie, or the vertiginous authenticity of the acting confused him and made him self-conscious of his own role in creating the fiction. Head's experiment, then, suggests that the theatrical problems that Darwin and Ferrier encountered in their experiments did not simply disappear with the 'negative state of attention'. Rather, the collusions of scientific observer and theatrical audience member re-emerged in circuitous and unexpected forms.

THE 'NEGATIVE ATTITUDE OF ATTENTION'

Head was born into a Quaker family in Stoke Newington in London on 4 August 1861, and was educated at Charterhouse before reading natural sciences at Cambridge.[4] Upon graduating, Head took up a research position in the laboratory of Ewald Hering (1834–1918), at the German University in Prague, whose work on the role of the nervous system in optical perception inspired Head's interest in the physiology of sensation. Returning to Britain, Head decided to train as a physician, taking up a post at the London Hospital in Whitechapel where he remained for the rest of his working life. Later, he claimed this decision to enter a clinical rather than research setting was motivated by his ambition to explore the uncharted waters of human sensation. At Whitechapel, Head would have unfettered access to a range of human subjects; as he reminded his scientific colleagues in 1912, 'for the study of sensation, man is necessary. For we must be able to hear from the percipient the consequences which follow stimuli.'[5]

In 1901, by now a specialist in nervous disorders, Head embarked on his first experiments in sensory disturbance using his patients, men, women, and children, most usually working-class inhabitants of the East End, as subjects. At this time, the physiology of pain was still, as William James had put it in 1892, an 'enigma'.[6] To try to understand the special collusion of skin, nerves, and brain which created a hot, stinging pain in the leg or a dull aching throb in the shoulder, Head began by studying the peculiar phenomenon of 'referred pain'. Patients suffering from a disease of an internal organ often experienced painful sensations in anatomically remote parts of the body that were themselves uninjured, for example a diseased lung may cause pain in the left shoulder. The 'reference of pain to the skin when the lesion affects an internal organ at first sight seems inexplicable', confessed Head, but by comparing the sensitive patches of skin to areas of the body affected by herpes zoster (more commonly known as 'shingles'), Head was able to show that the 'reference' of pain from the site of the injury to remote parts of the body was due to distortions caused by the disease in the traffic between skin, spinal cord, and cortex. In short, the misperception took place in the brain. This led Head to an important

[4] For full biographical details, see L. S. Jacyna, *Medicine and Modernism: A Biography of Henry Head* (London: Pickering and Chatto, 2008).

[5] Henry Head, 'The Afferent Nervous System', Page-May Lecture delivered at the Institute of Physiology at University College London, 1912, Wellcome Library for the History of Medicine, *Henry Head Papers* (PP/HEA), PP/HEA/B13. p. 5.

[6] William James, *Psychology: A Briefer Course* (London: Macmillan, 1892) p. 67.

principle that would determine his future research in sensation: 'the localisation of sensation is not a physical but a psychical phenomenon'.[7]

Head continued his research by focusing on the other pathological sensory distortions presented by his patients at the London Hospital. Their symptoms ranged from ordinary numbness or hypersensitivity of the limbs following accidents, to the bizarre occurrence of 'spontaneous sensation', today known as 'phantom limb syndrome'. In a quiet room, screened from the rest of the hospital, Head blindfolded these patients before applying various stimuli to the affected body parts, and telling the patient to 'call out whenever he experienced a touch, a prick, or any other sensation'. It was a frustrating process. The dangerous urban environment provided Head with an steady supply of patients, but the city's transience and poverty meant that patients might find it 'more convenient to attend some other hospital', might move house, or neglect appointments 'lest his employer should consider him unfit for work'. Head instituted Sunday clinics, and employed a skilled assistant to trace his patients, offering them generous compensation for time and travelling expenses, but 'many cases disappeared entirely'.[8] Moreover, Head believed his uneducated working-class patients were lacking in the sensitivity to be adequate as self-reporters: 'at his best he answers yes or no with certainty', Head complained, but 'such patients can tell little or nothing of the nature of their sensations'.[9]

Head's growing scientific interest in the intimate workings of the human sensorium took place against the emergence of the entwined cults of Decadence and Aestheticism in literature and art at the *fin de siècle*. Its chief exponents, Oscar Wilde, Arthur Symons, and Walter Pater, among them, privileged a highly refined capacity for sensory experience, and a 'fine instinct for beauty' in the beholder.[10] The rare and delicate gift of sensitivity was itself unambiguously feminized in their writing. As Walter Pater put it in his essay on the 'Bacchanals of Euripides' published in 1910, it is the women and 'feminine souls' who had the peculiar power of being able to 'experience most directly the influence of things which touch thought through the senses'.[11] Like Wilde and Pater, Head also subscribed

[7] Henry Head, 'On Disturbances of Sensation with Especial Reference to the Pain of Visceral Disease' *Brain*, 16 (1893), 1–130 (p. 123–4).

[8] Henry Head and James Sherren, 'The Consequences of Injury to the Peripheral Nerves in Man', *Brain*, 28 (1905), 116–338 (p. 118–9).

[9] Rivers and Head, 'A Human Experiment', p. 324. For a discussion of the relationship between class and the perception of pain, see Lucy Bending, *The Representation of Bodily Pain in Late Nineteenth-Century English Culture* (Oxford: Clarendon, 2000).

[10] Oscar Wilde, *The Picture of Dorian Gray* (1891), ed. Isobel Murray (London: Oxford University Press, 1974) p. 130.

[11] Walter Pater, 'The Bacchanals of Euripides', *Macmillan's Magazine*, 60 (1889), 63–72, repr. in *The Works of Walter Pater* (Cambridge: Cambridge University Press, 2011) pp. 53–80 (p. 57).

to a hierarchy of sensitivity, believing that only a few particularly cultivated people possessed the ability to fully appreciate the sensory world in all its rich complexity. Only a handful of his patients, Head believed, could both access the most delicate transitions in their sensations and were equipped with the verbal skills to report them. For example, whilst working as a physician at Netley Hospital during the First World War, Head was delighted to encounter one Colonel M. whom he regarded as 'an unusually intelligent man of intellectual tastes' and therefore 'an excellent subject for examination'.[12] If Darwin's girlish flinch from the lunging puff adder amused the distinguished man of science, Head himself was happiest cast in the role of one of these particularly sensitive 'feminine souls'. As his biographer Stephen Jacyna has noted, Head, who was part of London's cultural elite at the *fin de siècle*, a member of the experimental theatre society the Pharos Club, and well versed in French poetry, believed himself among the lucky few who possessed the 'highly refined sensibility' required for his investigations.[13] Perhaps, then, it is not altogether surprising to find that within two years of commencing his research on the physiology of feeling at the London Hospital, Head came to the conclusion that he himself would make the ideal experimental subject.

Thus, on 25 April 1903, aged forty-two and in perfect health, Head embarked on his self-experiment. 'I shall know a great deal about pain by the time this experiment is over', he wrote to his fiancée Ruth Mayhew, a headmistress at a school in Brighton.[14] At the home of a surgeon named Mr Dean, Head underwent an operation in which the radial nerve of his left arm was severed, a tiny sliver excised and the two ends sutured back together again with fine silk, ensuring the nerve fibres would eventually regenerate. When Head came to, he was 'delighted to find' that while 'deep sensibility' or sensitivity to being prodded or poked remained, his hand was now 'insensitive to stimulation with cotton wool, to pricking with a pin, and to all degrees of heat and cold'.[15] After testing the hand with a variety of stimuli, Rivers outlined the affected area with a sinuous black ink line and took the first of many photographs documenting the gradual, faltering return of sensitivity over the next five years (Figure 14). Head described the process of testing to Mayhew in a letter dated 15 May 1903: 'we sit at the large table with my left arm exposed between us, my

[12] Henry Head, *Studies in Neurology* ii, quoted in Jacyna, *Medicine and Modernism*, p. 131.

[13] Jacyna, *Medicine and Modernism*, p. 7.

[14] Letter from Henry Head to Ruth Mayhew, 21 July 1903, PP/HEA/D4/15/512.

[15] Rivers and Head, 'A Human Experiment', p. 325.

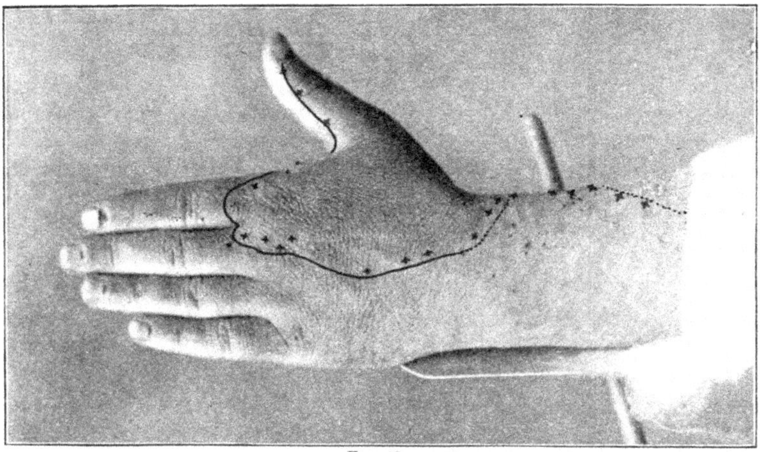

FIG. 49.

To show the extent of the loss of sensation produced by the operation.

The anæsthesia to cotton wool and to von Frey's hairs is bounded by the black line. The analgesia to prick and other cutaneous painful stimuli lay within the red crosses.

The darkness of the affected area is due to its deep red colour compared with the rest of the hand.

Fig. 14. 'Photograph of Head's hand showing the loss of sensation on 26 April 1903', W. H. R. Rivers and Henry Head, 'A Human Experiment in Nerve Division', in Henry Head, *Studies in Neurology*, i, 2 vols. (London: Hodder & Stoughton, 1920) pp. 225–329 (p. 227, Fig. 49).

The Bodleian Libraries, University of Oxford, 1534 d. 291

eyes are closed and he touches or pricks it in various ways recording his stimulus and my answer. Otherwise, no word passes between us and the silence is only broken by the scratching of his pen and my ejaculations.'[16] Rivers tickled the skin lightly and then brushed it more forcefully with cotton wool, pricked it with needles using the pressure-aesthesiometer and spring algesimeter, tested its 'passive movement' under electrical stimulation, applied different pressures using the algometer, and pressed test tubes of boiling and iced water to it (Figure 15).[17] At times, these tests were acutely painful, at which point Head cried out and withdrew his hand, his carefully worded self-reports interrupted by what Elaine Scarry has called 'an immediate reversion to a state anterior to language, to the cries a human being makes before language is learned'.[18] On at least one occasion, 'the pain was so excessively unpleasant that H. cried out and started

[16] Letter from Henry Head to Ruth Mayhew, 15 May 1903, PP/HEA/D4/14/495.

[17] Head, 'Methods of Examining Sensation', *Studies in Neurology*, pp. 12–34.

[18] Elaine Scarry, *The Body in Pain: The Making and Unmaking of the World* (Oxford: Oxford University Press, 1985) p. 4.

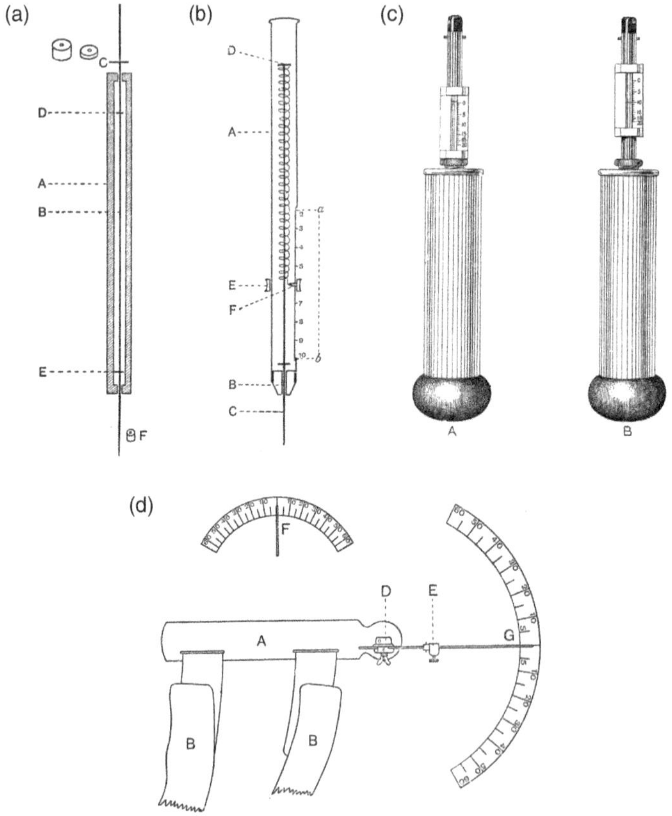

Fig. 15. Instruments used by Head and Rivers to measure sensation: (a) the Pressure Aesthesiometer; (b) the Spring Algesimeter; (c) Algometer Before and After Use; (d) The Instrument Devised by Dr. Gordon Holmes. 'Methods of Examination', W. H. R. Rivers and Henry Head, 'A Human Experiment in Nerve Division', in Henry Head, *Studies in Neurology*, i, 2 vols. (London: Hodder & Stoughton, 1920) pp. 12–46, (p. 18–20; p. 31).

away'.[19] Nonetheless, Head endeavoured to describe the sensations he felt, sometimes with a simple 'yes' or 'no', sometimes pointing to the location of the sensation on a photograph of his hand, at other times trying to describe the exact nature of the sensation with words such as 'burning', 'tickling', or 'stinging'.[20]

[19] Rivers and Head, 'A Human Experiment', p. 390.
[20] Rivers and Head, 'A Human Experiment', p. 334; p. 368.

To report on these experiences, Head entered the trance-like state he called a 'negative attitude of attention'. 'I must detach myself from the idea that experiments are in progress', he wrote to Mayhew, 'and with my eyes closed try to let my thoughts flow by like clouds on a windy day':

> Suddenly, in this flowing sea of thoughts there appears a flash of pain a wave of cold or the flicker of heat—It should appear with the suddenness of a porpoise, attract attention and again disappear leaving the untroubled sea to its onward flow.[21]

It was only by relaxing completely and entering this hazy, meditative state which the two men variously termed a 'negative attitude of attention', a state of 'detachment', a 'quiet state of internal absorption', or a 'state of passivity' that Head believed himself able to simultaneously feel and report the sensations aroused.[22] Most importantly, Head believed these trance-like states protected against the distorting effects of being too aware of his own performance in the experiment. The fact that the subject's self-consciousness could interfere with experimental results was well known by psychologists. In his bestselling popular book on psychology *The Story of Mind* (1899), the American psychologist James Baldwin explained that laboratory workers were continually adjusting their experiments so as to prevent subjects becoming embarrassed, awkward, or clumsy with self-consciousness. 'There is', he wrote, 'an important difference in the length of a person's reaction time according to the direction of his attention during the experiment'. If, for example, an experimental subject is responding to a signal by pressing a button, but is instructed to pay attention to his own finger during the process, the subject 'grows embarrassed, and his reaction time becomes very irregular and much longer'.[23] For similar reasons, Rivers noted that 'under no circumstances was H. allowed to know at the time whether his answers were right or wrong. For if he was told he had answered wrongly, he was roused to an intense determination to do better', leading him unconsciously to guess at the 'correct' results. Inevitably, the harder Head tried to describe the stimulus 'correctly', rather than simply describe what he felt, the more likely he was to get it wrong. In fact, the two men observed that as absorption passed into somnolence, Head was able to identify the stimuli with increased accuracy. 'Occasionally, especially after exercise in the open air, this condition of detachment would pass into sleep', the two men reported: 'we noticed that the answers seemed to improve up to the point at which H. ceased to reply'.[24]

[21] Letter from Henry Head to Ruth Mayhew, 27 November 1903, PP/HEA/D4/16/547.
[22] Rivers and Head, 'A Human Experiment', p. 345; p. 352; p. 343.
[23] James Mark Baldwin, *The Story of the Mind* (London: George Newnes, 1899) p. 146.
[24] Rivers and Head, 'A Human Experiment', p. 343.

This condition of sleepy detachment was, as the two men observed, rather woefully, one 'which H. has never succeeded in producing surrounded by the multifarious interruptions of home'. Instead, Head and Rivers decided to conduct the experiment in the relatively peaceful and contemplative environment of Rivers's study in Cambridge, where the neurologist could experience an 'absolute freedom from all external appeal to responsible action'.[25] Although the University of Cambridge already had a small psychological laboratory, established by Rivers himself in 1897, the two men chose to work in Rivers's college rooms. Recalling the domestic spaces in which experiments had been conducted in the middle of the nineteenth century, their decision also reminds us that alongside the new professional laboratories, scientists continued to work in diverse spaces. Indeed, Head and Rivers believed their choice of location played an important role in facilitating the experiment and the quiet state of 'internal absorption' it required. Cambridge not only seemed a different world to the rush and responsibility of Head's hospital work in London, it also removed Head from what in 1903 Georg Simmel had called the 'intensification of nervous stimulation' of the city. If in the mid nineteenth century, the city was characterized as a place of persistent shocks, its inhabitants starting and flinching from dangerous and new technologies, by the beginning of the twentieth century metropolitan dwellers were seen to be increasingly desensitized and inured, developing a 'blasé attitude' and a 'blunting of discrimination'.[26]

Each Saturday Head left London at lunchtime, tired from a morning's work with his patients at the London Hospital, and travelled by train to the relative peace of Cambridge. By the time he turned in for bed in his old college Trinity, Head and Rivers had planned their tests for the following day, had dined and socialized, and Head was thoroughly relaxed. The following morning, as church bells rang out, Head strolled from Trinity to St John's, through the first court and into the second, the heart of the college where nestling under the roof in the Old Court lay Rivers's rooms. 'A large low sitting room with a window in each side' led into a 'small square bedroom' and what Head described as 'the writer's work room'.[27] It was in this sanctuary, 'absolutely quiet and undisturbed, free from the petty worries of a busy life'—including, presumably, those of a university laboratory—that Rivers prodded and poked, stung, scratched, tickled, and burnt Head's

[25] Rivers and Head, 'A Human Experiment', p. 354.

[26] Georg Simmel, 'The Metropolis and Mental Life' (1903) repr. in *Art in Theory, 1900–1990: An Anthology of Changing Ideas* ed. Charles Harrison and Paul Wood (London: Blackwell, 1993) pp. 130–4 (p. 132).

[27] Letter from Henry Head to Ruth Mayhew, 15 May 1903, PP/HEA/D4/14/495.

arm, and Head carried out the formidable task of observing the minute changes in the sensations he experienced.[28]

Head and Rivers undertook their work at a time when scientific psychology, with its appeal to an objective knowledge about the mind, was in its infancy. In the same year that Rivers established a psychological laboratory at Cambridge, a Readership in Mental Philosophy was endowed at Oxford. The following year, 1898, James Sully opened an experimental psychological laboratory at University College London committed to the development of quantitative methods in the study of the human mind.[29] To legitimate this new science of psychology, it was vital to distinguish between a casual onlooker and the psychological observer trained in methods of observing human mind and behaviour. As Sully, a pioneer in the field of developmental psychology, put it in his introduction to *Studies of Childhood* (1896) there was a vast difference between the 'pretty anecdotes of children which tickle the emotions' and observations of the fleeting and subtle changes of a child's emotional expressions made by 'specially qualified workers' armed with knowledge and skill. Through their 'special knowledge which comes from studying the principles of science', psychological investigators could achieve what sentimental mothers could not—a 'cool and impartial process of scientific observation'. Though he was at pains to cast professional scientific observation as a unique category of objective looking, Sully did not turn to predictable comparisons between the scientific human eye and a measuring machine to shore up the distinction. Rather than compare his results to those obtained by those precision instruments that crowded the physiological laboratories at UCL, Sully offered a far more intriguing metaphor. 'The observer of children', he writes, 'must be a diviner, a sort of clairvoyant reader of their secret thoughts'. Only those with a special ability to 'get into touch with children' could capture the mercurial and fugitive transformations in their behaviour. Indeed, though Sully had dismissed mothers as serious observers bemoaning their sentimental attachment to their offspring, he also was willing to concede that women might be potentially better scientific observers of children given 'their higher gift of sympathetic insight'.[30]

[28] Rivers and Head, 'A Human Experiment', p. 342.

[29] Geoffrey C. Bunn, 'Introduction, Psychology in Britain', in *Psychology in Britain: Historical Essays and Personal Reflections* ed. G. C. Bunn, A. D. Lovie, G. D. Richards (Leicester: BPS Books, 2001) pp. 1–33 (pp. 1–3).

[30] James Sully, *Studies of Childhood* (New York: D. Appleton, 1896) pp. 14–15. For a discussion of the role Sully assigned to mothers, see: Sally Shuttleworth, *The Mind of the Child: Child Development in Literature, Science and Medicine 1840–1900* (Oxford: Oxford University Press, 2010) pp. 279–80.

'Sympathetic insight', 'getting into touch with', 'diviner', and 'clairvoyant' are not words and phrases we'd expect to find sitting alongside talk of the 'cool and impartial' processes and special training of scientific looking in the early part of the twentieth century. Daston and Galison have been influential in arguing that mechanical objectivity was the dominant discursive model through which scientific looking was constructed by the end of the nineteenth century.[31] Yet, in Sully's description of psychological observation, the study of the mind is brought together with talk of extrasensory perception, second sight, and sympathetic bodily vibrations. The connections running back and forth between scientific investigators, stage magicians, and clairvoyants from the middle of the nineteenth century up until the 1920s, have been explored in detail by Roger Luckhurst, Richard Noakes, and Martin Willis.[32] On the one hand, the public fascination with spiritualism provided psychologists, who visited séances to witness flying chairs, ecotoplasm, and wandering spirit hands, with a distinctive set of mental phenomena to investigate. At the same time, scientists collaborated with stage conjurors—including the great escapologist Harry Houdini himself—to debunk the fraudulent claims of mediums.[33] The close ties between the worlds of science and spiritualism remind us that even at the beginning of the twentieth century, scientists were not confined to the university laboratory, but moved between diverse environments to create scientific knowledge, spaces which in many cases were themselves already deeply embedded in the period's wider performance culture; in this way theatricality was always already inseparable from the scientific knowledge it helped to create. But for Sully, writing at the end of the nineteenth century, the links between magic and science ran even deeper than these examples suggest. For Sully, a peculiar unconscious communing could be found at the heart of the process of scientific looking itself.

The role of altered states of consciousness in scientific observation, and particularly introspection, was a particularly important problem for Head to grapple with. While in the eighteenth century, philosophers of mind Hume and Locke had practiced intuitive introspections, Head dryly noted that in the early twentieth century 'a man can no longer sit in his study and spin out of himself the laws of psychology by a process

[31] Daston and Galison, 'The Image of Objectivity', pp. 82–3.

[32] Roger Luckhurst, *The Invention of Telepathy: 1870–1901* (Oxford: Oxford University Press, 2002); Richard Noakes, 'Spiritualism, Science and the Supernatural in Mid-Victorian Britain', in *The Victorian Supernatural*, ed. Pamela Thurschwell, Carolyn Burdett, and Nicola Brown (Cambridge: Cambridge University Press, 2004); Martin Willis, *Vision, Science and Literature*. See also: Watt Smith, 'Cardboard, Conjuring and a Very Curious Experiment'.

[33] Willis, *Vision, Science and Literature*, p. 207.

of self-examination'.[34] As was discussed in Chapter One, the nineteenth century had witnessed an ongoing debate over the validity of introspection in the emerging sciences of mind. Nonetheless, in the 1870s, the German physiologist Wilhelm Wundt working at Leipzig argued that a truly scientific study of one's own mind was possible. According to Kenton Kroker, Wundt agreed that 'some mental phenomena as dreams, episodes of madness, or thought, were beyond the pale of experimental control'.[35] But under certain conditions, he believed observers could be trained to report on their own visual and aural perceptions in response to stimuli. Wundt developed rigorous techniques and specially adapted instruments for the task, and in his laboratories, researchers were required to undergo hundreds of hours of training in a set of codified techniques before they were allowed to practice *innere Wahrnehmung* ('inner perception'). Inspired by Wundt's success, between 1900–1920, the British psychologist Edward B. Titchener at Cornell took a similar approach. He argued that 'an introspective attitude and introspective capacity are not the common property of anyone who cares to exercise them', but techniques through which psychologists 'trained by long and arduous practice' learnt to report changes in feeling free from interpretation and inference.[36]

In Britain too, introspection was utilized as an experimental practice by a new generation of scientifically minded psychologists. Head was not alone in believing himself to be a scientifically 'trained observer', whose capacity for self-observation was based on his having a particularly refined sensibility.[37] In the 1890s, the British novelist and psychological investigator Vernon Lee had conducted experiments with the Scottish artist Kit Anstruther-Thomson in art galleries and churches across the continent, publishing the results in an extended essay on aesthetic experience, 'Beauty and Ugliness' in 1897.[38] As Carolyn Burdett has described, Anstruther-Thomson's extreme sensitivity both to artworks and spaces, from the soaring architecture of cathedrals to the bulges of a Grecian urn, as well as to the minute changes of her own visceral responses, fascinated Lee. 'As Lee encouraged her to scrutinize and record these sensations and feelings,

[34] Henry Head, 'Sensation and the Cerebral Cortex', *Brain*, 41, 2 (1918), 58–202 (p. 177).

[35] Kenton Kroker, 'The Progress Of Introspection in America, 1896–1938', *Studies in History and Philosophy of Biomedical Sciences*, *34* (2003), 77–108 (p. 78).

[36] Edward B. Titchener, *Lectures On The Experimental Psychology of The Thought-Processes* (New York: The Macmillan Company, 1909) pp. 276–7, quoted in Kroker, 'The Progress of Introspection', p. 82.

[37] Head, *Studies in Neurology*, i, p. 12.

[38] Vernon Lee and C. Anstruther-Thomson, 'Beauty and Ugliness' (1897) repr. in *Beauty and Ugliness and Other Studies in Psychological Aesthetics* (London: John Lane, 1912) pp. 45–76.

Anstruther-Thomson became increasingly able to distinguish changes in breath, balance and muscular tension as reactions to the observed form, seemingly amounting to a type of unconscious mimicry of it', writes Burdett. 'These bodily changes in turn caused emotional feelings—pleasant and harmonious ones, or constrained and uncomfortable ones . . . Lee concluded that these emotional feelings were actually the source of what is experienced as "beauty".'[39] As Burdett points out, many have found Lee's experiments 'faintly risible', but in fact they reflected Lee's deep engagement with the latest psychological research from the continent, in particular her interest in Theodor Lipps ideas of *Einfuhlung*, later translated as empathy, and Karl Groos's theory of *innere Nachahmung*, or inner mimicry.[40] Moreover, Lee did not only engage with the latest psychological ideas, but her research methods reflected those already established in Heidelberg by Wundt, and would also anticipate Head's own efforts to scrutinize his own sensory and emotional responses in Rivers's study and at the theatre. Indeed, when Wilfred Trotter and H. Morriston Davies replicated Head's self-experiment in 1918, they took for granted the reliability of an introspective method—although did not repeat the idiosyncrasies of the 'negative attitude of attention'—and offered advice to 'anyone contemplating similar work'.[41] For psychologists working in Britain, Europe, and America at the turn of the century, then, introspection had hardened into an objective method which avoided 'statements of personal opinion' and the interference of the onlooker in the process.[42] The trance-like negative attitude of attention, which Head believed allowed him to commune directly with his own sensations, to divine them (to echo Sully's words), catching hold of each fleeting change without the mediating and distorting effects of interpretation and self-consciousness, thus became a strategy for objective looking. According to Head and Rivers, a condition of 'reverie' or 'negative attitude of attention' was one of the many habitual 'precautions and safeguards customary in the psychological laboratory' that they employed.[43]

[39] Carolyn Burdett, ' "The subjective inside us can turn into the objective outside": Vernon Lee's Psychological Aesthetics', *19: Interdisciplinary Studies in the Long Nineteenth Century*, 12 (Spring 2011), 1–31 (p. 3).

[40] Burdett, ' "The subjective inside us can turn into the objective outside", p. 5. See also: Susan Lanzoni, 'Practising Psychology in the Art Gallery: Vernon Lee's Aesthetics of Empathy', *Journal of the History of the Behavioral Sciences*, 45, 4 (2009), 330–54 (pp. 344–51).

[41] Wilfred Trotter and H. Morriston Davies, 'Experimental Studies in the Innervation of the Skin', *Journal of Physiology*, 38 (1909), 134–246 (p. 140).

[42] Rivers and Head, 'A Human Experiment', p. 324.

[43] Head, *Studies in Neurology*, i, p. 12.

ELEANORA DUSE'S FLINCH

Conditions of reverie or 'negative attention' seem unlikely candidates for a study of passionate, gestured spectatorship in the long nineteenth century. But in many ways, dreamy states of internal absorption were partly self-conscious performances too. If introspection was a distinctive scientific practice in the early part of the twentieth century, it was also a pattern of looking increasingly associated with performers and audiences of the new avant-garde drama. Among the papers Head kept until his death, now archived at the Wellcome Library, is a clipping of a theatre review by *The Times* critic A. B. Walkley. It describes a performance given in London in 1900 by the Italian actress Eleanora Duse. Head may or may not have attended this production, but as entries in his scrapbooks reveal, the neurologist certainly did admire the actress. According to Walkley, watching Duse perform was like watching someone 'acting for herself and by herself'. She does not 'force a single cry, prolong a single gesture or exaggerate a single point in order that she may be the better understood by audiences' but rather seemed 'to stand somewhat aloof'.[44] If Strindberg had insisted in his preface to *Miss Julie* that the actor should not enter 'into direct contact' with the audience 'outside the frame of the set', Duse seemed to disavow any relationship between spectator and performer altogether.[45] Hers was a 'rapt absorption' in character, and a 'timid, depreciatory air' out of it.[46] So fully absorbed was Duse in her feelings that, at the curtain call, the threshold of the theatrical fiction, Duse flinched—or at least, seemed to—from the reappearance of the audience. Just as Wilde's Dorian Gray 'started and drew back' from the lilac blossoms when Lord Henry placed a hand on his shoulder, so Duse was startled out of her reverie by the apparent discovery that all along, she has been watched.[47] 'She seems half startled by bursts of applause', wrote Walkley, and 'gets through the unavoidable business of "bowing her acknowledgements" with evident impatience'.[48]

Duse was a formative figure in theatre's turn away from theatricality at the *fin de siècle*. 'Revolted by the falseness of the theatrical milieu', writes Jonas Barish in his book about the history of anti-theatricality, Duse shied

[44] A. B. Walkley, 'Eleonora Duse in *La Dame aux Camélias*', 16 June 1900, *The Times*. Clipping found among Henry Head's personal papers, PP/HEA/E4.

[45] Strindberg, *Miss Julie* (Preface) p. 67.

[46] Walkley, 'Eleonora Duse'.

[47] Wilde, *The Picture of Dorian Gray*, p. 20

[48] Walkley, 'Eleonora Duse'.

away from theatre's need 'to externalize', to fix 'our gaze on surfaces', to engage with what George Bernard Shaw had decried as theatre's 'art of pleasing'.[49] 'All London calls her no actress' Head scribbled enthusiastically in his scrapbook.[50] She is 'natural, simple, sincere, a real woman', in the midst of 'all this sham', wrote Walkley. Duse's insular intoxication provided a libidinous, even louche, frisson for her audiences, sending 'a faint shiver of pleasure' through them.[51] John Stokes has contended that a recurring topos in fictional representations of theatre at the *fin de siècle* is one in which the actress 'becomes so involved in what she is doing that she appears "possessed" by it, controlled by and yet inhabiting her role as if in a dream'. In turn, this absorption made her audience perilously over-attentive, producing 'an intoxicating or hypnotic effect'.[52] Edmond de Goncourt's *La Faustin*, 1882, Gabriele D'Annunzio's *The Flame of Life*, 1900, and Proust's *Within a Budding Grove, Remembrance of Things Past*, 1919 are all cited by Stokes for their depiction of this intoxication on both sides of the footlights.

Other works of this period, however, call the straightforward sincerity of the actor's—and the audience's—absorbed reverie into question. The singing heroine of George du Maurier's *Trilby*, for example, becomes an international celebrity for her pure voice and unvarnished performances. She sings of the most 'terrible and pathetic of all possible human tragedies' without 'dramatic or histrionic exaggeration of any sort'. With her voice slight, subtle, and 'simple as a child's', she holds her audience entranced 'beneath the spell', their flesh creeping, eyes weeping and pulses made to race.[53] As the novel progresses, however, we discover that Trilby's naturalness is rather more complicated than at first it seemed. Though she performs whilst in a trance, hers is a very peculiar state of consciousness, a hypnotic condition contrived through the interventions of her mesmerist husband Svengali. In this way, du Maurier plays with the ideal of naturalness on stage, revealing the purity of Trilby's performance to be simultaneously a romantic expression of a pure subjectivity and the product of outside influence and manipulation.

Walkley's description of Duse's flinch from her applauding audience emphasized the actress's sincerity in the midst of theatrical sham. But on closer inspection, it also betrayed a momentary hesitation, a queasiness

[49] Barish, *The Antitheatrical Prejudice*, p. 329; p. 343.

[50] Henry Head and Ruth Mayhew, 'Rag Book', iiiA, August 1903, pp. 28–32, PP/Hea/E3/5, p. 28.

[51] Walkley, 'Eleonora Duse'.

[52] John Stokes, 'Varieties of Performance at the Turn of the Century' in *The Cambridge Companion to the* Fin de Siècle, ed. Gail Marshall (Cambridge: Cambridge University Press, 2007) pp. 207–22 (p. 210).

[53] George du Maurier, *Trilby* (London: Osgood, 1895) pp. 309–10.

about the authenticity or spontaneity of the gesture. Twenty years earlier, Ferrier, in his laboratory notebooks, had admitted he could not always be sure whether Monkey F had flinched, or merely twitched: she 'seems to start, but other times pays no attention'.[54] Likewise, for Walkley sitting in the auditorium, Duse's gesture was rather ambiguous: she '*seems* half startled by bursts of applause' (my italics). Though her surprise at the curtain call apparently suggested a trance broken by spectators she'd forgotten were even there, it may have also been a sham, a knowing pose. Schooled in theatre's dark arts, Duse knew her flinch would thrill and delight her audience, giving them the satisfaction of believing what they had witnessed was not mere *acting*, but unencumbered emotional truth.

While absorption could be deployed as part of a deliberate theatrical sham among actors, for audience members, self-consciousness complicated the transitions in and out of reverie too. In the early twentieth-century theatre, it seems, absorption and theatricality, the two states which Michael Fried has argued to be profoundly incompatible, existed on a more subtle continuum.[55] In fact, Fried's 1967 essay 'Art and Objecthood', though famously antagonistic towards theatre, offers one way of thinking about how theatricality might linger and reassert itself in a theatrical culture drawn towards states of sublime, intoxicating reverie.[56] Rather than absorbing the viewer in a complete illusion, Fried argued that theatricality involves the viewer in a degree of self-consciousness about their own participation, making them aware of their own body during the act of viewing. Theatricality is therefore apparent in the moments when an artwork's complete illusion falters, and when the spectator is made intensely aware of attempts to seduce or solicit a response, and their own responsibility to provide it. As Ridout has persuasively argued, it is precisely in moments of spectatorial self-awareness, or the audience's own stage fright, that the theatrical relationships between performers and spectators—arrangements which are disguised by naturalistic conventions—seep into view. For Ridout, theatricality emerges in accidents or failures when the smooth surface of the naturalistic representation jars and the audience's own presence, as well as their role in creating the fiction, is awkwardly revealed to them.[57] In light of this more nuanced reading of the theatrical encounter

[54] Appendix A, 7 July 1881.

[55] Michael Fried, 'Absorption and Theatricality' (1967), repr. in *Art and Objecthood: Essays and Reviews* (Chicago: University of Chicago Press, 1998) pp. 148–72.

[56] Michael Fried, *Absorption and Theatricality: Painting and Beholder in the Age of Diderot* (Berkley: University of California Press, 1980) p. 100. See also: Postlewait and Davis 'Theatricality: An Introduction', p. 20.

[57] Ridout, *Stage Fright*, pp. 1–2.

as an event during which spectators are continually moving in and out of self-consciousness, the possibility of a thoroughly intoxicated audience seems an unlikely prospect.

Indeed, for Head, managing to enter a trance-like state of absorption whilst at the theatre was a rare and coveted event. 'I got it once,' he wrote, whilst *reading* a play—it was Ibsen's *The Wild Duck*—alone one evening in the fading light of a Prague beer garden. 'The daily world around me seemed unreal,' he wrote. 'I felt as if I had gone through some colossal personal experience of which the memory could only end with death.' He witnessed others enjoy such exhilaration in the theatre. 'I have seen others get it with a play of Ibsen's, once in a memorable instance where a man took me to see *Little Eyolf* in order to talk business between the acts.'[58] But for Head, when it came to actually going to the theatre, the 'daily world' more stubbornly persisted. On 11 December 1898, Head wrote of a trip to the theatre to see Forbes Robertson and Mrs Patrick Campbell in *Macbeth*, complaining that he had been 'particularly unfortunate' as to be seated near a man who was insistent on explaining the entire plot of the play to his female companion. 'He began by stating it was a Scotch play and told her that he thought Macbeth was a Scotch king.' Exasperated, Head intervened, but to little effect: 'When I asked him to be silent he apologized saying she had never seen the play and I told him the book of words was published. He was then quieter but she clamoured for explanations'.[59] Jim Davis and Victor Emeljanow have rightly cautioned against describing late nineteenth-century audiences as a homogenous unit, reminding us that accounts of the demonstrative behaviour of earlier audiences were often overplayed, and that diverse audience styles persisted well into the twentieth century: while the West End audiences might have been famous for their indifference, 'batches of rampant, hooting boys' still inhabited the gallery at the Pavilion Theatre in Whitechapel Road.[60] However, it is also worth remembering that middle-class audiences at West-End productions of Shakespeare plays were also capable of disrupting the illusion with a cacophony—or, to echo Rancière, a choreography—of programme-rustling, coughing, shushing, tutting, and shifting about in their seats.

It was not only irksome whispering neighbours that frustrated Head's attempts to attain a quiet feeling of total absorption at the theatre. So too did the uncomfortable relationship between untrustworthy appearances

[58] Head and Mayhew, 'Rag Book', pp. 28–32 (p. 30).

[59] Letter from Henry Head to Ruth Mayhew, 11 December 1898, PP/Hea/D4/3/89.

[60] Davis and Emeljanow, *Reflecting the Audience*, p. 58.

and the ever-elusive real on stage. In 1903, shortly before embarking on the self-experiment in nerve regeneration, Head saw Duse perform the title role in *Hedda Gabler*. On returning home, he wrote in his scrapbook, in language that echoed Walkley's, of the 'extraordinary feeling of emotional reality that Duse gives me'.

> I say 'emotional feeling' advisedly, for in ordinary life this is a state that is foreign to me. With me the sense of reality is intellectual—I say 'I know that to be true because...' Rarely in my life, after times of great emotion, I seem to have become convinced of something not by reason but emotionally as a revivalist may become 'convinced' of sin. This feeling Duse nearly always gives me and never have I been more conscious of its existence than when I saw her play in *Hedda Gabler*.

In Head's account of watching Duse, the psychologist experiences a quasi-spiritual conversion. For Head, it was his fervent emotions, rather than his rational mind, that brought him into close contact with the moral world of Ibsen's play, just as a revivalist might seek out an immediacy of the Holy Spirit through evangelical song and ecstatic prayers. At the same time, even though he was able to attain this sublime state, it seems the connection was somewhat short-lived. Only a few lines later in the same diary entry, Head reveals that he had in fact been concentrating so hard on Duse's 'emotional reality' that he became distracted and confused by it. Just as a word becomes peculiar when we repeat it too often, so when Head focused too much on Duse's authenticity, the boundaries of her performance started to blur. 'I knew I was in a theatre watching an actress', explains Head, but as the play progressed, Head noticed that the actress embodied 'the very ticks of speech' of a woman he had once known—a woman who had, at the time, filled him 'with vivid interest as a scientific observer'. And so, rather than concentrate on Duse's performance, the uncanny similarity led Head's mind to amble off into another world altogether. Sitting in the dark of the auditorium, Head was distracted by nagging doubts: 'Had the original I saw reproduced on stage been one of my patients?—How did she come into my life? These were the questions that constantly cropped up in my mind.'[61] During this incident, as with the one with the noisy neighbouring audience member, Head's aesthetic pleasure and the transcendence he so desired, lay tantalizingly out of reach.

Head's accounts of theatre-going describe an experience of vacillation in the auditorium, in which spectators slip in and out of states of absorption, attention, and distraction. Precisely because theatres are places of live encounter between performers and spectators, distractions abound. The

[61] Head and Mayhew, 'Rag Book', pp. 31–2.

critic Walkley who had so admired Duse's naturalness, made a professional virtue out of swerving between absorption and distraction, sometimes managing the impossible-sounding task of attaining both at the same time. In a lecture delivered at the Royal Institution in February 1903, Walkley described theatrical audiences as 'peculiarly inattentive'. Asking us to cast our eyes around the playhouse, he introduces a cast of familiar culprits: 'The millionaire in the stage box is politely stifling a yawn behind his kid glove; Miss in the stalls is whispering to her Mamma that Sir Toby Belch seems very tipsy, and that anyhow it isn't half so funny as *Charley's Aunt.* The pit are shuffling their feet, and the gallery boy is shouting "boo!" In a later piece, Walkley echoed G. H. Lewes's depiction of the theatrical audience as self-watchers, by arguing that the theatrical 'crowd finds itself an interesting spectacle'. 'From the moment of its formation it becomes self-conscious, self-assertive', he wrote, so that 'to absorb its attention—that is to say, to make it forget its own existence—is an extremely difficult feat'. For Walkley, women, 'the less attentive sex', were to blame, forming as they did the majority of the 'modern theatrical audience'; so too were the working classes at fault for becoming too easily distracted and in turn distracting others, for their 'power of attention is naturally low'. Becoming absorbed in the fiction through this gauze of inattention, or from behind a lady's '*matinée* hat' through which one might 'occasionally glimpse' the play, would have required a special aptitude indeed.[62]

Amid these competing distractions, one might expect the theatrical critic to regard himself as a paragon of focus and concentration. Indeed, he ought to possess a rare capacity to transcend the social world of the auditorium to commune directly with the drama. In fact, whilst at the theatre, Walkley entered what he described as 'a rather complicated state, a state of double consciousness'. It is a phrase redolent of the technique of self-watching which, as the first chapter of this book described, Irving, following Diderot, had attributed to actors in the 1870s, and G. H. Lewes had found in the task of psychological introspection.[63] For Walkley, the ideal theatrical spectator should strike a delicate balance between absorption and attentiveness. While inattentiveness was the curse of the modern auditorium, both absorption and over-attention were also troubling. For Walkley, a 'wholly sympathetic absorption' in the fictional world could lead spectators into a state of 'complete delusion'.[64] Stories, some almost certainly apocryphal, of over-invested audience members were not unfamiliar to Victorians. One famous anecdote involved a group of sailors

[62] A. B. Walkley, *Dramatic Criticism* (London: John Murray, 1903) p. 13; pp. 27–30.
[63] Walkley, *Dramatic Criticism*, p. 34.
[64] Walkley, *Dramatic Criticism*, p. 32.

who, on shore-leave, visited a theatre where they 'happened to see a representation of a mutiny on board ship, and were so excited that they rushed on the stage and took sides with the authorities in quelling the movement'.[65] Walkley provides a further example with an anecdote featuring Sir Roger de Coverley who, while watching a performance of *The Distrest Mother*, became so greatly concerned for the heroine that from his seat in the stalls he loudly and vociferously egged her on to escape her captor, shouting 'ay, do it if you can!' At the other extreme, were spectators who frustratingly experienced 'absolute non-illusion'. Either because the acting was so singularly unpersuasive, or because they were too familiar with the secret workings of the stage paraphernalia, some spectators failed to achieve the all-important 'suspension of disbelief'. Walkley cites the example of the novelist Leo Tolstoy, who once described feeling entirely detached and 'unsympathetic' during a performance of Wagner's opera *Siegfried*. In this production, the title role was taken by a man whose 'white, weak, genteel hands', poor sword skills, false beard, and flabby stomach 'revealed the actor'.[66]

According to Walkley, finding a middle ground between emotional absorption with detached attentiveness was the demanding but specialized task of the professional theatre spectator.

> There is a French proverb which says that you cannot at once join in a procession and look out of the window. Yet it is a feat of that kind which the ideal theatrical spectator has to accomplish, for remember that he is not only taking in pleasure with a complete self-surrender, he is also commanding himself so as to estimate the quality of his pleasure—while it is coming in.

For Walkley, then, the 'ideal spectator' balanced the extremes of complete absorption and unsympathetic detachment. The theatre critic therefore was 'not the most passionate' spectator, but instead entered into a 'double consciousness' in which he simultaneously experienced and monitored his emotional responses to the drama.[67] If the phrases 'double-perspective' and 'double-consciousness' recall Diderot's and Irving's descriptions of acting, they also echo techniques attributed to audiences of sensation theatre in the 1870s.[68] Like these audiences, the early twentieth-century critic was as interested in the spectacle as in his own emotional responses. Here, where acting and looking elide in Walkley's description of professional theatre watching, his 'rather complicated state of double consciousness' crosses paths with scientific self-observation. Not least, it recalls the

[65] Sully, *Studies of Childhood*, p. 314.
[66] Walkley, *Dramatic Criticism*, pp. 32–3.
[67] Walkley, *Dramatic Criticism*, p. 34.
[68] Diderot, *Oeuvres Esthétiques*, p. 195; Irving, 'The Art of Acting', p. 56.

trained psychological introspector Head, who sitting in Rivers's rooms in Cambridge, estimated the quality of his own sensory responses as they were 'coming in'. Like Head, Walkley attributed his ability to achieve a 'double-consciousness' to a special training and superior sensitivity. As Walkley put it, 'this by no means easy mental process requires not only an effort of the will, a special motive, but training and special aptitude'.[69] Like the actress Duse, then, the 'ideal theatrical spectator' and the introspecting psychologist were both neither wholly immersed in their feelings nor entirely dispassionately self-conscious about them, but moved back and forth between the two states.

Paying attention to the effects of Duse's acting as if noting the sensations aroused by the spring algesimeter, Head claimed to 'know as a psychologist skilled in self analysis, that she produces in me an effect I can not otherwise obtain from acting'.[70] As the scrapbooks that Mayhew and Head jointly kept (they called them 'rag-books') reveal, Head was interested in assessing the psychological changes that occurred in him as he watched theatrical performances. Theatre-going, writes Jacyna, was 'an intensely personal experience which offered him exceptional opportunities to pursue the introspective study of his own psychic processes'.[71] Exercising his special skill of 'double-consciousness', however, though a professional interest for Head, may also have been a hazard when it came to enjoying being at the theatre, and his desire for states of reverie. One wonders whether Head's theatrical experiments left him feeling a little like Proust's young hero Marcel, the 'inspired student' of *Guermantes Way*. Going to see his favourite actress, La Berma, Marcel craves transcendental experiences. Instead, the visit is deeply disappointing, and woefully distracting. The earnest student finds that when the lights dim and the actress appears on stage, a querulous voice arrives in his head. It asks: 'Is that good? Is it admiration I am feeling? Is this what is meant by richness of colour, nobility, power?' In response to his anxious questioning, Marcel hears a stranger's voice in his head with its despotic 'high-pitched voice' and 'oddly questioning tone'. In Marcel's experience of a doubled consciousness, trying to appraise feelings as they are coming in, in order to 'name things and our thoughts', becomes exasperating.[72] As Marcel discovers, the critic's ideal act of spectatorship, amounts—at least, for those not trained, or paid, to do it—to a profoundly unsatisfying aesthetic experience.

[69] Walkley, *Dramatic Criticism*, p. 34.

[70] Head and Mayhew, 'Rag Book', p. 31.

[71] Jacyna, *Medicine and Modernism*, p. 211.

[72] Marcel Proust, *The Guermantes Way* (1920) *In Search of Lost Time*, iii, 6 vols. trans. Mark Treharne (London: Penguin, 2002) p. 47.

Several years later, Marcel returns to the theatre to see La Berma once more tread the boards. 'I set no great store by this opportunity of seeing La Berma perform, which a few years earlier, had thrown me into such a state of over-excitement', Marcel confesses. Despite, or perhaps because, of his weary attitude, Marcel unexpectedly notices a creeping sense of pleasure and delight. La Berma's art had become 'pathetically thin, it was no longer inhabited by a profundity of soul', and yet, because of her insubstantiality and Marcel's lack of interest, rather than the exercise of his earnest 'critical mind', Marcel begins to enjoy the show. For Marcel, close attention to his own sensations inhibits the pleasures of aesthetic contemplation. In contrast, inattention, boredom, and distraction turn out to be agreeable conditions for watching actors and their 'pathetically thin' art, which, in this half-light accrue the appearance of dimension and depth. Thus, he concludes, it is the 'society people' sitting languidly and nonchalantly in the boxes, yawning like Walkley's millionaire, who alone 'would have had the clarity of mind to attend to the play, if only they had had minds'.[73] Just as during his experiment, Head's ability to ascertain the correct temperature of the water splashing his hand improved as he neared sleep, at the theatre being distracted and inattentive was the prelude to a thoroughly enjoyable evening.

FEELING INTERRUPTED

States of attention, reverie, and distraction have begun, in recent years, to play an increasingly important part in wider debates around nineteenth-century visuality. In *Suspensions of Perception*, Jonathan Crary describes how from the 1870s, in Britain and Europe, there was an 'explosion of research and debate' on the topic of attention.[74] Though it quickly became a key site of scientific scrutiny, it remained an unstable category and was subject to shifting, often contradictory, explanations. For example, in 1880, the British psychologist James Cappie described attention as the 'bringing of the consciousness into focus in some special direction', continuing that 'without it meaningless reverie will take the place of coherent thought'.[75] In Cappie's definition, to bring one's attention to something was an intentioned and effortful endeavour, aimed at extracting a distinct

[73] Proust, *The Guermantes Way*, pp. 34–7.

[74] Jonathan Crary, *Suspensions of Perception: Attention, Spectacle and Modern Culture* (Cambridge, MA: MIT, 2001), p. 23.

[75] James Cappie, 'Some Points in the Physiology of Attention, Belief and Will', *Brain 9* (July 1886), 201, quoted in Crary, *Suspensions of Perception*, p. 17.

and quiet focal point from the busy world which assaults our senses. For Cappie, attention and reverie were rivalrous: to quote Crary, attention was seen as 'a disciplinary defence against all potentially disruptive forms of free association'. Over the next two decades, the meanings attached to attentiveness expanded, and the boundaries between efficacious attention and incoherent distraction began to blur. There was particular interest in the overflow of attentiveness into states of trance or autohypnosis, and attention and distraction began to be seen as not two 'essentially different states' but as part of a 'single continuum... a dynamic process, intensifying and diminishing, rising and falling, ebbing and flowing according to an indeterminate set of variables'.[76] As Crary points out, by the early twentieth century, attention occupied a somewhat paradoxical position. On the one hand, attention was a precondition of learning and creative experience. On the other, it was increasingly seen as a vital strategy of social discipline and control: from factory floor to cinema auditorium, attention was the mode through which individuals could engage productively and efficiently with the world around them.

Yet, reverie was not always seen as disruptive, even by the psychologists who seemed most invested in the study of attention, and for whom vigilance and concentration were preconditions of professional observation. Crary has suggested that the techniques utilized in the study of attentiveness themselves functioned as disciplinary instruments: attention was 'not just one of the many topics examined experimentally by late nineteenth-century psychology' but was also 'the fundamental condition of its knowledge'.[77] Yet, at the same time, as Martin Willis has suggested, laboratory instruments and techniques for looking were also capable of undermining the authority of the scientific observer, highlighting his 'fragility'.[78] Indeed, Head's introspective process offers a counterpoint to the idea that attention was a privileged form of engagement among scientific observers of this period. Parallels can be drawn between Marcel's discovery that a focused attentiveness may not be the most productive way to enjoy theatre, and Head's assertion that a 'negative state of attention' best allowed him to experience his own sensations. In one unusual session, Rivers was surprised to find Head repeatedly identifying correctly the space between two points of a compass that rested on the back of his hand. The two men associated this exceptional set of results with a 'complete wandering of attention from the manipulations'. Head was 'completely absorbed' by thoughts of a book he had been reading, until 'recalled by

[76] Crary, *Suspensions of Perception*, p. 17; p. 47–8.
[77] Crary, *Suspensions of Perception*, p. 25.
[78] Willis, *Vision, Science and Literature*, p. 2.

R.'s question'.[79] The ebb and flow of attention, absorption, and distraction which Head associated with theatre-going, also featured in his psychological introspection. At the same time, this also meant that the theatrical problems which irritated Head on his trips to see plays and inhibited his attempts to achieve pure absorption in the fiction—the noisy neighbours and programme-rustlers and disturbing confusions between actors and patients—also crept into the refuge of Rivers's workroom. After all, the experimental setting of Rivers's workroom was, like the theatres Head frequented, characterized by the co-presence of a spectator and performer, both of whom were, in different ways, trying to forget they were being watched.

Head and Rivers claimed that entering a 'negative state of attention' was a technique of a trained self-observer, a discipline that Head soon 'learnt to adopt at will'.[80] On closer inspection, however, it is a claim they rather overstated. As the compass test incident suggested, Head's 'complete wandering of attention from the manipulations' was often quite haphazardly achieved, not intentional at all. Moreover, Head's ability to envelop himself in a hazy reverie was often frustrated. In one letter to Mayhew, Head revealed that in winter, the coldness of the Cambridge study rendered him 'stubborn', unable to comply with the siren's call of his own 'sea of thoughts'.[81] At other times, his exhaustion (rather than sleepiness), the result of a busy week treating patients at the London Hospital, meant that the sensation in his hand 'went all to pieces'.[82] One cannot help imagining that, when Head flinched in pain from the instruments that stung and burnt his flesh—'the pain was so excessively unpleasant that H. cried out and started away'—he awoke with a start from his reverie, suddenly alert to his surroundings.[83] The late nineteenth-century interest in attention did not only explore volitional states of concentration and focus, but also the role of the reflexes in suddenly bringing a threat or danger to attention. Flinching—from the shot of a pistol, the bite of a lizard, or a sudden darting movement in the corner of one's eye—was already associated with the involuntary sharpening of attention: as Darwin had put it in 1872, 'we naturally desire, when startled, to perceive the cause as quickly as possible; and we consequently open our eyes fully, so that the field of vision may be increased, and the eyeballs moved easily in any direction'.[84] Head's alert response to the cause of his surprise shattered his 'internal absorption',

[79] Rivers and Head, 'A Human Experiment', p. 353.
[80] Rivers and Head, 'A Human Experiment', p. 343.
[81] Letter from Henry Head to Ruth Mayhew, 11 December 1903, PP/HH/D4/15.
[82] Letter from Henry Head to Ruth Mayhew, 8 March 1904, PP/HH/D4/18/581.
[83] Rivers and Head, 'A Human Experiment', p. 390.
[84] Darwin, *The Expression*, p. 281.

almost certainly making it harder to resume. Occasional reminders of the outside world—a knock at the door, a noise outside, or a stranger entering the room—would distract Head. 'R.'s servant entered our workroom in the middle of an almost perfect series of answers', wrote Head, complaining that at once his reports 'became less accurate'.[85] As it was when he sat next to the whispering couple during *Macbeth*, the insistent murmur of the outside world brought Head from his 'quiet state of internal absorption' into an awareness of the outside world and his performance within it. In his accounts of the experiment, as in those of his theatre-going, Head moved in and out of states of absorption—in which he could forget he was both watched by Rivers, and indeed watching himself—to theatricality, a condition in which he became alert to his own responsibilities before the presence of an audience.

Sometimes Head became aware of having an audience of real people—Rivers, the servant, even himself: after all, like Darwin, Head was observing his own responses. But there were others who, by simply traipsing in and out of Head's imagination, further distracted him. On 27 November 1903, Head revealed to Mayhew that she too had trespassed onto his thoughts:

> No dearest, you did not guess the curious way in which you were with me as I sat with closed eyes on Sunday under the tests of J. Rivers, '*Vision qui derange et trouble l'horizon de ma raison*' [sic]. Now have you guessed? If not, I will tell you tomorrow when we are together.[86]

Through his allusion to the poetry of Paul Verlaine, famous both as a sensuous poet and lover of Arthur Rimbaud, Head's 'strange visions' hint at an erotic fantasy too racy to be committed to paper. Head's sexual fantasies 'derange and trouble the horizon' of his 'reason', intruding on his reverie and preventing him from paying attention to his sensations. Later in the same letter, the intimations of this erotic fantasy dissolve into a more conventionally expressed 'longing', but nonetheless, Head's daydreams about his fiancée made him 'neglectful of the stimuli that flashed into consciousness so preoccupied was I with the warmth of your dear presence'.[87] While his absorption in a novel left Head able to answer the tests

[85] Rivers and Head, 'A Human Experiment', p. 353.

[86] Letter from Henry Head to Ruth Mayhew, 27 November 1903, PP/HEA/D4/16/547. The original lines are: *étrange/Vision qui dérange/Et trouble l'horizon/De ma raison* (strange/visions which derange/and trouble the horizon/of my reasoning) from Paul Verlaine, 'A Clymène' in *Selected Poems, Paul Verlaine*, trans. C. F. MacIntyre (Berkeley and London: University of California Press, 1948) pp. 73–4.

[87] Letter from Henry Head to Ruth Mayhew, 27 November 1903.

more accurately, thinking of his fiancée during the experiment left him distracted and discombobulated.

According to Jacyna, Head's negative state of attention was symptomatic of a larger modernist sensibility, a 'recoil from the vulgarity and constraint of bourgeois norms' and his 'withdrawal into an inner world'. Indeed, Jacyna characterizes it as itself a kind of flinch, 'a retreat from the demands of the world into the inner life of Head's own sensations'.[88] But reading Head's introspections alongside his attempts at reverie in the theatre, and placing them in the context of a wider preoccupation with attentiveness at the *fin de siècle*, gives a rather more complex account of the psychologist's inward absorption. In this alternative reading, it becomes clear that for Head an enthralled 'interior absorption' was by no means a static condition, but a process that intensified and faded, oscillating between attention and reverie, between inside and outside, almost never quite able to fully inhabit either. Perhaps it is the photograph for which Rivers and Head posed in the Cambridge workroom, which brings these strange fluctuations between absorption and theatricality most starkly into view. Like Duse, in her performance of rapt concentration, Head adopted a pose of reverie in the *tableau*. Perfectly self-conscious, his eyes closed, his face tilted upwards, for this photograph, as for the experiment as a whole, Head was engaged in what Fried calls a 'fiction of aloneness'.[89] At the same time, Head may, whilst the photographer fussed around about the lighting and position, have slid into one of those listless comas of absent-mindedness which, as Crary reminds us, may happen when we concentrate for too long on any task. As Dorian Gray, whilst being painted, slips over into a reverie, so might have Head, whilst attempting to stay still before the camera, have found himself sliding in and out of rapturous, dreamy absorption and tense, embarrassed self-awareness: 'Mr Gray, come over and look at yourself', said Lord Henry admiring the finished painting: 'The lad started, as if awakened from some dream.'[90]

A PRIMORDIAL FLINCH

On the morning of 4 May 1903, nine days after the operation that severed the nerve of Head's hand, the two men noted an unexpected development. On the day following the operation, the area surrounding the wound had been fully analgesic—insensitive to pinpricks, wire 'hairs', hot and cold

[88] Jacyna, *Medicine and Modernism*, p. 4; p. 7; p. 125.
[89] Fried, 'Absorption and Theatricality', p. 109.
[90] Wilde, *The Picture of Dorian Gray*, p. 24.

test tubes and tickling with wisps of cotton wool. This insensate area was demarcated in black ink and photographed. However, nine days later, the two men discovered that a thin band of hypersensitive skin, approximately two millimetres wide, had developed around the numb area (Figure 14). At this strange no-man's land, Head's responses were extremely 'vivid', 'abnormally painful', and 'intensely disagreeable'. The 'prick of a pin', for example, produced pain 'far in excess of anything experienced on normal parts' and Head 'could not refrain' from flinching, 'from crying out and withdrawing his hand'. These disproportionately painful feelings appeared at a higher threshold than usual: on the area of Head's hand not affected by the experiment, a pinprick felt painful when the algesimeter measured a pressure of 25°, but in the border area, the force required was almost double, around 40°. Moreover, when a test tube of boiling water was applied to his hand, Head was unable to identify the point of contact, as the painful sensations radiated widely across Head's arm and hand. Similarly, when ice was applied to the hypersensitive band on the forearm, 'a sensation of coldness was produced in the thumb'.[91] With these violent and apparently disconnected sensations of pain, the neurologist's somatically responsive body became strange and unpredictable to him.

Head had studied the phenomenon of referred pain among his patients at the London Hospital, so the idea that painful sensations might wander across the body in cases of injury or disease was not unfamiliar. However, the emergence of a band of excessively sensitive skin during the recovery of his own severed nerve led Head and Rivers to reconsider the significance of these sensory peculiarities. They suggested that such excessive and non-specific pain responses were residues from earlier periods of human evolution which lingered in the nervous system. 'The conception of man as a created being has long passed away', proclaimed Head, a decade after his human experiment had ended, 'but the manner of regarding sensation, to which it gave rise, still dominates'. It might appear, he continued, that touch, pain, heat, and cold are each produced by a 'special set of end-organs' on the surface of the body, analogous to the ear for hearing and the eye for sight. Those who had studied the sensorium through 'anatomical or post-mortem examination' with its reliance on 'topographical details', came to view the nervous system as 'something stable', 'fixed and unalterable in its action'. Yet for Head, who experienced the nervous system in all its unpredictability, the body's proximal senses were not 'arranged on so simple a plan'.[92] Rather, over the course of the experiment Head and Rivers observed what they believed to be a palimpsestual

91 Rivers and Head, 'A Human Experiment', p. 368.
92 Head, *Studies in Neurology*, ii, p. 639.

nervous system, in which vestiges of earlier stages of animal development lingered between the lines of a later, and more highly evolved set of nervous mechanisms. After an accident or disease which damaged the more highly evolved system, this earlier network of feeling would erupt across the body's sensory landscape rendering its responses strange and unfamiliar. Just as Darwin's recoil from the puff adder at the London Zoological Gardens dramatized the accretion of emotional habits over millennia, so when Head cried out and withdrew his injured hand from a pin-prick, his flinch revealed a limb temporarily returned, in its earliest stages of recovery, to a primordial sensibility. Far from 'fixed and unalterable in its action', then, Head and Rivers proposed that the proximal sensorium was malleable and contingent, the relationship between the feeling body and the tactile world not eternal, but temporal, mediated by unreliable physiologies and vulnerable to illusion.

The band of hypersensitive skin soon spread outwards, and within ten weeks of the operation, covered the whole hand, producing 'extremes of pain and pleasure unknown in the normal state'.[93] It was only in the final year of the experiment that a finer, more graduated sensibility started returning to the hand, and even at the end of five years when the two men concluded the experiment, a small area between the knuckles of first and middle fingers remained in this earlier stage of recovery.[94] Head and Rivers concluded that there were two distinct systems at work, an older one they called 'protopathic' which was insensitive to fine or delicate stimuli, and a more recently evolved, higher 'epicritic' system, which could more easily discern between the subtle locations and strengths of stimuli. These entwined nervous systems, they argued, corresponded to two distinct areas of the brain. The more ancient optic thalamus, they linked to the 'affective aspects of sensation' and the newer cerebral cortex provided the 'discriminative and relational dimensions'. The idea of 'lower' and 'higher' sensory regimes proved an important and enduring one for Head, and he repeatedly emphasized their hierarchical arrangement. For Head, the epicritic system, organizing, inhibiting, and honing the impetuous impulses of the lower protopathic, was the history of humanity made flesh. For according to Head, 'the aim of human evolution is the domination of feeling and instinct by discriminative mental activities'.[95]

Head was certainly not alone in his belief that feeling and intellect were competing spheres, and that rational mental life contained and curtailed

[93] Head, *Studies in Neurology*, ii, p. 639.

[94] Head and Rivers, *A Human Experiment*, p. 382.

[95] Henry Head and Gordon Holmes, 'Sensory Disturbances From Cerebral Lesions', *Brain* (1911), 102–254 (pp. 190–1).

the dangerous impulses of primitive man. The idea of a doubled or split self, in which alongside the civilized man lurked a beast-like other, had been from the 1880s onwards a mainstay of popular fiction. In one of the most famous examples, Robert Louis Stevenson's *Strange Case of Dr Jekyll and Mr Hyde* (1888), the upright Scottish physician and scientific investigator Dr Jekyll discovers, through a self-experiment performed in his private laboratory, 'that man is not truly one, but truly two'. Realizing he is beset by a 'thorough and primitive duality', he sets about teasing apart the 'two natures that contended in the field of my consciousness'.[96] Famously, while Jekyll retains morality, self-control, and rationality (all qualities which might be associated with Head's term the 'epicritic'), his spiteful impulses, and self-serving egomaniacal drives are split off into Hyde. Repeatedly described as 'savage' and 'apelike', it is the cruel and murderous Hyde who is associated with bestial, lower impulses (the 'protopathic') belonging to an earlier evolutionary stage.[97] If Head's flinch from a pinprick during the experiment startled him, made his nerves tremble and brought him into a heightened, edgy self-awareness, his overpowering automatic response also reminded him that his body was nonetheless in thrall to ancient, hidden impulses.

Head's and Rivers's distinction between the epicritic and protopathic has since been discredited, regarded today as an 'unjustified and unsophisticated biological assumption, since it proposed a sort of animal which would seem to have very little chance of ordinary biological success'.[98] Yet its assumption, as historians of science including Jacyna, Roger Smith, and Jonathan Miller have emphasized, is historically significant for the way it inscribes nineteenth- and early twentieth-century ideas about hierarchy and emotion in the body. In his study of the term 'inhibition' in nineteenth-century medical discourse, Smith compares Head's two-tier system to wider anxieties about the 'latent power of disorder to break out unless restrained by the watchful eye of the ordering power', a rhetoric that staged dramatic battles between ordering and disordering principles, between 'spirit and flesh, head and hand, culture and nature, male and female, and the higher classes and the masses'. The evolution of an 'epicritic' system prevented humans from being merely mechanical creatures, mere flinchers. As Smith put it, 'if we responded constantly and inevitably to all impulses from peripheral end-organs, we should be automata, the victims

[96] Robert Louis Stevenson, *Strange Case of Dr. Jekyll and Mr. Hyde* (London: Longmans, 1886) p. 108.

[97] Stevenson, *Strange Case of Dr. Jekyll and Mr. Hyde*, p. 24; p. 138.

[98] Jonathan Miller, 'The Dog Beneath the Skin', *The Listener* (20 July 1972), pp. 74–6, PP/HEA/d4a5, p. 76.

of indiscriminate relations'.[99] Turning to the emergence of psychoanalysis in the early decades of the twentieth century, Miller sees in Head's distinction between an epicritic and protopathic sensibility a reflection of the psychoanalytic topography of repression and control, and the language of ego, id, and superego. Miller interpolates the relationship between epicritic and protopathic as a battle between dynamic, irrepressible, 'jack-in-the-box' emotions and a secretly active inhibitory function, whose aim is to 'sit on and suppress'. The level of 'concealed inhibition', writes Miller, keeps down the 'dynamic, springy, antique version of the animal which is concealed under this evolutionary heap of subsequent development', the epicritic suppressing an 'older protopathic animal that was crouched like a monster, like a dog beneath the skin'. Like Smith, Miller points out that the idea of a protopathic and epicritic nervous system resonated, in the long shadow of the French Revolution, with fears about 'the incoherent, violent, ungraduated energies of the mob', for whom 'mimesis and kinds of copying is very significant'.[100] According to Jacyna, Head's distinction was deeply embedded in the colonialist discourse of the early years of the twentieth century of 'the triumph of civilization over savagery in human history'. In Jacyna's reading, epicritic modes of feeling are aligned to the emotional self-mastery ascribed to European explorers and missionaries, and the protopathic to the brute or animalistic feelings ascribed to the 'primitive cultures' they sought to civilize. Thus, writes Jacyna, Head believed he had 'identified the physiological basis of the dichotomies in human nature between the emotional and the rational, the corporeal and the intellectual, and the civilized and the savage'.[101]

Head and Rivers quickly marshalled further evidence to support their belief that a dynamic battle between refined control and brute emotions raged at the heart of the nervous system. The two men turned to other body parts they believed might betray 'protopathic' characteristics. In spite of his poetically erotic daydreams, it probably comes as no surprise to discover that Head believed his penis to be the least evolved part of his body. Gamely, the two men embarked on a new series of tests. The *glans penis* responded to cutaneous stimuli with 'remarkable peculiarities', the published article reports. While entirely insensitive to cotton wool, prodding with wire hairs produced 'a characteristic diffuse boring or stinging pain much more unpleasant than over the skin of the penis or foreskin'. When tested with the algesimeter, Head was conscious straightaway of the needle, but no painful sensation was produced until 20°, at which point

[99] Roger Smith, *Inhibition* (London: Free Association Books, 1992) p. 2; p. 173.
[100] Miller, 'The Dog Beneath The Skin', p. 76.
[101] Jacyna, *Medicine and Modernism*, p. 131.

it was 'excessively unpleasant' and Head 'cried out and started' at a pain that radiated widely and seemed to be situated in the urethra as well as in the glans. An uninterrupted electric current placed on the glans caused an 'aching, tingling sensation' which was 'extremely unpleasant'. Tests were also done to assess the responsiveness to heat and cold. For these, a series of drinking glasses were filled with water at a range of temperatures. 'H. stood with his eyes closed, and R. gradually approached with one of the glasses until the surface of the water covered the glans but did not touch the foreskin'. From 0°–21° the sensation of cold 'seemed "colder" than over the skin of the penis'; between 21°–26° Head 'did not recognize that he had been stimulated'; at 38° he complained of a 'slight ache'; at 43° it was 'extremely painful'; and at 45°, a curious phenomenon they termed 'paradox cold' emerged (as it had also on the hand), where an extremely hot stimulus was experienced as extremely cold.[102] The men concluded from these tests that the *glans penis* was the only organ that in its ordinary state was endowed exclusively with a protopathic sensibility.

While Head linked the pleasurable excesses of sex to the more primitive protopathic sensorium, he also, and perhaps more surprisingly, identified the re-emergence of older indiscriminate sensory experience with certain aspects of creativity. Indeed, though Jacyna thinks of Head primarily as a man of epicritic sensibility, able to finely pinpoint the delicate and fleeting changes in his own sensations, Head also wrote about the aesthetic possibilities of protopathic sensibility with great excitement. One month into the self-experiment, while his hand was almost entirely in a protopathic state, Mayhew visited Head in London. Later he wrote to her, effusively reporting that his left arm 'tingled' when she walked into any room he was in. In the same letter, he also confided that his arm felt warm and started tingling during spells of creativity whilst writing poetry, and in particular at moments when the neurologist experienced total and almost transcendent absorption in his creative task: 'During the period on Saturday morning when I knew both by my internal feelings and by the fact that the lines were coming rapidly that my mood was lyrical, the left arm glowed and tingled.' One might almost compare his arm here to a vibrating divining rod, a physiological index of Head's lyrical mood. It seemed that under certain heightened conditions, the part of his body still in a protopathic condition resonated in sympathy with his emotions. A decade later, the connection between damaged nerves and an increased artistic sensitivity continued to intrigue Head. During the First World War, Head treated a sergeant for an injury. The patient suffered extensive nerve damage on

[102] Rivers and Head, 'A Human Experiment', pp. 389–90.

the right-hand side of his body, which had left it extremely responsive to both pleasurable and painful stimulation. Head noted that the patient's entire right-hand side was in the protopathic stage of recovery, and quoted the following testimony of the patient as evidence: Since the attack, the patient claimed he had become 'more amorous'; 'I crave to place my right hand on the soft skin of a woman. It's my right hand that wants the consolation. I seem to crave for sympathy on my right side.' The sergeant concluded with the observation: 'My right hand seems to be more artistic.'[103]

In contrast to the emotionality of the protopathic, Head linked epicritic feelings to rationality. While his protopathic arm tingled when Head was in a lyrical mood, when re-reading and editing his poems Head noticed that 'the pleasure it has given me to see the finished lines on paper leaves my arm quiet' and is 'obviously only intellectual'.[104] Like the trance-like absorption he experienced whilst reading alone in the beer garden in Prague, or whilst watching Eleanora Duse in the theatre, for Head the protopathic state was rare and sought-after. The epicritic, however, was all too familiar. A month after the 'tingling arm' incident, Head wrote another letter to Mayhew. In it, he described a frustrating outing to the theatre with his mother, with whom it seems, the psychologist had a complicated relationship. In the foyer, while the pair were waiting to take their seats, Head found himself compelled—he knew not why—to subject his mother to a forensic cross-examination. He describes his thirst for 'cold-blooded scientific truth', his eagerness to unpick his mother's own fanciful allegations towards his father. Such behaviour is his 'nemesis', he writes, despairingly. 'I develop a vile genius for dissecting her and her marriage', he reports. His language recalls the cruelties of the vivisector Dr Moreau—Head describes his delight on seeing the 'paralysed struggles' with which his mother received his incisive observations. For his next guilt-ridden metaphor, Head moves from monstrous vivisector to laboratory measuring device. 'She has only talked to a horrible recording machine', he admits, 'that registered and classified her as a psychological phenomenon'.[105] The letter, though it almost certainly betrays some of the struggles of Head's double life as poet and scientific psychologist, also reminds us that for Head, the intellectual and rational were not always straightforwardly superior.

While theatrical techniques played an important role in Head's scientific method, problems long associated with theatre audiences also shaped Head's interpretation of his results. For Head, one of the distinctive aspects of protopathic sensitivity was the way sensations and emotions wandered

[103] Head and Holmes, 'Sensory Disturbances From Cerebral Lesions', p. 136.
[104] Letter of Henry Head to Ruth Mayhew, 24 May 1903, CMAC, PP/HEA/D4/13.
[105] Letter from Henry Head to Ruth Mayhew, 24 June 1903, PP/HEA/d4/14/505.

across disparate body parts, even reaching out beyond the boundaries of an individual's skin to mingle with others. And though Head's hierarchical distinctions between protopathic and epicritic gave scientific succour to already entrenched ideas about race and class, they also reflected what by the first decade of the twentieth century was a rapidly expanding scientific interest in the question of empathy. Throughout the eighteenth and much of the nineteenth century, the language of sympathy articulated the strange capacity for bodies to resonate with one another and flinches were often prime examples of an innate fellow feeling or shared response. As Adam Smith put it in the *Theory of Moral Sentiments*, 'we naturally shrink and draw back our own leg' when we witness another about to be injured, 'and are hurt by it as well as the sufferer'.[106] For William Godwin, writing in 1853, the people 'in whom my sensations are by a kind of necessity echoed and repeated', who feel the pain from which he recoiled, were 'part of myself'.[107]

By the end of the nineteenth century, the discourse around sympathetic or shared visceral responses was beginning to shift. As Carolyn Burdett and Susan Lanzoni have both described, in the first decade of the twentieth century the older moral discourse of sympathy was reimagined in the light of new scientific psychological research in the field of aesthetics.[108] In 1909, the psychologist Edward Titchener coined a new word to describe this scientific account of fellow feeling—empathy, a translation of the German word *Einfühlung*. Empathy described 'feeling oneself into' something, and prioritized reflex and unconscious bodily movements over willed moral intention. As T. H. Huxley had put it in 1894, it is 'by purely reflex operation of the mind' that we 'take the hue of passion of those who are about us, or, it may be, the complementary colour'. Such involuntary responses called into question the moral dimension of sympathetic suffering, thus according to Huxley, Smith's idea that we 'put oneself in the place' of another gave excessive importance to deliberate substitutions, and placed too little emphasis on the unwilled, unexpected, and 'primitive' aspects. 'It is not by any conscious "putting one's self in the place" of a joyful or a suffering person that the state of mind we call sympathy usually

[106] Smith, *The Theory of Moral Sentiments*, p. 4. As David Marshall has described, Smith's theory of morality is deeply implicated in the imagery of the theatrical encounter: David Marshall, *The Figure of Theatre. Shaftesbury, Defoe, Adam Smith and George Eliot* (New York: Columbia University Press, 1986), p. 172.

[107] William Godwin, *Fleetwood, or, the New Man of Feeling* (1805) (London: Bentley, 1853), p. 179.

[108] Carolyn Burdett, 'Is Empathy the End of Sentimentality?' *Journal of Victorian Culture*, 16, 2 (2011) 259–74 and 'The subjective inside us can turn into the objective outside' pp.13–20; Lanzoni, 'Practising Psychology in the Art Gallery'.

arises; indeed it is often contrary to one's sense of right, and in spite of one's will, that "fellow feeling makes us wondrous kind", or the reverse,' he wrote.[109] Head continued to use the word 'sympathy' rather than empathy, but his example of the arm involuntarily tingling when Mayhew entered a room, or the sergeant's right side impelled to seek consolation, are part of this period's wider shift towards finding the physiological basis for fellow feeling. For Head, vicarious feeling resided in the protopathic nervous system, which, in times of injury, worked to unpick the boundaries between self and other. The damaged skin was no longer, to quote Steven Connor, thought of 'in the fixated terms of surface, boundary, or container', but as the delicate 'mingling' of that which 'touches almost without touching'. Even when no physical contact occurred, the skin tingled as though fingers had reached out across the empty space to stroke it.[110]

Throughout the nineteenth century, theatre audiences repeatedly served as an important example for the dangers of this kind of emotional contagion, and as the final chapter of this book will explore, the risks posed by such groups of individuals were increasingly of interest to psychologists in the early decades of the next. In the 1890s, Gustave le Bon in France and Gabriel Tarde in Italy became the most vociferous proponents of what was fast becoming known as crowd psychology. Their interest turned on the transmission of feelings through groups, and in their writing they revived, and attempted to give scientific explanation for, anxieties that had been freely circulating for much of the nineteenth century. As the previous chapter described, worries about the dangerous contagions of lust, fear, and horror between spectators had erupted in the midst of the debates on anti-vivisection. Frances Power Cobbe, for example, invoked the terrifying spectre of meek audience members turned unwittingly into bloodthirsty monsters when they stumbled into the throng.[111] Le Bon and Tarde built on these ideas, arguing that when an individual joined mobs, crowds, or groups they became regressed, returned to a primitive condition of emotional susceptibility, in turn becoming a homogenous unit. 'Crowds are not intelligent', wrote le Bon, but rather, 'the sentiments and ideas of all the persons in the gathering take one and the same direction, and their conscious personality vanishes'.[112]

[109] T. H. Huxley, *Prolegomena, Evolution and Ethics* (1894) (Princeton, NJ: Princeton University Press, 1989) p. 86.

[110] Steven Connor, *The Book of Skin* (London: Reaktion Books, 2004) p. 282.

[111] Cobbe, 'The Education of the Emotions', p. 238.

[112] Gustave le Bon, 'The Mind of Crowds', in *The Crowd: A Study of the Popular Mind* (London: T. Fisher Unwin, 1896), repr. in *The Fin de Siècle: A Reader in Cultural History, c.1880–1900*, ed. Sally Ledger and Roger Luckhurst (Oxford: Oxford University Press, 2000) pp. 54–6 (p. 54).

Head's description of a physiological protopathic system reflected this wider surge of interest in the regressive, wandering, and merging of affects, as it was explored in the contexts of both psychology and theatre. For le Bon, one of the clearest examples of this regressive loss of autonomy in the group mind was the theatre audience. 'Nothing has a greater effect on the imagination of crowds of every category than theatrical representations', he wrote, and in the auditorium 'the entire audience experiences at the same time the same emotions'. He went on to report the story of a theatre manager who was obliged every night to stand at the stage door in order to protect one of the actors (who habitually played villains) 'against the violence of the spectators, indignant at the crimes, imaginary though they were, which the traitor had committed'.[113] While Walkley emphasized the diversity of the theatrical crowd, and complained at how very hard it was to absorb the audience in the drama, le Bon offered a rather different picture. It was not only certain types—the innocent country girl, the knight, the uneducated sailors—whose conscious minds could be derailed by theatre's fiction. It was not simply, as Head and Rivers observed, that among the injured sensations were liable to wander freely between bodies. Anyone stumbling into a crowd might become susceptible to the feelings ebbing and flowing through it. The idea of a 'group mind' even appealed to Walkley, who suggested in his later work on audiences that 'the collective mind, the mind of the crowd approximates rather to the mind of primitive man'.[114] If Head and Rivers observed that among the injured, sensations were liable to wander freely between bodies, so on entering the theatre auditorium, a similar regressive breakdown of the spectator's individual boundaries was seen to occur.

THE 'HUMAN EXPERIMENT' AND ITS HEIRS

Head and Rivers's 'human experiment' eventually drew to a close when the two men ascertained that the recovery process had reached its end. Epicritic sensation had returned to the hand, except for one small part that for the rest of Head's life remained in a protopathic state, a reminder of the lengths he had gone to uncover the secrets of the human sensorium. Two years after Head concluded his experiment, two British psychologists Wilfred Trotter and H. Morriston Davies embarked on an attempt to replicate his results. Like Head, they chose the route of self-experimentation, but criticized his use of only a solitary subject, and a single area of sensory

[113] le Bon, 'The Mind of Crowds', p. 55.
[114] Walkley, *Dramatic Criticism*, p. 27; p. 26.

loss. Instead, the two men underwent seven operations between them, dividing cutaneous nerves in the knee, sternum, arm, and thigh in an attempt to gather a greater spread from which to draw their results. Trotter and Morriston Davies confirmed Head and Rivers's observations, but they did call into question the earlier experimenters' conclusion that two distinct mechanisms, the epicritic and protopathic, were at work in the nervous system. Moreover, though like Head they did insist that the success of the experiment depended on a 'trained observer as subject', one capable of 'exceptionally delicate introspective analysis', they made no mention of his eccentric-sounding 'negative attitude of attention' as a reliable technique.[115]

By the 1920s, introspection was beginning to falter as an accepted psychological practice. This gradual loss of confidence can even be detected in Trotter and Morriston Davies's accounts of their experiments, which though supported the idea of introspection in principle, acknowledged it would inevitably be subjective: 'It is clear', they wrote, 'that in the investigation of the problem of sensation by any method whatsoever, the value of the observations is never free from the serious qualification that no objective measure or record of a sensation can be made'.[116] The American psychologist and former student of Titchener, Edwin G. Boring also went on to replicate Head's experiment as one of the requirements for his doctorate. In 1912, Boring divided one of the cutaneous nerves on his forearm and traced the return of sensitivity over the following four years, but emerged with results that differed from both English experiments, and, like Trotter and Morriston Davies, skirted around the issue of the 'negative attitude of attention'.[117] Later, Boring reflected that 1920, the year Wundt died, marked the end of scientific psychology's use of introspective methods. Nonetheless, he was quick to point out self-reporting practices continued to be part of life in the experimental laboratory 'under various aliases', for example, in the verbal report, and in psychoanalysis.[118] In 1920, when Head collected his articles on sensation together in two large volumes, he admitted that the method of his experiment had fallen out of favour, but was moved to defend introspection as a trustworthy practice which could yield 'measurable results'.[119] After such an

[115] Trotter and Davies, 'Experimental Studies in the Innervation of the Skin', p. 136; p. 138; p. 96.

[116] Trotter and Davies, 'Experimental Studies in the Innervation of the Skin', p. 143.

[117] Edwin G. Boring, 'Cutaneous Sensation after Nerve-Division', *Quarterly Journal of Experimental Physiology*, 10 (1916), 1–95.

[118] E. G. Boring, 'A History of Introspection', *Psychological Bulletin*, 50, 3 (1953), 169–89 (p. 167).

[119] Head, *Studies in Neurology*, i, p. 12.

arduous and painful five years, it must have been trying, to say the least, to find his experiment dismissed. All the same, by the time he died aged 78 of Parkinson's disease, Head had received four nominations for the Nobel Prize for physiology, had been granted a knighthood, and had remained highly influential both as the editor of *Brain* and as an experimenter and lecturer.

In the history of the emergence of psychology as a scientific discipline at the end of the nineteenth century, Head's trance-like reveries might appear at first glance like a quaint historical anomaly, a bump in the road to the cultivation of scientific objectivity. In fact, Head's introspection was firmly embedded in an already established repertoire of experimental techniques. For almost fifty years, introspection was one of the local practices through which scientific objectivity in psychological investigation was constituted. This episode reminds us of the historical contingency of the ideal scientific gaze, that objectivity itself was not a stable idea but one constantly under formation. Moreover, the connections running back and forth between Head's introspective strategies and the techniques and problems of late nineteenth- and early twentieth-century theatre audiences also underline the fact that these mutating patterns of scientific objectivity were themselves deeply implicated in wider cultural practices of looking. As this book has so far explored, the models of scientific observation and passionate, theatrical spectatorship were deeply enmeshed, yet though they echoed and repeated one another, their proximity was often disavowed by the men of science themselves. Though it may be surprising to find theatricality creeping into the heart of Darwin and Ferrier's experiments on emotions and reflex responses, in Head's study of the sensorium, theatre seems perhaps even more out of place. After all, Head's 'negative attitude of attention' emphasized privacy and inwardness, and required a disavowal of staged face-to-face experimental encounters. It was a strategy premised on the possibility of forgetting one's self-consciousness as a scientific performer-observer, in order to commune directly with inner sensory experience.

Nonetheless, Head's experiment collides with early twentieth-century theatre precisely at the point of this attempted retreat from sociality. If Head's introspection sought to banish problematic self-consciousness, so in the playhouse the theatricality of live, face-to-face encounters was being deliberately forgotten too. While Eleanora Duse pretended she was not watched by an audience, and cringed from the applause at the curtain call, spectators attempted to ignore the fellowship of the auditorium in order to enjoy a private and transcendental communion with the performer on stage. Moreover, this emphasis on individual reverie was not confined to the auditorium, but appeared in descriptions of sensory experience in the work of novelists, poets, and critics too. It is striking, however, that in both Head's experiment and his accounts of theatre-going, such a retreat from self-consciousness was, in practice, almost impossible to sustain. Exploring his flinches may help us find new connections between the worlds of scientific endeavour and theatrical pleasure, but the neurologist's winces and recoils also point up moments in which his much-desired reverie floundered, marking the transitions between private inwardness, and outward-facing performance. Head's 'negative attitude of attention' failed with each flinch from a sudden stab of pain, or surprised start and when the servant entered the room, his body's involuntary responses bringing Head to attention. With each start or cringe, he became newly consciousness of his role, discovering, once again, that he was being observed and observing himself too. Rather than sustaining reverie, then, Head's experience was one of wavering between reverie and theatricality, between a listless, forgetful absorption and the stark awareness of playing his part.

At the same time, Head's flinches draw attention to a larger transition occurring in the fortunes of the perceiving body at the beginning of the twentieth century. From the predictable and uniform portrait of reflex responses drawn by Marshall Hall, within a century the human sensorium had become something unreliable and susceptible to illusion. When Head drew his hand away from the prick of a needle, or recoiled because extremely cold water on his finger seemed to burn his elbow, his flinches testified to the enduring presence of older evolutionary nervous system at work. Extending Darwin's understanding of flinching as part of an evolved, and evolving, repertoire of an emotional expressions, and Ferrier's description of the body as mechanistically performing involuntary responses of surprise and fear, Head's investigations into pain dramatized a radically unstable sensory body. Through his work, it became clear that between external physiological stimuli and sensory experience lay a complex chain of transformations. In the connections running between skin, spinal cord, and brain, many distortions might occur, leaving the sensory body susceptible to manipulation and capable of misperception. As the next chapter will explore, this newly malleable relationship between the sensory body and the world it perceived came under greater scrutiny amid the horrors of the First World War, when physicians attempted to understand, and treat, the seemingly inexplicable epidemic of shell shock.

4

A Convalescent Recoils

In the Autumn of 2008, I found myself in a secluded corner of the Wellcome Library for the History of Medicine, London, before me a small TV monitor, wired up to a VHS player, loaded with an unmarked video cassette. I pressed 'play' and the screen wobbled into life, flecked with silver. White letters appeared:

> War Neuroses
> Netley, 1917
> Seale Hayne 1918[1]

The title card trembled for several long seconds, before a second card appeared:

> Pte. MEEK, aged 23 Feb. 1917, complete retrograde amnesia, hysterical paralysis, contractures mutism and universal anaesthesia dating from Feb. 1916 (00:18)

Next, a sequence taken in a single shot with a static camera. It shows a man, presumably Pte. Meek, dressed in flapping hospital blues and sitting in a wheelchair before an imposing neoclassical stone building. His upper body is wrapped snake-like around itself, his legs stiff and extended (Figure 16). A brisk nurse in a white apron waves a doll in the air, as if trying to gain the attention of a small child. Meek recoils from her in spasms and jerks. The following sequence shows Meek receiving physical manipulations. The card reads:

> He is completely unaware of the vigorous efforts to overcome the rigidity of his ankles (00:42)

[1] Arthur Hurst and J. L. M. Symns, *War Neuroses*, Netley Hospital 1917, Seale Hayne 1918, Wellcome Moving Image and Sound Collections, 2042F. There are four surviving versions of *War Neuroses*, kept at the Wellcome Library, The Imperial War Museum, Pathé Archives, and the British Film Institute. The version referred to here is the one held by the Wellcome Library which can be viewed online at <http://catalogue.wellcome.ac.uk/record=b1667864~S8%29>. Hereafter all references to *War Neuroses* will be to this version, and will be identified in seconds in parenthesis in the text.

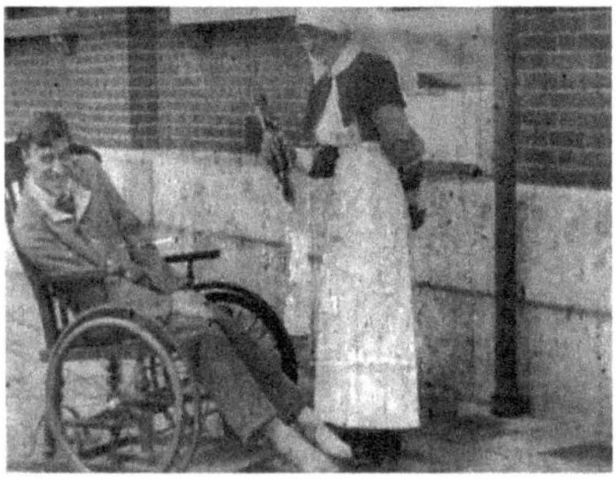

Fig. 16. Pte. Meek (00:18), Arthur Hurst and J. L. M. Symns, *War Neuroses*, Netley Hospital 1917, Seale Hayne 1918.

Wellcome Library, London

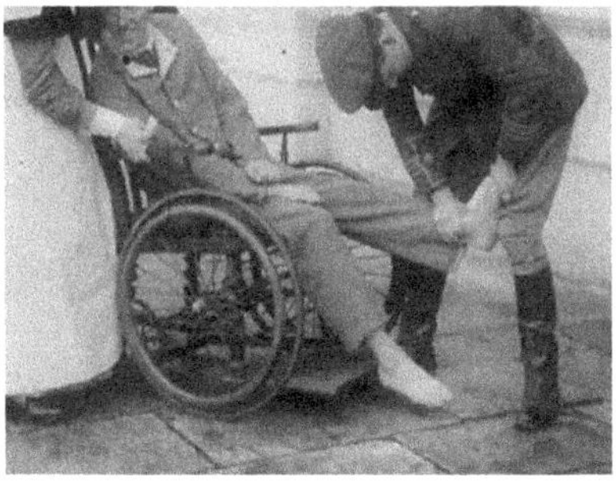

Fig. 17. Pte. Meek receiving treatment (00:42), Arthur Hurst and J. L. M. Symns, *War Neuroses*, Netley Hospital 1917, Seale Hayne 1918.

Wellcome Library, London

A military doctor grasps each of Meek's ankles in turn, strenuously twisting and pulling at them, as if trying to release an object stuck under layers of ancient accumulated dirt. The legs, however, remain stiff and unyielding (Figure 17). The third title card announces that the invalid has undergone an astonishing transformation:

> Sudden recovery of memory Nov. 1917, with gradual recovery of body functions. June, 1918 teaching basket-making—his peacetime job (01:18)

Apparently shot almost a year and a half later, the footage depicts Meek walking, albeit stiffly, across a farmyard towards five men wearing military uniforms who sit around a table weaving wicker baskets. With a quick sideways glance towards the camera, as if seeking encouragement or direction from whoever stands behind it, Meek picks up a half-finished basket and tugs at its handle to test its construction (Figure 18). In Meek's next and final scene, the soldier appears before a stone building wearing a suit.

September, 1918 Complete recovery—2½ years after onset (01:55)

Meek runs swiftly down the flight of steps. When he gets to the bottom, he re-adjusts his position to face the camera, as he had no doubt been directed to do. He then rotates his arms in large circles above his head, before running back up the stairs, a choreographed sequence demonstrating the invalid's fitness to return to military service (Figure 19).

The film *War Neuroses* was made over two years, 1917 and 1918, at the Netley (Hampshire) and Seale Hayne (Devon) Military Hospitals by the physician Arthur Hurst (1879–1944) and with the assistance of a second doctor J. L. M. Symns (dates unknown). Shot by the commercial

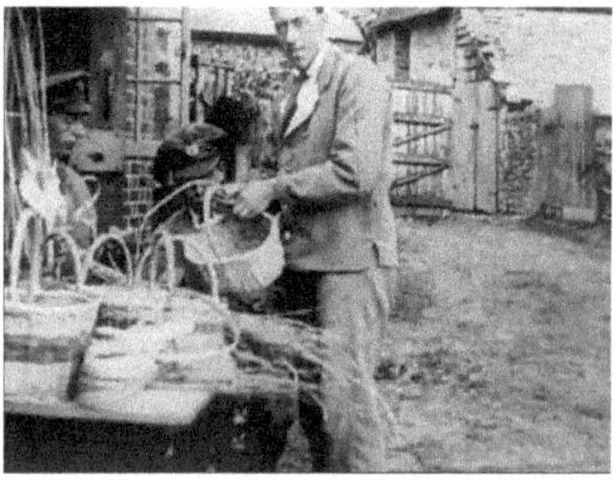

Fig. 18. Pte. Meek teaching basket weaving (01:18), Arthur Hurst and J. L. M. Symns, *War Neuroses*, Netley Hospital 1917, Seale Hayne 1918.

Wellcome Library, London

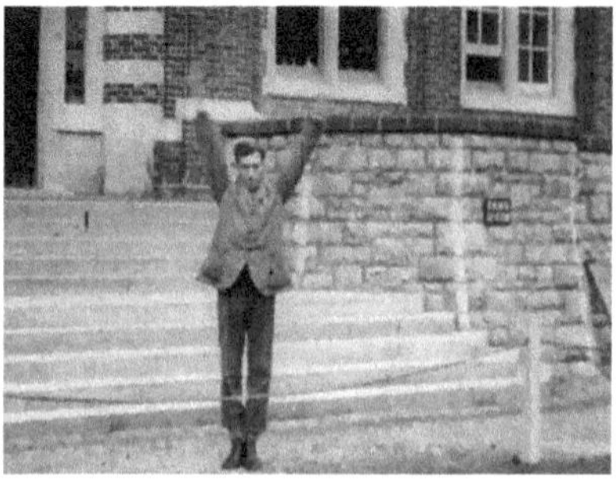

Fig. 19. Pte. Meek demonstrating his fitness (01:55), Arthur Hurst and J. L. M. Symns, *War Neuroses*, Netley Hospital 1917, Seale Hayne 1918.

Wellcome Library, London

film company, the *Pathé Frères*, and commissioned by the Royal Army Medical Corps and the Medical Research Committee, which had been set up in 1913 to fund research into public health, the black and white silent film demonstrates the experimental therapies pioneered by Hurst to treat soldiers suffering what was, by this time, widely referred to as 'shell shock'. Eighteen minutes long, the film documents the symptoms and 'rapid recoveries' of twenty-one patients, of whom Meek appears first. Pte. Preston, aged nineteen, has been diagnosed with 'amnesia, word blindness, and word deafness', except to the word 'bombs', so that on hearing this trigger, Preston dives for cover under the hospital bed (02:32) (Figure 19). Thirty-five years old, Pte. Ross Smith exhibits a 'facial spasm' with rapid eye movements and a twitching ear (02:52). Pte. Read, who was buried by a shell on 2 August 1917, demonstrates a fitful, fidgety, 'hysterical gait', swaying from side to side as he attempts to traverse Netley's walkway, obsessively wiping some imagined stain from his nose (04:33). Pte. Sandall is jittery and restless, unable to stand or talk without hopping from one foot to the other, all the while flapping his hands at his sides (08:22). Among the numerous symptoms Hurst treated at Netley were exaggerations of 'the flinch-reflex'. 'The patient jumps violently and

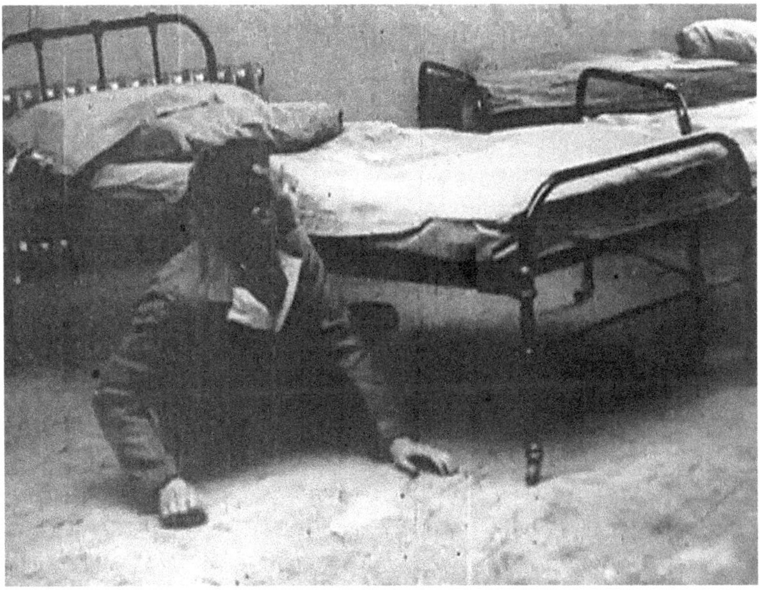

Fig. 20. Pte. Preston (02:32) Arthur Hurst and J. L. M. Symns, *War Neuroses*, Netley Hospital 1917, Seale Hayne 1918.

Wellcome Library, London

trembles from head to foot at the slightest sound', wrote Hurst describing one of the most characteristic signs of shell shock. 'He raises his arm as if to protect his face from a blow.' These men had no obvious physical injury, rather their symptoms were regarded by the physicians who filmed them to be 'hysterical' in origin, the result of 'auto' or 'hetero-suggestion' under conditions of extreme and relentless strain.[2]

After their symptoms had been recorded, Hurst set to work treating his patients with a method he called 'simple persuasion and re-education'.[3] It seemed to be an astonishingly successful technique. Within a few months, weeks, days, and in some cases, mere hours, of treatment, the hysterical symptoms had remarkably disappeared, and the men's renewed capacity for callisthenics, field-ploughing, and chicken-feeding recorded for perpetuity on celluloid. However, Hurst's claims to have discovered the key to ensuring soldier's 'rapid recovery' from shell shock ultimately proved unwarranted. As the Southborough Committee, which reported on medical and military responses to shell shock at the end of the war, noted, as soon as the soldiers were discharged 'they began to decline' and had 'usually developed new symptoms by the time the train away from Seale Hayne arrived in Salisbury'.[4] Despite the ultimate failure of his treatment, Hurst's film offers an important insight into a distinctive early twentieth-century therapeutic approach. One of the significant characteristics of Hurst's method was his liberal and unabashed use of a range of theatrical practices, and in particular his deliberate choreographing of both patients and medical staff as emotional and self-conscious audiences. While the experiments discussed so far in this book involved one or two observers and their subjects at most, this final chapter investigates the relationship between theatrical and scientific looking in a large experiment with many participants. Unexpectedly, it was through the deployment of a new film technology at Netley—a technology that would come to replace theatre as the mainstay of popular entertainment—that the persistence of theatrical techniques and problems in the *folie à plusieurs* of Hurst's treatment came to the fore.

Part medical documentary, part propaganda, part exercise in self-aggrandizement, *War Neuroses* has provided the history of shell shock

[2] Arthur Hurst, *Medical Diseases of the War*, 2nd edn. (London: Edward Arnold, 1918) p. 42; p. 21.

[3] A. F. Hurst and J. L. M. Symns, 'The Rapid Cure of Hysterical Symptoms in Soldiers', *The Lancet*, 192 (1918), 139–41 (p. 140).

[4] HM Stationery Office (HMSO), *Report of the War Office Committee of Enquiry Into 'Shell-Shock'* (London: HMSO, 1922) p. 80.

with some of its most memorable iconography. One of the most frequently requested films in the Wellcome Library's archives, it is also still shown to medical students as part of their study of post-traumatic stress disorder. Yet the conditions of the film's production, and the part the film-making played in the therapy it celebrated, has received surprisingly little scholarly attention. *War Neuroses* is not only a (sometimes unreliable) record of the symptoms of shell shock. For Hurst, the film also played a vital therapeutic role, because it facilitated a set of peculiarly theatrical relationships between recovering performers and suffering spectators that sustained an 'atmosphere of cure'. If Hurst emphasized the inherent theatricality of war neuroses—he believed it to be the result of a regressed compulsion to imitate—he also argued that theatre was central to the patient's recovery. At Netley, medical staff and patients took turns in acting and watching. Hurst staged sham operations and orchestrated battle recreations. An 'atmosphere of cure' was created through the self-consciously upbeat performances of medical staff and patients. While some convalescents displayed their symptoms and recoveries, others became passionately performing audience members whose susceptibility to imitation made a similarly miraculous recuperation possible. It was through the creation of *War Neuroses* that all these techniques came together and were recorded for posterity. It is for this reason that watching *War Neuroses* at the beginning of the twenty-first century is a peculiarly uncomfortable task. Encountering the hundred-year-old footage in the Wellcome Library, surrounded by the trappings of professional scholarship, I found myself sinking deeper into my chair, turning aside from the shuddering invalids on the screen. Unable to bear to watch, unable quite to tear myself away, I cringed in a horrified, embarrassed silence. Perhaps most of all I was ashamed. Simply by watching, I had become folded into Hurst's grand theatrical project: by giving my audience I had become complicit. I tried to turn aside, but like Leontius I was drawn towards the ghosts of the past, my own act of spectatorship leaving me feeling exposed.

THEATRE IN THE ASYLUM

As early as September 1914, when Britain had been at war for only a month, soldiers displaying a collection of bizarre and inexplicable symptoms began returning to Britain.[5] Some men were paralysed, others trembled, spasmed, jerked, and twitched, some were rendered mute, others unaccountably deaf. Some were found wandering far from the trenches

[5] Anthony Babington, *Shell Shock: A History of the Changing Attitudes to War* (London: Cooper, 1997) p. 43.

having lost all memory of their circumstances, others experienced nightmares, from which they woke in cold sweats, or daydreams in which horrors they had witnessed were endlessly replayed. Excessive jumpiness and unwarranted flinches were common: 'the patient is abnormally sensitive to sound', wrote Hurst, and 'sudden noises often frighten him' reminding him 'of the bursting of shells'. He flinches 'whenever anybody, even the patient's friends and relations, comes near' and 'hides his head under the bedclothes when anybody approaches him'.[6] In the early months of the war, many of these men, with their 'stammering, disconnected talk' were executed for malingering and cowardice.[7] However, by early 1915, physicians in the Royal Army Medical Corps, whose specialisms ranged from psychology and neurology to ophthalmology and surgery, argued that such erratic conduct might be symptomatic of a nervous illness, not the result of a 'demonstrable organic lesion', but of a 'wound of consciousness'.[8] How to treat this mass-outbreak of hysterical symptoms, however, was a challenge for which the Medical Corps, as the many historians of shell shock have documented, were profoundly unprepared.[9]

Arthur Hurst, who at the outbreak of war had changed his name from the Germanic Hertz, is overlooked by many charting the British response to shell shock, most probably because his methods were ultimately dismissed by his contemporaries.[10] Born in Yorkshire on 23 July 1879 and educated in grammar schools in Bradford and then in Manchester, Hurst graduated from Magdalen College, Oxford in Natural Sciences in 1901, before continuing his medical studies at Guy's Hospital. In 1907, he was

[6] Hurst, *Medical Diseases of the War*, p. 43.

[7] Siegfried Sassoon, 'Survivors' in *Collected Poems, 1908–1956* (London: Faber and Faber, 1984) p. 90. Originally published in *Counter-Attack and Other Poems* (London: Heinemann, 1918); Babington, *Shell Shock*, p. 101.

[8] J. H. Parsons, 'The Psychology of Traumatic Amblyopia Following Explosions of Shells', *Proceedings of the Royal Society of Medicine (Neurological Section)* 8, 2 (1915), 55–65. Quoted in Tracey Loughran, 'Shell Shock and Psychological Medicine in First World War Britain', *Social History of Medicine*, 22, 1 (2009) 79–95 (p. 84).

[9] For accounts of the British response to shell-shock see: Babington, *Shell-Shock*; Joanna Bourke, *Dismembering the Male: Men's Bodies, Britain and the Great War* (London: Reaktion Books, 1996); Peter Leese, *Shell Shock: Traumatic Neurosis and the British Soldiers of the First World War* (New York: Palgrave, 2002); Ben Shephard, *A War of Nerves: Soldiers and Psychiatrists 1914–1994* (London: Jonathan Cape, 2000); Elaine Showalter, *The Female Malady*; M. Stone 'Shell-Shock and the Psychologists', in *The Anatomy of Madness: Essays in the History of Psychiatry, i: People and Ideas*, ed. W. Bynum, R. Porter, and M. Shepherd (London and New York: Tavistock, 1985) pp. 242–71.

[10] Hurst, who was knighted in 1937, was well regarded for his work in the fields of gastroenterology. However, as his obituarist noted of his contributions during the war, he was unable to see the 'limitations' of persuasion, and treatment of war neurosis was 'one of the few directions in which he broke no new ground'. Anon., 'Obituary, Sir Arthur Hurst', *British Medical Journal* (26 August 1944), 292–3 (p. 292).

appointed assistant physician in charge of the neurological department at Guy's, and at the outbreak of war, he was sent as medical adviser to the British forces to Salonika in Greece, where he oversaw a serious epidemic of dysentery. On returning to Britain in 1915, he was appointed as a Medical Officer at the Royal Victoria Military Hospital, Netley, near Southampton. Completed in 1863, Netley hospital was a town in its own right, with a water supply, gas works, electricity-generating station, post office, railway, laundry, school, fire station, bakery, shops, stables, storehouses, swimming pool, anthropological museum (nicknamed 'Skull Alley'), and a theatre.[11] Situated on an outcrop between the Itchen and the Hamble rivers—locally known as 'Spike Island'—soldiers wounded in Europe arrived by boat at Southampton Docks, and were then transferred by 'ambulance train' to the grounds. Between August 1914 and December 1918, twelve hundred such trains arrived at Netley.[12] Hurst was placed in charge of Netley's isolated D-Block, the Military Lunatic Asylum, where soldiers suffering what was by then widely known as 'shell shock' were sent.

Early attempts to explain shell shock were imprecise, with physicians disagreeing over the part played by the will, the conscious mind, and the nervous system in the outbreak and treatment of symptoms.[13] On the one hand were those who subscribed to predominantly materialist explanations. Charles Samuel Myers, who coined the term 'shell shock' in 1915, argued, for example, that the seemingly inexplicable symptoms of paralysis, mutism, or twitching could be explained by microscopic lesions in the brain caused by the impact of nearby exploding shells.[14] On the other hand, psychologists such as W. H. R. Rivers, who was broadly sympathetic to the psychoanalytic writings of Sigmund Freud, believed shell shock originated in the unconscious mind, caused by a profound and overwhelming recoil from the horror of war or a 'flight into illness'.[15] Elaine Showalter has suggested that these competing etiologies came to be rooted in assumptions about the differing sensitivities and emotions of people of different classes and genders, although Peter Barham has

[11] For further information about Netley Hospital, see: Philip Hoare, *Spike Island: The Memory of a Military Hospital* (London: Fourth Estate, 2001) p. 114.

[12] Hoare, *Spike Island*, p. 188.

[13] Loughran, 'Shell-Shock and Psychological Medicine in First World War Britain' (p. 84).

[14] C. S. Myers, 'A Contribution to the Study of Shell-Shock', *The Lancet* 1, 13 (February 1915), 316–20.

[15] Sigmund Freud, 'Some General Remarks on Hysterical Attacks' (1909), trans. D. Bryan, *The Standard Edition of the Complete Psychological Works of Sigmund Freud*, x, pp. 227–34 (p. 231). For the 'flight into illness' in British psychological contexts see: Jessica Meyer, 'Shell Shock as a Self-Inflicted Wound, 1915–1921', in Salisbury and Shail (eds.) *Neurology and Modernity*, p. 235.

argued the situation was more complex than Showalter allows.[16] Broadly speaking, officers with their 'more complex and varied' mental life, were deemed to experience 'neurasthenia' (equivalent to today's stress or anxiety). Their symptoms could be relieved through talking and writing therapies, such as those cultivated by Rivers at Craiglockhart Hospital for Officers near Edinburgh where the poets Siegfried Sassoon and Wilfred Owen were both treated. By contrast, working-class privates were often diagnosed 'hysterical' and subjected to a range of physical interventions and tactics of 'persuasion'. Using faradization (the application of electric shocks to stimulate muscles) and solitary confinement, alongside a repertoire of even more barbaric punishments such as burning a mute patient's tongue with cigarettes to force him to speak, doctors believed that hysterical patients might be persuaded out of their symptoms through suggestion, shock-tactics, and bullying threats.[17]

When Hurst first came to Netley, he experimented with a range of punishing 'therapies' aimed at forcing his patients to relinquish their symptoms, including applying electric shocks, withdrawing food, and isolation. However, he quickly abandoned these methods in favour of what he called 'simple persuasion and re-education'.[18] In Hurst's view, hysterical shell shock was the consequence of the erosion of the inhibitory system as a result of the excessive strain of fighting, the persistent hunger, wet, cold, and 'fearful tension and apprehension'. This ongoing stress lowered the nervous system's 'vital resistance' leaving it open to more primitive impulses, not least those of imitation and suggestion.[19] The idea that the imagination could be powerful enough to initiate changes in the body and call forth its reflex responses was not an entirely new one. In the middle of the nineteenth century, the proto-psychologists Thomas Laycock and William Carpenter investigated what the latter termed 'ideo-motor activity'—the phenomenon of bodily movements being invoked simply by the power of a suggestive idea. In 1845, Laycock described the case of a hydrophobic patient in an asylum, whose fear of water was so extreme that when shown a glass of water he 'recoiled, gasped, and started up'. However, Laycock was fascinated to discover that the patient did not only flinch at the sight of actual water, but behaved in a similar fashion 'when

[16] Peter Barham, *Forgotten Lunatics of the Great War* (London and New Haven: Yale University Press, 2007).

[17] Lewis Yealland was particularly noted for such cruel approaches, see Showalter, *The Female Malady*, p. 175

[18] Hurst and Symns, 'The Rapid Cure of Hysterical Symptoms in Soldiers', p. 139.

[19] Frederick W. Mott, 'The Effects of High Explosives on the Central Nervous System', *The Lancet*, 187 (1916), 331–8 (p. 331).

it was *suggested* to the patient that he shall drink' (my italics).[20] In a lecture he gave at the Royal Institution seven years later on 12 March 1852, William Carpenter suggested that in certain states of 'reverie' brought on by hypnotic environments such as séances, the subject's voluntary control is suspended, and he or she becomes a 'mere thinking automaton', or 'biologized subject', whose 'whole course of ideas is determinable by suggestions operating from without'.[21] For Hurst, writing over sixty years later, soldiers were placed in a similarly vulnerable condition when their inhibitions were weakened by the relentless strains of life in the trenches. Susceptible to their imaginations and surroundings, the soldiers developed the paralysis, mutism, and twitches that characterized the neuroses of war either through 'auto-suggestion' or 'hetero-suggestion'. After his legs were buried in an explosion, Pte. Read developed 'a hysterical gait, swaying movement and nose-wiping tic' (04:36). Even though no physical harm had been sustained, the soldier's legs became stiff and unyielding due to his belief that he had suffered a devastating injury on being buried, a vivid example of what Hurst called self- or auto-suggestion. By contrast, nineteen-year-old Pte. Sandall, who was already suffering from hysterical facial tics when he arrived in a field hospital in France in September 1917, developed 'additional symptoms' including gait and speech impediment 'by imitation', when he met and befriended another patient Pte. King (07:52, Figure 20). Suggestible to his surroundings and the symptoms of others patients, Pte. Sandall's case was an example of hetero-suggestion.

For Hurst, distortions and mis-performances of the flinch reflex provided clear examples of how seemingly intractable hysterical symptoms were produced—and might be reversed. Some patients performed wildly exaggerated starts and recoils, continuing to do so even 'after the cause of their exaggeration has disappeared'.[22] Others started in the silence of a hypnosis session or flinched in their sleep. In cases such as these, the startle reflex—the compulsion to withdraw or recoil when alarmed or in pain—appeared strangely pliable. At the beginning of the nineteenth century, Hall had described flinches as part of a predictable and uniform reflex arc, stable and enduring in its performance. However, by the beginning of the twentieth century, it was becoming clear that our bodily reflexes were not organized on so simple a plan. In 1906, the neurologist Charles Scott Sherrington published a series of lectures he had

[20] Thomas Laycock, 'On the Reflex Functions of the Brain', *British and Foreign Medical Journal*, 19 (1845), 298–311.

[21] William B. Carpenter, 'On the Influence of Suggestion in Modifying and Directing Muscular Movement, Independently of Volition', *Proceedings of the Royal Institution* (1852), 147–54.

[22] Hurst, *Medical Diseases of the War*, pp. 41–2.

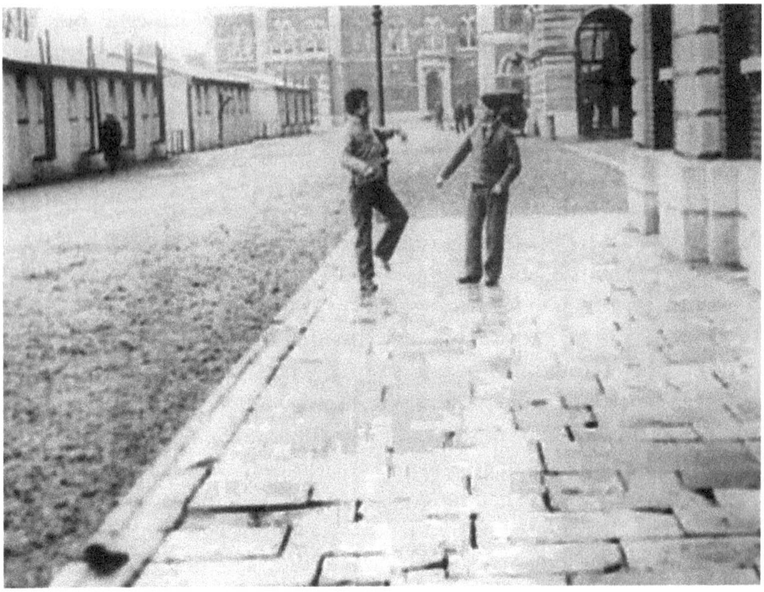

Fig. 21. Ptes. King and Sandall, 'Stump Orators' (07:52), Arthur Hurst and J. L. M. Symns, *War Neuroses*, Netley Hospital 1917, Seale Hayne 1918.

Wellcome Library, London

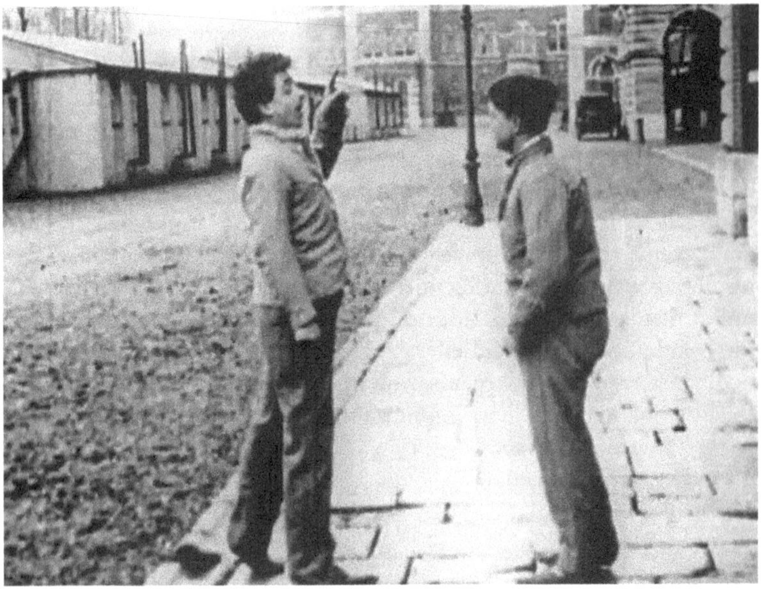

Fig. 22. Ptes. King and Sandall, 'Stump Orators' (07:28), Arthur Hurst and J. L. M. Symns, *War Neuroses*, Netley Hospital 1917, Seale Hayne 1918.

Wellcome Library, London

presented at Yale University two years earlier, in a book entitled *The Integrative Action of the Nervous System.* The collection was dedicated to David Ferrier, whose demonstration of Monkey F he had seen at the 1881 International Medical Congress, and whose work had subsequently inspired Sherrington to focus on neurology. In particular, Sherrington was interested in the relationship between brain and spinal reflexes. Moving away from Hall's description of a simple spinal reflex, Sherrington described the link between brain and spinal cord as a 'whole chain of structures—receptor, conductor, and effector'. The notion of a separate simple spinal reflex, universal and predictable in its action, was he claimed 'probably a purely abstract conception because all parts of the nervous system are connected together and no part of it is probably ever capable of reaction without affecting and being affected by various other parts'. Continually working, responding and reacting, the reflex system was 'never absolutely at rest'. More importantly, reflexes could continually reinvent themselves by assimilating new stimuli and forming new aggregates: 'the main secret of nervous co-ordination', he wrote 'lies evidently in the compounding of reflexes'.[23] Sherrington's understanding of a fully integrated nervous system, in which a network of sensory and motor pathways acted reciprocally on one another, gave a physiological basis to the idea that even our most basic reflexes could be vulnerable to outside influence and prey to illusion.

The Great War provided unambiguous evidence of Sherrington's insight, showing clearly that reflex responses could be re-educated. As Hurst himself pointed out, among those who had never fought in the trenches, there was a clear distinction between flinching and jumping. The 'flinch reflex' involved 'the assumption of a crouching attitude; the arm is raised in front of the face and the eyes blink'. 'It has the object of hiding the individual and defending him from attack', wrote Hurst. A 'jump reflex', on the other hand, consisted in 'a sudden movement of the limbs and trunk, and is associated with blinking of the eyes and dilation of the pupils; it is caused by sudden sounds, and is really the preparation of immediate activity, which would be displayed if the individual obeyed his instinctive desire to save himself by flight'. According to Hurst, both flinching and jumping were transformed under the special conditions of trench warfare. For example, he noted that soldiers returning from the Front, when startled by a sudden noise, rather than leaping up as most civilians tended to do,

[23] Charles Scott Sherrington, *Integrative Action of the Nervous System* (New Haven: Yale University Press, 1906). These ideas were first laid out in the Silliman lectures Sherrington gave at Yale University in 1904.

automatically ducked their heads.[24] One of Hurst's patients Pte. Preston (aged 19), who arrived at Netley suffering from amnesia, an inability to read, and deafness to all words except for the word 'bombs', displayed a particularly distressing example of this transformation. In *War Neuroses*, Preston is seen sitting quietly on a chair in his ward. A doctor sits next to him in officer's garb, on a bed specially angled towards the camera for the occasion. Suddenly, the doctor utters the trigger-word 'bombs'. Preston knocks his chair backwards and throws himself under the bed. After a few moments, crawls out, blinking, cautiously, looking confused at the camera crew that greets him (Figure 20). Like Darwin, who could not help swerving from a snake firmly encased in glass, Preston is compelled to re-perform his responses to dangers encountered in other times and places, a once efficacious adaptation now heartbreakingly out of place. Unlike Jack Wilton in *The Unfortunate Traveller* who flinched off the battlefield, these soldiers flinched *with* it, their nervous systems and the battleground coming to constitute a single field.

If the body, made increasingly pliable in the unique conditions of modern warfare, could be bent into one shape through imitation and suggestion, then Hurst believed that the same psychological processes could be harnessed to simply bend it back again. If suggestion and imitation explained the peculiar contagiousness of shell shock among members of the same battalion, it also, according to Hurst, provided the key to reversing the symptoms. The cornerstone of Hurst's treatment at Netley was the creation of what he called a 'proper atmosphere of cure', an enforced optimism that took on the status of an almost quasi-religious belief:

> After admission the sister encourages the patient to believe that he will be cured as soon as the doctor has time to see him. If paraplegic or mute, two or three patients in the ward who have been rapidly cured of paraplegia or mutism tell him of their cure. The medical officer sees him some hours later, and after examining him and coming to the conclusion that the condition is hysterical he tells him as a matter of course that he will be cured the next day. By the following morning the patient is fully convinced that the hoped-for cure will take place.[25]

It was essential to the atmosphere of cure that both doctors and patients should believe. The patient must be 'fully convinced that the hoped-for cure will take place', but also the medical officer too should be 'equally convinced that he will cure the patient'. No transcripts exist of the precise exhortations Hurst and the medical team at Netley uttered in their capacity

[24] Hurst, *Medical Diseases of the War*, p. 41.
[25] Hurst, *The Diseases of the War*, p. 140.

as 'persuasionists', but it is clear that they not only involved mantra-like repetitions of reassuring and motivating phrases ('he will be cured') to rapidly inculcate belief ('the patient is fully convinced'), but also required the patients to participate by staging themselves and watching one another on their road to recovery. New arrivals were introduced to convalescing patients who told of their transformation. 'The presence in the ward of three men recently cured of paraplegia', wrote Hurst, 'helped to convince' one patient that he would as a matter of course be cured. Another, a man recovering from violent tremors was reportedly 'shown' to a new arrival, in an ad hoc theatre created in the ward where convalescents were both actors and audience members.[26]

As Teresa Brennan has suggested, 'the *deliberate* creation of an atmosphere' is a 'theatre' (orig. italics), but the 'atmosphere of cure' was only one of a cluster of theatrical techniques Hurst deployed at Netley.[27] If Netley's medical staff were exhorted to perform optimism, at other times they were, quite literally, turned into actors, directed in fictional scenarios enacted in the operating theatre. After the war, Hurst recalled treating two men who arrived at Netley completely deaf. Unsure whether this was genuine hysterical illness or malingering, Hurst subjected both patients to sham operations. The first:

> Was given enough ether to make him excited, and two small cuts were then made behind his ear; a hammer was banged on a sheet of iron during the 'operation'. The moment after the incision had been made, the patient jumped off the table with his hearing restored. The second patient was unwilling at first to undergo an operation, but finally consented as he was naturally impressed by the recovery of the first patient, who was in the same ward and had been deaf for a much longer period. The same 'operation' was performed and complete recovery occurred in exactly the same way. The joy shown by the patients on their recovery whilst in the theatre and on returning to the ward was so obviously unfeigned that there could be no doubt about the genuineness of the deafness.[28]

Such an approach was not new. As Mikkel Borch-Jacobsen has argued, before the turn of the twentieth century 'it was taken for granted that one could both grow ill and heal through the influences of imagination, sympathy, imitation, or strong emotions'.[29] The '*traitment moral*' (or 'moral treatment') as it was practiced by the French physician Phillippe Pinel

[26] Hurst and Symns, 'The Rapid Cure of Hysterical Symptoms in Soldiers', pp. 140–1.
[27] Brennan, *The Transmission of Affect* (Ithaca: Cornell University Press, 2004) p. 16.
[28] Hurst, *Medical Diseases of the War*, pp. 120–1.
[29] Mikkel Borch-Jacobsen, *Making Minds and Madness: From Hysteria to Depression* (Cambridge: Cambridge University Press, 2009) p. 206.

(1745–1826) during his time as chief physician at the Salpêtrière provides a particularly vivid example of what Foucault has termed a therapeutics by 'theatrical representation'. Rejecting the bleeding and purging practiced by his contemporaries, Pinel made his patients unwitting participants in immersive theatrical productions, a 'complicity of the unreal with itself'. A tailor, for example, who, in his manic delusions, believed himself to be awaiting the death sentence for murder, was acquitted in a mock trial complete with judge and jury, and at once gave up the delusion. In another case described by Pinel's contemporary M. Hulshorff in Berlin, a delirious patient believing he was dead, refused to eat, and thus was at risk from dying of starvation:

> A group of people who had made themselves pale and were dressed like the dead, entered his room, set up a table, brought food, and began to eat and drink before the bed. The starving "dead man" looked at them; they were astonished that he stayed in bed; they persuaded him that dead people eat as much as living ones. He readily accommodated himself to this idea.[30]

Pinel called such stagings 'pious frauds' or 'innocent ruses', which turned the patient's own impressionable nature, powerful imagination, and deeply passionate nature (all three understood to contribute to the causes of the malady) to therapeutic advantage. According to Jan Goldstein, the theatricality of the treatment is 'underscored textually by Pinel's frequent use of the word *appareil*—that is, display, show, pomp, appearance'.[31] At Netley, too, madness and its cure were a *folie à plusieurs*, the treatment capitalizing on the looping effects of its patient's self-conscious performances of both illness and recovery for therapeutic effect.[32]

Re-education was already a well-established technique among those who treated tics and hysterical contractures of the limbs. Yet this practice too had a strongly theatrical element, in which physicians and patients took turns at performing and spectating. A physical intervention, 're-education' involved massaging stiffened limbs and holding trembling hands still, but most of all it involved encouraging the patient to re-learn the 'proper' movements through copying. Cpl. Anderson, who came to Netley in March 1917, suffering with a hysterical 'dancing' gait (10:02), was one patient cured through re-education by imitation. Anderson's gait,

[30] Michel Foucault, *Madness and Civilization: A History of Insanity in the Age of Reason*, trans. Richard Howard (London and New York: Routledge, 2002) p. 174; p. 177; p. 179.

[31] Jan Goldstein, *Console and Classify. The French Psychiatric Profession in the Nineteenth Century* (Chicago and London: University of Chicago Press, 2001) pp. 83–4.

[32] As Borch-Jacobsen has put it, the physician is always engaged 'in the field that they describe', so that 'madness is always a *folie à deux*, or rather a *folie à plusieurs*', Borch-Jacobsen, *Making Minds and Madness*, p. 11.

Hurst concluded, had initially come about because the patient had been suffering severe leg pains, and had devised his ingenious 'gait' to avoid putting too much pressure on the affected limbs.

> I explained to him that the gait which had been the means of saving him from pain had now become a habit, and that he must try to cure himself by copying every movement I made when I walked. He did this for ten minutes, at the end of which he could walk fairly well. By the next morning, greatly to his delight, he was walking quite normally and now found it difficult to reproduce his old dancing gait.[33]

Through rehearsal and repetition, the patient would appropriate the doctor's performance. For the French neurologists Henri Meige and Eugene Feindel, in their landmark 1902 work on motor and sensory disturbances *Tics and their Treatment*, the techniques of re-education are described in a language suffused with the theatrical idiom. The physician must 'modify the patient's attitudes. If he has been comfortably seated during the opening performances, try him when he is standing, and as soon as he has accomplished this, vary the position of his head, arms, trunk, and legs, repeating the *séance* [sitting] in each case.' While copying the physicians, the patients monitored their own 'performances' and 'attitudes' by observing their reflection, like the readers of Darwin's *Expression*, in the mirror: 'the repetition of the prescribed exercises should take place in front of a looking-glass whereby the patient may be exactly informed of any mistakes in gesture or attitude.'[34]

'Curiously and regrettably', writes Elizabeth Cowie in her analysis of the film, *War Neuroses* 'does not show the process of suggestion used with the soldiers'.[35] Yet, it seems to me that Hurst's treatment through the suggestive 'atmosphere of cure' was expressed precisely through the making of the 'kinematographic records'. By the time Hurst began treating the war-wounded at Netley, the idea that asylums might play host to theatrical entertainments, and that acting and visiting the theatre might have some therapeutic advantage, was already firmly established. For example, in 1837, the Scottish alienist W. A. F. Browne, published a series of lectures entitled *What Asylums Were, Are and Ought to Be* in which he advised that excursions to the theatre, as well opportunities for patients to collaborate on staging dramas, could be a useful tool for rehabilitation: 'they are thus

[33] Hurst, *The Diseases of the War*, pp. 82–3.

[34] Henri Meige and Eugene Clement Louis Feindel, *Tics and Their Treatment*, trans. S. A. K. Wilson (London: Sidney Appleton, 1907) p. 318.

[35] Elizabeth Cowie, 'The Spectacle of Actuality', in *Collecting Visible Evidence*, ed. Jane M. Gaines and Michael Renov (Minneapolis: University of Minnesota Press, 1999) pp. 19–45 (p. 35).

gradually prepared to resume their station in society.'[36] Later, as superintendent at the new Crichton Royal Hospital, Browne oversaw many visits to the Dumfries Theatre, and the playbills of numerous in-house productions, such as the staging of the farce *Raising the Wind* by patients in December 1844, survive in the records.[37] Browne argued that such recreations created a 'healthy tone' which 'pervades the establishment during the whole of the theatrical season'.[38] Part of the 'healthy tone' Browne envisaged was undoubtedly born out of the excitement and anticipation at an imminent theatre trip, and the eager spirit of joint endeavour with which asylum patients themselves rehearsed their own productions, a focal point in what could be a monotonous existence. If Browne's 'healthy tone' was created by theatrical shows, then film-making offered Hurst a similar opportunity to create an 'atmosphere of cure'. In 1917, film-making, a relatively new phenomenon, was still something of a spectacle in its own right. Throughout *War Neuroses*, curious passers-by who have stopped to gawk at the proceedings, are accidentally caught at the edge of the shot (Figure 23). The appearance of the professional *Pathé Frères* camera crew on Spike Island would almost certainly have created excitement and anticipation. Moreover, the opportunities to participate in the film as actors may have delighted many of the asylum patients. At the very least, the patients' commitment to the process is clear in a short film they made, which appears at the end of *War Neuroses*.

'Directed, photographed and acted by convalescent war neurosis patients' (24:31), *The Battle of Seale Hayne* enacts an imaginary campaign. The film, which lasts only a few minutes, owes its name and visual iconography to the by now infamous feature documentary *The Battle of the Somme* (1916), whose graphic depiction of British troops on the front line horrified audiences at home. *The Battle of Seale Hayne* opens with two men running down a country road to warn of an imminent attack. The squadron of ten men jump to their feet with their rifles over their shoulders and march to meet the enemy. The following scene is a wide shot of a desolate landscape filled with smoke from mortar attacks. Men run across the hillside, hiding behind rocks and trees, firing at the enemy. In the final sequence, the men go 'over the top' of the brow of a small hill. One man falls, dead or wounded. Another, in an act of theatrical bravado, flings himself backwards and rolls the several metres down the hill. A group

36 W. A. F. Browne, *What Asylums Were, Are and Ought to Be* (Edinburgh: Black, 1837) p. 222.

37 A. C. Tait, 'History of Crichton Royal', *Medical History*, 16, 2 (1972), 178–84 p. 182.

38 W. A. F. Browne, 'The Moral Treatment of the Insane; A Lecture', *British Journal of Psychiatry*, 10 (1864), 309–37 (p. 318; p. 332).

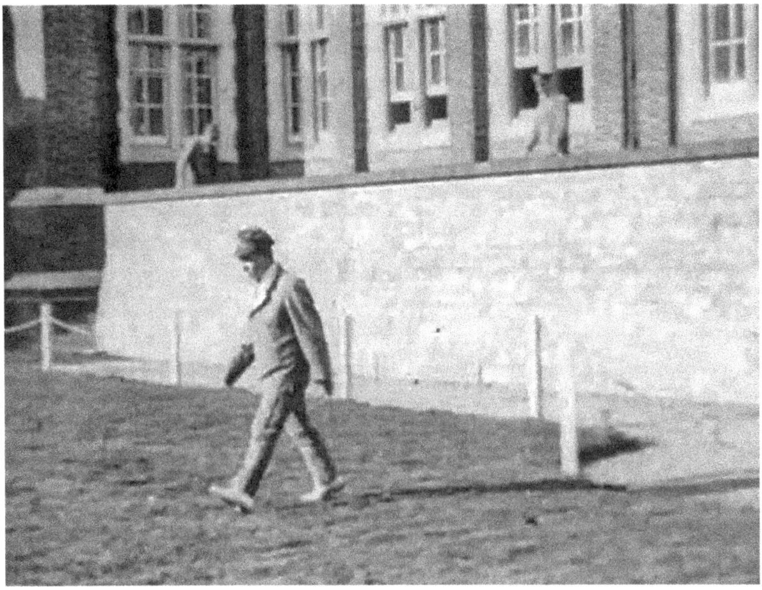

Fig. 23. 'Hysterical Gait Following Flesh Wound of Thigh. Before Treatment' (21:01), Arthur Hurst and J. L. M. Symns, *War Neuroses*, Netley Hospital 1917, Seale Hayne 1918.

Wellcome Library, London

of medics rush towards him carrying a stretcher, and the film concludes with his rescue. For Hurst it was important that patients were not passive recipients of the 'atmosphere of cure', but active participants in their treatment. Simple persuasion, he wrote, 'has the advantage of making the patient take an active part in his own cure'.[39] It might be tempting to read *The Battle of Seale Hayne* as a return to the site of original trauma, but to Hurst, the short film provided patients with an opportunity to mimic and embody discipline, heroism, and camaraderie, as well as to occupy themselves with a common task. It was a re-enactment of a military prowess that the patients would soon be called on to perform once again, this time in the theatre of war.

By 1917, Hurst was so confident in his 'atmosphere of cure' that he went so far as to say that 'the nature of the actual treatment is really immaterial' but that 'persuasion through the atmosphere of cure is the most powerful means of reversing the neurotic symptoms'.[40] By turning staff as well as

[39] Hurst and Symns, 'The Rapid Cure of Hysterical Symptoms in Soldiers', p. 141.
[40] Hurst and Symns, 'The Rapid Cure of Hysterical Symptoms in Soldiers', p. 140.

patients into actors, Hurst did create a powerful theatre through which, as *War Neuroses* testifies, profound neurotic symptoms disappeared with astonishing rapidity. However, like all theatrical transformations, once the play was over, the effects quickly vanished into dust. After the end of the war, the Southborough Committee claimed that Hurst's patients had merely submitted to his 'all-powerful will'.[41] Hurst, who suffered chronic asthma and was partially deaf, was known as a charismatic and forceful personality, rather dogmatic (he 'was either "always" or "never", with no penumbra of qualification') and attention-seeking—when bored at medical meetings, would ostentatiously 'switch off his hearing aid, open his bag, spill his papers over the floor and noisily tidy them up'.[42] He was, as his former pupil, the neurologist Charles Symonds recalled, 'a great showman', who was himself 'fond of the theatre'.[43] Yet, while the Southborough committee imagined the patients as a susceptible and passive audience, easily swayed by Hurst's showmanship, for Hurst himself the patient-spectators occupied a more complicated position in which watching was also a kind of performance. Indeed, the theatricality of Hurst's approach at Netley may come as no surprise when we consider the fact the illness of hysteria was, by the time Hurst began his work at Netley, already deeply embroiled in the language of theatrical self-display.

STAGE-STRUCK: HYSTERICAL PATIENTS AS AUDIENCE-MEMBERS

Over the last thirty years cultural theorists have been increasingly drawn to the theatrical imposture threaded through the nineteenth-century diagnosis and treatment of madness. As Elaine Showalter, Georges Didi-Huberman, Alison Winter, and Mark Micale, among others, have described, hospitals and asylums were not immune from the larger culture of theatrical scientific display in the nineteenth century. One vivid example, described by Alison Winter in *Mesmerized: Powers of Mind in Victorian Britain* highlights how patients were recruited as performers in dramatic demonstrations of new therapeutic techniques.[44] In 1837, two Irish sisters Elizabeth (aged 16) and Jane (aged 15) O'Key, both domestic

[41] HM Stationery Office (HMSO), *Report of the War Office Committee of Enquiry Into 'Shell-Shock'* (London: HMSO, 1922) p. 80.

[42] Anon. 'Obituary, Sir Arthur Hurst', *British Medical Journal*, 2, 292 (1944) 292–3 (p. 293).

[43] Charles Symonds, *Studies in Neurology* (Oxford: Oxford University Press, 1970) p. 10.

[44] Winter, *Mesmerized*, pp. 67–78.

servants, were admitted to University College hospital diagnosed with epilepsy and hysteria. They became, as Winter puts it, 'prima-donnas' of the medical stage, for their striking responses to treatment by the continental technique of mesmerism, otherwise known as animal magnetism. On 10 May 1838, their physician John Elliotson invited an audience of medics and other luminaries, including Charles Dickens and Michael Faraday, to the University College London anatomy theatre to witness the astonishing effects of magnetic treatment. In a trance-like state of altered consciousness, brought on by Elliotson's mesmeric passes, Elizabeth O'Key performed a repertoire of astonishing magnetic phenomena, including 'traction', in which she imitated the physician's gestures whilst blindfolded. She also bantered with the audience and mischievously flung insults at them, her performance taking on the flavour of a music hall comedienne. When she was finally woken, she quickly reverted to her demure ordinary self. *The Lancet* admired the transformations wrought in the magnetic sleep: the most 'accomplished actor that ever trod the stage', they claimed 'could not have presented the change with a truer show of reality'.[45] It was, however, an ambiguous, backhanded sort of praise. O'Key's transformation may have proved more scintillating than the simple mouthings of an average actress on the London stage, but an actress she was nonetheless.

The invention of photography created further opportunities for theatrical imposture and psychiatric ailments to collide. In the 1850s, the English alienist Hugh Welch Diamond (1809–1886), pioneered the use of asylum photography whilst Resident Superintendent of the Female Department of the Surrey County Lunatic Asylum, where he created numerous calotypes of patients suffering a mental disorders. The photographs, which served as means of identifying patients upon readmission and for diagnosing in accordance with physiognomic types, could also, Diamond believed, help effect cures. Photography was particularly useful in treating patients suffering delusions, who, when presented with their mirrored image, even when posed and dressed in costumes, came to realize their true identity.[46] Perhaps one of the most famous of these images is entitled 'Ophelia'. In her essay *Representing Ophelia*, Elaine Showalter has described a complex reciprocal relationship between psychiatric treatments of hysteria, female sexuality, and the cultural representations of Shakespeare's tragic heroine. A young woman might identify with Ophelia, the character's conflicting duties, bawdy songs, disordered appearance, and drowning giving

[45] Quoted in Winter, *Mesmerized*, p. 74.

[46] H. W. Diamond, 'On the Application of Photography to the Physiognomic and Mental Phenomena of Insanity', *Proceedings of the Royal Society*, 117 (1856). See also: S. L. Gilman, *The Face of Madness: Hugh W. Diamond and the Origin of Psychiatric Photography* (New York: Brunner-Mazel, 1976) p. 86.

outward shape to the inner torment the patient herself experienced. At the same time, the new practice of photographing asylum patients underscored this blending of psychological symptoms with theatrical archetypes. As Showalter puts it, 'where the woman themselves did not willingly throw themselves into Ophelia-like postures, asylum superintendents, armed with the new technology of photography, imposed the costume, gesture, props, and expression of Ophelia upon them'.[47] The photographs of female lunatics at the Salpêtrière in Paris, as well the dramatic and often erotically charged reproduction of hysterical symptoms under hypnosis in Jean-Martin Charcot's sensationalist Tuesday Lectures in the 1880s, are other frequently referred-to examples of the tangled relationships between female insanity and theatrical spectacle in the nineteenth century.

In these cases, the gazed-upon, often female body may be regarded as an object, her appearance manipulated and controlled by the physician in a play of power based on nineteenth-century divisions of gender and class. At the same time, as Mark S. Micale has described, it is unsurprising that asylum practices and discourses emphasized the theatrical aspects of hysteria. With its emotional excesses and flamboyant transformations, hysteria was 'a highly corporealized pathology in which psychological anxieties are played out on the stage of the human body. Self-dramatization is an inherent part of it.'[48] Those treating symptoms of hysteria were struck by the way bodily symptoms with no physiological basis could suddenly develop—and disappear—through the workings of imagination and emotion alone. Moreover, the mechanisms through which hysterical symptoms developed were themselves deemed theatrical. The compulsion to imitate and copy, to absorb one's surroundings and become distinctly vulnerable to all suggestions, was, according to W. H. R. Rivers, the co-architect of Head's protopathic/epicritic distinction, a 'throw-back, partly to the dramatic character of the activity of early life'.[49] At the same time, the proximity of hysteric to actress served to undermine the perceived sincerity of the patient's distress in real and damaging ways. As Didi-Huberman has described, female patients at the Salpêtrière were subject to a larger, stigmatizing anti-theatrical prejudice, one that assumed actors were 'the least sensitive, the least "affected within themselves", they have so little soul, if any'. Through their constant posing before the asylum's cameras, Charcot's

[47] Elaine Showalter, 'Representing Ophelia: Women, Madness and the Responsibilities of Feminist Criticism', in *Shakespeare and the Question of Theory*, ed. Patricia Parker and Geoffrey Hartman (London: Methuen, 1985) pp. 77–94.

[48] Mark S. Micale, *Approaching Hysteria: Disease and its Interpretations* (Princeton: Princeton University Press, 1995) pp. 149–50.

[49] W. H. R Rivers *Instinct and the Unconscious* (Cambridge: Cambridge University Press, 1920) p. 149.

patients were identified as histrionic, and like Diderot's *comédien*, found themselves caught up in an impossible paradox. Either the hysteric 'is truly in "sympathy" with her role—and isn't that because her own suffering proves to be so unsubstantial?—or else she is miming wholly deprived of affect (although with great virtuosity), and the pain she proclaims might also merely be mimed'.[50] The relationship between theatrical imposture and hysteria, already tangled, grew even knottier at the outbreak of the Great War. When certifying a patient, doctors were indeed making urgent life or death decisions, as shamming insanity, like intentional self-wounding, was an insubordination punishable by execution. Yet, as Hurst himself admitted, 'the diagnosis of hysteria from malingering is exceedingly difficult' since as a result of self-suggestion the hysteric might assume many of the characteristic, even clichéd, symptoms of the malady. In turn, this made their symptoms 'indistinguishable from the paralysis which the malingerer voluntarily assumes'. Like the theatre critic A. B. Walkley who could not be certain whether the actress Elenora Duse's flinch was truly spontaneous, as a medical observer Hurst found himself caught up in the queasy uncertainty experienced by theatrical audiences, unsure whether a frozen limb or twitching face was authentic or mere acting. Occasionally naïve or unskilled malingerers were caught out. 'The appropriate treatment for a paraplegic man, who is discovered walking in the ward when he thinks he is alone and unseen, is to send him to the military authorities for punishment.' However, examples of such wholesale pretence were rare, and Hurst believed it more common for soldiers to consciously or unconsciously prolong their incapacity and delay their return to the Front by exaggerating existing symptoms. Such minor embellishments might in time become absorbed by the actor, creating an ever more complex palette of neurotic symptoms. As Hurst put it, 'a man who pretends to be paralysed for a sufficiently long period may end up genuinely believing he is paralysed, just as the German people have repeated the official lies as to the cause of the war so frequently that many now doubtless believe in the truth of what they originally knew was untrue.'[51]

With the introduction of film cameras into hospitals and asylums, came new opportunities for recording symptoms, and like the hysterical women who posed for Diamond's and Charcot's cameras, the patients who made their appearances in *War Neuroses* gave strikingly theatrical performances. If the film is uncomfortable to watch today, it is surely because of the profound self-consciousness of its actor-convalescents. Mugging for

[50] Didi-Huberman, *The Invention of Hysteria*, pp. 228–9.
[51] Hurst, *The Diseases of the War*, pp. 28–9.

the camera, the patients walk up and down as they have been instructed to do, drop their walking sticks at agreed spots, lose their balance and fall as they have rehearsed, in order to demonstrate the stiffness of their legs or the compulsiveness of their tics. Rarely depicted in the wards, but rather against picturesque backdrops including a paved street, a majestic colonnade, and the hospital's manicured grounds, their quick sideways glances to the camera for reassurance or direction make it abundantly clear that for the most part, this choreography is not of their own devising. The theatricality of these images is not only unnerving because it seems to minimize the patients' agency and the sincerity of their suffering. The obviously rehearsed quality also poses important ethical questions about the processes through which such performances were extracted. One wonders about the ability of the patients, whose identities are only occasionally disguised, to freely consent to the filming process. Certainly, the demands of the film-making schedule frequently trumped those of treatment at Netley, and Hurst did not disguise the fact. Pte. Read's treatment, for example, was delayed for two days because the doctor 'wished to obtain a kinematograph record of gait and tic'.[52] In addition, symptoms were deliberately triggered for the camera. Pte. Preston, whose deafness and mutism make his fully informed consent extremely unlikely, was provoked into flinging himself to the floor and hiding under the bed (both frightening and potentially physically dangerous) by doctors who knowingly uttered the word 'bombs' for the cameras. Finally, and perhaps most astonishingly, in one sequence depicting the recovery of Sgt. Bissett, the similarities between 'kinematograph records' purportedly taken two months apart, is so striking—including the direction of the billowing smoke in the background, and the positions of three bystanders who watch in the shadow of a far-off building—that it is hard not to conclude that in some cases patients were asked to *re-create* their gaits and tics for the camera (14:15).[53] This was a sanctioned malingering, a particularly dangerous strategy in light of the fact it was devised by a doctor who believed that faking an illness could lead to the development of an actual one. Whether feigning symptoms, or otherwise performing them in carefully choreographed sequences framed in studiously selected *mise en scène*, the soldiers who made their appearances in *War Neuroses* entered a theatrical regime of the spectacle. Their bodies became simulacra, copies of ill bodies already deemed mere imitations.

[52] Hurst and Symns, 'The Rapid Cure of Hysterical Symptoms in Soldiers', p. 140.

[53] Edgar Jones has recently made a similar assertion. See: Edgar Jones, 'War Neuroses and Arthur Hurst: A Pioneering Medical Film about the Treatment of Psychiatric Battle Casualties', *Journal of the History of Medicine and Allied Sciences*, 67, 3 (2012), 345–73 (p. 367).

In their investigations of the theatricality of late nineteenth-century hysteria, Showalter, Winter, Didi-Huberman, and Micale have all identified the patient with *actresses* and the physicians with spectators, whose silent and immobile gaze fixes and objectifies the ill body. One might be tempted to read a similar relationship into *War Neuroses*. Yet, in fact, the film offers a more complicated relationship between audiences and performers, one in which patients and staff became part of the same 'choreographic community' of spectators.[54] On the one hand, the watching physicians, animated by the performers' furtive sideways glances, often take the position of silent outsiders who gaze from behind the cameras at the scene played out before them. Yet, this off-screen audience also occasionally stumbles into view, making their appearances alongside the patients they treat. For example, when Pte. Richards drops his walking sticks to demonstrate his inability to walk without them, a doctor rushes into shot to stop the patient falling (15:59). Elsewhere, members of Netley's staff are caught on camera by accident. In one scene, a passing doctor, noticing the spectacle of the filming and feeling curious, stops to gawp at the proceedings (21:01, Figure 23). Later in the film, two nurses, realizing they have wandered into the background of the 'kinematographic record' of Cpl. Anderson's 'dancing gait', dart quickly behind a pillar, their embarrassed recoil from the scene of looking reminiscent of Ferrier, who ducked out of the sight of his experimental monkey (10:29, Figure 24). The predicaments of these spectators blurs the line between watching and performing, the onlooker hoping to remain anonymously invisible becomes momentarily emotional and exposed.

Just as the medical onlookers became emotional performers, at Netley, hysterical convalescents were routinely thought of less as actors than as emotionally volatile and suggestible theatrical *audience members*. The 'atmosphere of cure' cast patients as participants in a carefully engineered environment, where they were immersed in cleverly orchestrated scenarios. They listened and absorbed the reassuring refrains of nurses. They bore witness to the rapid recoveries of their fellow patients. Indeed, *War Neuroses* documents many examples of the latter. While there are no on-screen witnesses to Cpl. Anderson's 'dancing gait', when it came to filming Anderson's 'improvement after re-education the same day', three watching patients were placed artistically in the shot. One leans casually against the wall, the other two sit with their arms folded on the steps, and all three of them watch as the grinning Anderson walks towards the camera, hardly any trace of his former 'dance' still visible (11:05). Another example of

[54] Rancière, *The Emancipated Spectator*, p. 5.

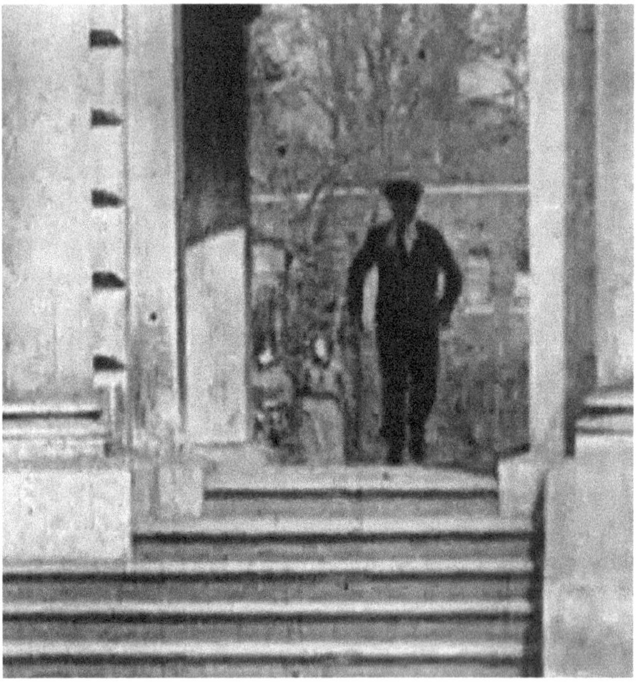

Fig. 24. 'Cpl. Anderson aged 27, Hysterical "Dancing" Gait' (10:29), Arthur Hurst and J. L. M. Symns, *War Neuroses*, Netley Hospital 1917, Seale Hayne 1918.

Wellcome Library, London

persuasion by theatre appears in the record of Pte. King's hysterical gait. To demonstrate King's improving gait, the doctors set up a temporary theatre on the steps of one of Netley's colonnades. Chairs, dragged out from the wards for the occasion, were set up in rows and a large number of patients called upon to participate. For this sequence, the audience was seated on the stage, while King entered from between them, the camera capturing both the performer and the reactions of his audience. It is an odd inversion of the usual theatrical logic, but one clearly chosen to place the reactions of the audience in the frame, to stage the patients as spectators as well as performers. In a bizarrely regal entrance, made bathetic by his gait, King sways, jerks, gesticulates, and apparently rants to himself, all the while jabbing his forefinger at the camera. The audience, perhaps they are supposed to be the King's court, perhaps a crowd of spectators at an evening's entertainment, seem to be laughing uproariously at the 'hysterical stump orator's' ludicrous appearance (06:53, Figure 25). Their response seems horrifying today, a species of that cruel mockery associated with visitors

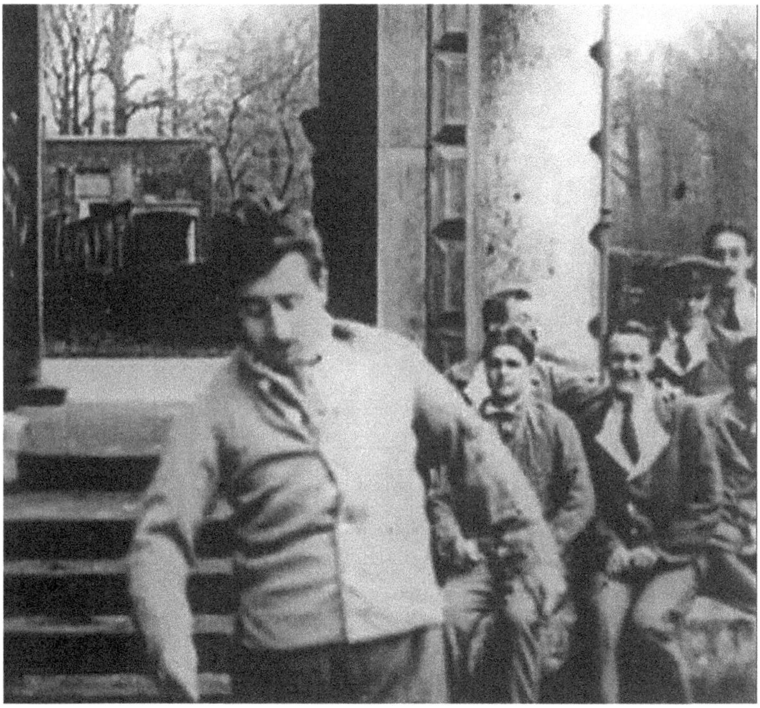

Fig. 25. Pte. King and his audience (06:53), Arthur Hurst and J. L. M. Symns, *War Neuroses*, Netley Hospital 1917, Seale Hayne 1918.

Wellcome Library, London

to the Bedlam in the eighteenth century. But in fact, at Netley, laughing at one's fellow convalescents was understood to serve an important therapeutic purpose.

Throughout the nineteenth century, alienists had repeatedly drawn attention to the curative effects of laughter on asylum patients. In 1837, Browne had suggested that theatrical amusements might play an important role in rehabilitating patients and returning them to ordinary society. As Juliet Foster has pointed out, by the end of the nineteenth century touring theatrical troupes, both professional and amateur, were frequent visitors to asylums, with farces, burlesques, vaudevilles, and other comedies clearly favoured by those in charge.[55] After two decades as superintendent at the

[55] J. L. H. Foster, 'Performance in Psychiatric Hospitals: A Case Study of Fulbourne, Bethlem Royal and Brookwood Hospitals', in *Considering Performance, Madness and Psychiatry: Isolated Acts*, ed. A. Harpin and J. L. H. Foster (Basingstoke: Palgrave, 2014) (in press).

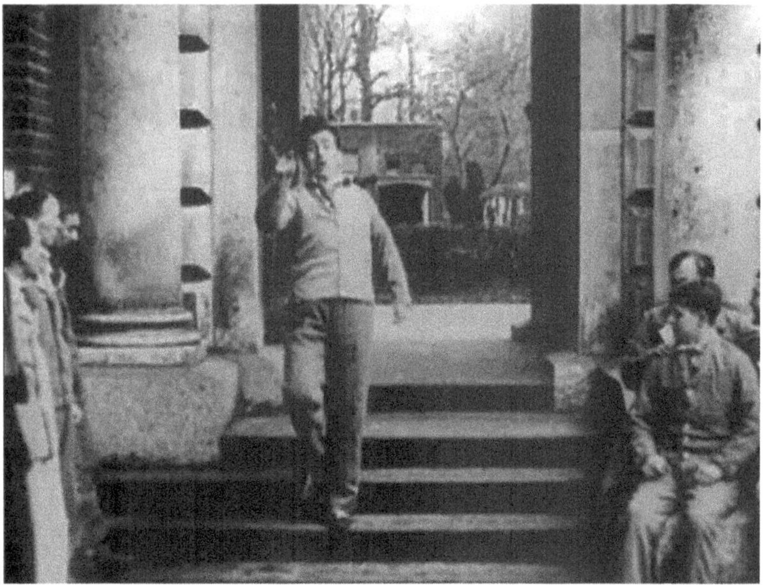

Fig. 26. Pte. King pointing (06:48), Arthur Hurst and J. L. M. Symns, *War Neuroses*, Netley Hospital 1917, Seale Hayne 1918.

Wellcome Library, London

Royal Crichton in which he oversaw a regime which included frequent trips to the theatre as well as in-house productions by patients, Browne expanded on the therapeutic benefits of drama. Entertainments offered rare pleasures: 'watch an assemblage of lunatics while national or cheerful airs are played', wrote Browne, 'and it becomes palpable that though dead to all else, they are alive to sweet and familiar sounds'. Similarly, 'large parties of the insane', when allowed to roam beyond the asylum walls, sought out 'amusement in the concert rooms and theatres of crowded cities'. At the same time, Browne believed that the mind was influenced through the senses, and that watching theatrical spectacles could have transformative effects. He cited an anecdote, well known at the time, of the poet Lloyd who 'was cured of melancholia by seeing a play'. Theatre created what Browne called a 'healthy tone', not least because it provided opportunities for the insane audience members to 'imitate the manifestations of the sound and strong'. It was a risky business. A play wrongly chosen could do more harm than good, as an unfortunate incident described by the French alienist Esquirol testified. Not long after the Revolution, whilst watching a political drama (whose name was long forgotten) representing the deposition of a king by his subjects, 'the audience, composed chiefly of patients, regarded the rebellious act as real and unjustifiable; rushed upon the stage with tumultuous indignation, vindicated legitimacy, and restored the ill-treated monarch'.[56] Anecdotes of naïve audience members interrupting the drama—from country bumpkins to sailors to over-excited knights—had peppered Victorian literature and psychological writing. However, Browne believed such effects could be harnessed for therapeutic ends, convinced that insane audience members were most likely to be susceptible to the looping effects of theatre. Farces and other comedies, so long as they were not too bawdy, provided a desirable model in which patients might lose themselves and, by imitating 'the sound and strong', become transformed. It is not clear whether Hurst had read Browne's work, but he certainly drew liberally on similar techniques, not only generating an optimistic 'atmosphere of cure' (like Browne's 'healthy tone') which made light of the patient's symptoms, but also creating opportunities for imitating recovered, or recovering, patients through watching them.

The idea that sensitive individuals, whilst at the theatre, might experience deep changes of both body and temperament, was a theme also explored by novelists of the late nineteenth century. H. G. Wells's short tale, *The Sad Story of a Dramatic Critic* (1897), explores the strange transformations wrought on a particularly impressionable spectator through repeated visits to a late nineteenth-century playhouse.[57] The hero, Egbert Craddock Cummins is a rather shy, slightly stuttering, and easily embarrassed young journalist, who has never set foot inside a theatre fearing its dangerous effects on the advice of his now-deceased Aunt Charlotte. It comes as something of a shock then, when Cummins is called into his editor's office and informed he has been appointed the paper's new dramatic critic. Cummins protests that he is unfit for the part, but the editor will not be swayed, and being a man of 'yielding disposition', the journalist returns home to dress for his first assignment. That evening, as the bell rings for the final call, Cummins finds himself lost 'in a lot of red plush passages', and ends up taking a seat in the gallery when he should have been in the stalls. It is the first of a series of comically embarrassing and confusing effects of his trip to the theatre. As the curtain rises on a modern-day scene, Cummins is gripped by an encroaching feeling of alarm. He is surprised and increasingly horrified by the phenomenal unnaturalness of the acting before him: the 'fantastic gestures, the flamboyant emotions, the weird mouthings, melodious snortings, agonising yelps, lip-gnawings, glaring

[56] W. A. F. Browne, 'The Moral Treatment of the Insane', p. 318; p. 332.

[57] H. G. Wells, 'The Sad Story of a Dramatic Critic', *The Plattner Story and Others* (London: Methuen, 1897), pp. 262–73.

horrors, and other emotional symbolism of the stage' appalls him. 'Purple with indignation', Cummins returns home to file his review, believing it his duty to reform these horrible excesses. That night, he dreams of actors, 'actors glaring, actors smiting their chests, actors flinging out a handful of extended fingers, actors smiling bitterly, laughing despairingly, falling hopelessly, dying idiotically'.

The following morning, standing before the bathroom mirror, Cummins notices that he has himself assumed a most peculiar gesture. 'I had flung up the left arm (fingers fully extended) and clutched at my diaphragm with my right hand.' Disconcerted, he repeats the gesture over and over again in the mirror, wondering what had made him do it. From that day forward, now going to the theatre almost every evening, Cummins's whole demeanour begins to change. He catches himself 'bowing ineffably' when he meets his most confused fiancée, Delia, 'stooping in an old-fashioned, courtly way over her hand'. At work, he notices himself 'doing "nervous business" fingers on teeth' when asked a difficult question, and clasping his hand to his brow during petty arguments. Cummins is confused by his own behaviour—'no one could be more keenly alive to the arrant absurdity of the histrionic bearing'—but gradually begins to understand what has been happening:

> The acting, I saw, was too much for my delicately strung nervous system. I have always, I know, been too amenable to the suggestions of my circumstances. Night after night of concentrated attention to the conventional attitudes and intonation of the English stage was gradually affecting my speech and carriage. I was giving way to the infection of sympathetic imitation. Night after night my plastic nervous system took the print of some new amazing gesture, some new emotional exaggeration—and retained it.

Like hysterical patients across Europe at the end of the nineteenth century, Cummins finds himself to be highly suggestible, the 'vivid impressions' of the actors leaving their traces on his nervous system turning his limbs and expressions into a carousel of theatrical postures and tics. He calls it a disease, a 'matter of contagion', and blames it squarely on the theatre: 'I have heard of stage-struck people before, and thought it a figure of speech.' For Wells, theatre, rather than the theatrical asylum, provides a suggestive metaphor for the bodily contagions of behaviour, and the transformations they engender. But for Cummins, the result is not merely temporary, but as intransigent as a hysterical illness. Alarmed by his own artificiality, he discovers it is not simply a character he can put on and take off like a coat, but that his new persona has grafted on to him, even transforming his involuntary reflexes, all the while leaving him acutely self-aware of the dislocation, the gap between the way he would like to behave and the movements he is compelled to perform. Self-conscious of the ludicrous gestures he enacts—'I grinned, and capered, and scowled and posed' he writes 'and knew—with what voiceless agony!—that I did it all the time'—Cummins is entombed in his 'dramatic casing'. His predicament calls into question the very possibility of an authentic being: 'a kind of theatrical veneer threatened to plate over and obliterate my private individuality altogether', he laments.

First published in 1897, Wells's story recalls a case study recorded by the French physician Gilles de la Tourette. His patient, a hysteric named O., reported, 'I have always been conscious of a predilection for imitation. A curious gesture or bizarre attitude affected by any one was the immediate signal for an attempt on my part at its reproduction, and is still.' As a result, O.'s symptoms were a 'veritable debauchery of absurd gesticulations, a wild muscular carnival' of odd gestures and unusual attitudes.[58] For both Cummins and O., watching led to imitation, and in turn, to the audience becoming the kind of spectators who also make theatrical spectacles of themselves. If theatrical audiences were part of the discourse around hysteria, so it seems that a hysterical compulsion to imitate was also part of an emerging anxiety about theatrical audiences. Following Tarde, who had declared in the 1890s that 'society is imitation, and imitation is a species of somnambulism', others working in the burgeoning field of crowd psychology believed theatrical audiences to be mobs, already primed to imitate.[59] In an article entitled *The Psychology of Theatre Audiences*, which drew liberally on le Bon and Tarde, the American drama critic Clayton Hamilton explained that 'even the most cultured and intellectual of men, when he forms an atom of a crowd, tends to lose consciousness of his acquired mental qualities and to revert to his primal simplicity and sensitiveness of mind'. This phenomenon, he continued, explained the practice of hiring claques at theatrical performances to amplify the audience's responses ('applause begets applause in the theatre, as laughter begets laughter and tears beget tears'), for above all, theatrical audiences could be defined by 'their credulity, their sensuousness, their susceptibility to emotional contagion, their incapacity for original thought'.[60] Hamilton's ideas were echoed in the work of the American psychologist George Elliott Howard, who argued in his article 'Psychology of the Spectator' (1912), that 'the spectator's emotions are highly suggestible' which in turn leaves them 'particularly exposed to the sway of suggestion-imitation', further arguing that

[58] Quoted in Meige and Feindel, *Tics and Their Treatment*, p. 2.

[59] Gabriel Tarde, *The Laws of Imitation* (1890), trans. Elsie Clews Parsons (New York: Holt, 1903) p. 87.

[60] Clayton Hamilton, *Theory of the Theatre: And Other Principles of Dramatic Criticism* (New York: Henry Holt and Company, 1910) pp. 30–58.

a 'mass of closely communicating individuals' might even be capable of forming 'without presence'.[61]

To contend that the patients at Netley were, like O. and like Cummins, first and foremost audience members rather than actors might seem to split hairs—after all, both O and Cummins end up actorly. Nonetheless, it is important to recognize that by the beginning of the twentieth century, the hysteric's predilection for imitation was allied not so much with being on stage, where the performer might enjoy some control over his or her mimicry, as being off it, where the spectator, like Cummins lost in the maze of plush, red passages in the theatre, was understood to be disorientated, susceptible, and regressed. Yet, this did not mean looking was understood to be an entirely passive experience either. For Hurst, being an audience in the 'atmosphere of cure', did not only mean being a piece of clay to be moulded in imitation of 'the sound and the strong'. It also required onlookers to participate in its delicate emotional ecosystem of optimism and nonchalance, to respond to scenes of terror and agony, not with cringes of empathy or horror, but with bright and encouraging smiles. As Hurst knew, the audience did not only experience theatre's transformative effects, it created them too.

POINTING AND LAUGHING: THE UNSYMPATHETIC SPECTATOR

Throughout the nineteenth century, the practice of displaying medical curiosities for an intrigued, and sometimes horrified, paying public, underwent a dramatic transformation. From travelling anatomy demonstrations and freak-shows, to shops like that described by Dickens in *Our Mutual Friend*, where 'Bones, warious. Skulls, warious. Preserved Indian baby', were jumbled up for sale, the relationship between commerce, entertainment, and the body came to be viewed with increasing suspicion by the medical establishment. By the second half of the century, hospital museums increasingly sought to distance themselves from these seedy commercial enterprises, envisaging a new kind of audience, one who did not gawp in curiosity or cringe in disgust, but gazed in quiet, sober, and learned contemplation. Some collections of morbid anatomies closed their doors to the public altogether. Others, as the historian Sam Alberti has described, attempted to condition the behaviour of visitors by

[61] George Elliott Howard, 'Psychology of the Spectator', *The American Journal of Sociology*, 18, 1 (1912) 33–50 (p. 38).

guards and guides and numerous signs instructing in appropriate behaviour. Body parts formerly available for palpating, poking, and even sniffing were now secured behind glass, and where previous visitors, repulsed and enthralled, had 'trembled with fear or winced in empathy', the new breed of visitor was now expected to perform an emotionally restrained and silent style of looking.[62] Just as across the channel, German-speaking nations distinguished between the excitable *Schaulustige* and the still gaze of the educated elite, in Britain to legitimately look at the suffering of others was also to gaze dispassionately, to be neither seen nor heard.

The story of the 'civilizing process' of anatomy museums in the nineteenth century is of course more complicated than this potted history suggests, not least because as Alberti reminds us, actual visitors to museums undoubtedly subverted these new conventions and broke the rules.[63] But the part played by the invention of cinematography in the display of medical artefacts adds another layer to this narrative of a fall from fleshy, multi-sensory engagement to a new 'scopic regime'. On the one hand, the display of unusual symptoms, growths, tumours, and even operations on film, might be understood to privilege the eye over the other senses, further distancing the spectator from the fleshy reality itself and creating opportunities for immobile 'gazing'. At the same time, however, it is clear from close attention to *War Neuroses* that the kind of spectatorship anticipated by this new amalgam of cinema and the pathologized body was far from straightforward. Indeed, in its layering of various competing representational schema, and in turn, the diverse medley of audience and emotional styles it seemed to expect, *War Neuroses* has more in common with the mix of business and pleasure in Mr Venus's taxidermy shop than any newly reorganized anatomy teaching collection.

On 12 March 1918, Hurst presented his finished film alongside a lecture on the treatment of shell shock to the Neurological Section of the Royal Society of Medicine. As if offering up a diseased limb in formaldehyde, or a photograph of a tumour, Hurst presented his film as 'a permanent record' of war neuroses, hoping that his 'kinematographic records' might serve future physicians in diagnoses and yield other 'results of

[62] Samuel J. M. M. Alberti, 'The Museum Affect Visiting Collections of Anatomy and Natural History', in Fyfe and Lightman (eds.) *Science in the Marketplace: Nineteenth-Century Sites and Experiences*, pp. 371–404 (p. 394).

[63] As Alberti notes, disgust and horror were certainly common responses to the morbid anatomies on display. One visitor confiding in his diary that a woman's corpse 'was horrible to look at', while another, in 1874, wrote to a colleague that the Hunterian's display of pathological stomachs was 'not very pleasant to contemplate'. See Alberti, 'the Museum Affect', p. 391.

scientific value'.[64] Hurst was not the first physician to have experimented with the cine-camera since its invention in 1895. In the laboratory, specially adapted lenses had given remarkable pictures of the kinetic dances of organisms too miniscule to be seen by the human eye. In hospitals too, doctors were able to document disorders of movement for the first time, and from 1899, films depicting patients started to appear alongside lectures in teaching hospitals and at international conferences.[65] Nonetheless, some of the practices around early forays into the use of film in the hospital were dubious to say the least. Hurst's request that the Netley convalescents should sham symptoms for the camera, was not without precedent: in 1905, the Boston neurologist Walter Greenough Chase had gone even further when, whilst documenting his epileptic patients at a colony near New York, he deliberately induced their seizures in order to capture them on film.[66] As Edgar Jones has pointed out, films were still an experimental medium in this period, and 'the ethics of their use for medical research and training had yet to be codified'.[67]

Nonetheless, a shared, one might say 'official', visual language was beginning to emerge by the 1910s. In a form reminiscent of Eadweard Muybridge's studies in human locomotion and Chase's neurological studies, many of the patients in Hurst's film appear stripped of any emotional or narrative context, and specimen-like, their naked, symptomatic bodies are the sole objects in the frame. These patients (there are only two out of the twenty-one cases recorded) are introduced not by name or history, but by diagnosis alone. 'Hysterical pseudohypertrophic muscular paralysis' is naked, except for a loin cloth. He circles an empty ward (the beds have been pushed to one side), his contorted body picked out against the featureless, whitewashed wall as he staggers and falls to the ground (17:52). In 'Hysterical contracture of hand persisting 35 months after wound near elbow', an intransigently clenched fist, its nails digging into the flesh of its owner's palm, is ghostly-white against in black screen (21:52, Figure 27). It is a style which recalls the German neurologist Max Nonne's own war neuroses film, in which trembling, semi-naked patients appear as almost

[64] Arthur Hurst, 'Cinematograph Demonstration of War Neuroses', *Proceedings of the Royal Society of Medicine*, 11 (1918) 39–42 (p. 39).

[65] Hanna Landecker, 'Microcinematography and the History of Science and Film', *Isis*, 97 (2006), 121–32 (p. 122); Rachael Low and Roger Manvell, *The History of the British Film, 1906–1914*, ii, 6 vols. (London: Allen and Unwin, 1973), p. 36.

[66] For a discussion of the techniques used by Walter Greenough Chase, see Lisa Cartwright, *Screening the Body: Tracing Medicine's Visual Culture* (Minneapolis: University of Minnesota Press, 1995) pp. 47–71.

[67] Jones, 'War Neuroses and Arthur Hurst', p. 347.

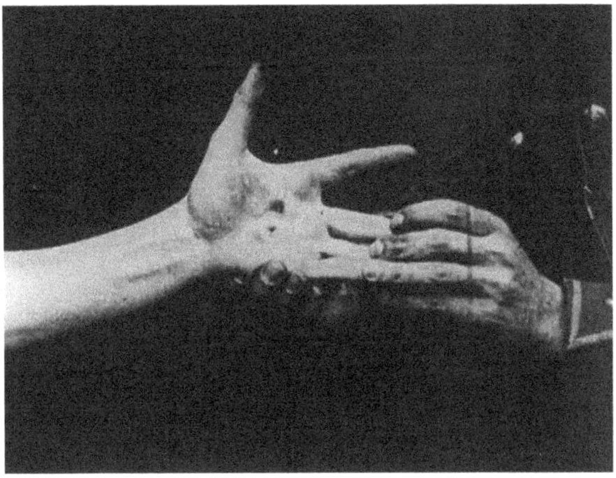

Fig. 27. 'Hysterical Contracture of the Hand' (21:52), Arthur Hurst and J. L. M. Symns, *War Neuroses*, Netley Hospital 1917, Seale Hayne 1918.

Wellcome Library, London

abstracted silhouettes.[68] In their use of stark pictorial conventions, as well as lack of information about the individual patient and the circumstances of his injury, these sequences invite an unsentimental relationship with the bodies on display. One might argue that, in the context of very early films, a lack of sentiment was always an impossibility. For early cinema audiences, the simple fact that a camera could capture such dynamic physiological movements evoked curiosity and excitement. In 1894, one of the first motion pictures, an advertisement for Edison depicting a close-up of an employee named Fred Ott sneezing, was released. *The Sneeze*'s success traded off the thrill of simply being able to witness a convulsive body caught on film: it was this sense of novelty and excitement which has led Tom Gunning to dub these early documentaries a 'cinema of attractions'.[69] By 1917, however, the initial excitement had presumably waned, the audience, for the most part, more au fait with cinema's magic.

[68] Max Nonne, *Funktionell-motorische Reiz und Lähmungs Zustände bei Kriegsteilnehmern und deren Heilung durch Suggestion und Hypnose*, Psychiatrische Klinik Hamburg-Eppendorf 1916. For further information about Nonne's film, see Paul Lerner, 'Hysterical Cures: Hypnosis, Gender and Performance in World War I and Weimar Germany', *History Workshop Journal*, 45 (1998), 79–101 (p. 79).

[69] Edison Kinetoscopic Record of a Sneeze (or 'Fred Ott's Sneeze'), 1894. Tom Gunning, 'The Cinema of Attraction: Early Film, it's Spectator and the Avant-Garde', *Wide Angle*, 6, 2 (1986), 63–70.

Yet, *War Neuroses* is far from cleansed of medical cinema's links with the world of entertainment. As the footage makes abundantly clear, Hurst sought to generate feelings of pleasure and amusement in the hearts and minds of those who encountered his 'kinematographic records'. *War Neuroses* bears many of the hallmarks of the jaunty government propaganda films, that were intended to shore up public support for the war, support that by 1916 was rapidly dwindling. Invalided soldiers, on their road to recovery, often appeared in these short pieces of persuasion—indeed, Hurst's patients were not the first to appear before the Pathé's cameras on Spike Island. In 1916, the company made *'Crocked' but Cheerful* (1916), an upbeat newsreel depicting amputee soldiers laughing uproariously whilst performing a parodic 'route-march', pushed along in wheelchairs and stretchered on the back of wagons. In a similar vein, '*Dr Thames begins his Summer Treatment*' (1916) shows a jolly band of war-wounded joking about whilst clambering aboard a boat for a restorative river trip. It is not entirely clear whether *War Neuroses* was ever intended to be shown to a general public: four separate and slightly differently edited versions of the footage survive. The fact that in one the words 'Pathé Weekly Pictorial' appear along the bottom is evidence that a wider distribution was at least considered, though it is clear that the film was never shown outside the medical establishment. Perhaps it was deemed too disturbing by censors at the Ministry of Information's Cinematograph Department to be shown to a public that, like Hurst's patients, were viewed as a highly suggestible and emotionally volatile mass.

But whether or not *War Neuroses* was intended as propaganda, its unnerving juxtaposition of illness and levity was for Hurst a core part of his programme of treatment at Netley. Arguing that 'sympathy which is misplaced is most harmful', Hurst encouraged a playful, even humorous response to his patients' symptoms.[70] He believed that laughter and fun could diffuse the war-wounded's obstinate pessimism about the possibility of recovery, and help cultivate a belief in the possibility of change. One example of Hurst's attempts to introduce levity is a series of ludicrous nicknames given to the lurching, wheeling gaits of the patients. It is a move that bizarrely foreshadows Monty Python's Ministry of Silly Walks. Cpl. Anderson's symptoms are introduced as a 'hysterical "dancing" gait': the patient appears to be jigging and tapping (10:29). Demonstrating his 'hysterical "wire spring" gait', Sgt. Peters' legs compress and then send him shooting forward (12:32). Hurst dubs Pte. Williams's case a 'hysterical "slippery ice" gait', and indeed, the patient appears to be negotiating a

[70] Hurst, *Medical Diseases of the War*, p. 235.

frozen pavement (13:01). These caricature nicknames, with their pleasurable frisson of recognition, certainly diminish the seriousness of the men's symptoms and frame their demonstrations of pathological gaits as slapstick turns.

Of course, all the convalescents who appear in *War Neuroses* are, in very real sense, acting. They make their exits and their entrances as they have been instructed to do, carrying out a self-conscious choreography of gestures and routines that keep their bodies centre-frame in the camera's immobile gaze. But in some cases their performances explicitly reference routines that would have been familiar to audiences of early twentieth-century music halls. Depicted walking and talking together, Ptes. King and Sandall are dubbed 'hysterical "stump orators"', ludicrous simulacra of already laughable rhetoricians whose symptoms developed in imitation of one another. As they slowly make their way towards the camera along a small paved street replete with an iron lamppost and Netley's belching gas works in the background, the pair are reminiscent of a comic double act, drunkenly staggering around on a street in a Victorian factory town. Like all good comedy duos, their skit relies on an incongruous play of status: King, who is older and rotund, wags his finger and lectures Sandall, all the while ridiculously slipping off the kerbstone; Sandall, who seems younger and lower-status than his blustering companion, meanwhile, jigs up and down, attempting to interrupt the diatribe (07:28, Figures 21 and 22). The film-maker Jean Epstein described Charlie Chaplin's performance of the Tramp (first recorded in the films *The Tramp* and *The Bank*, both 1915) as a choreography consisting entirely of 'the reflex actions of a nervous, tired person'.[71] As *War Neuroses* testifies, this relationship was in fact a two-way street, the depiction of reflex disorders in 'kinematographic records', and the comic skits of the music hall and later silent film, mutually constituted.

If Hurst encouraged an 'air of practical cheerfulness' among staff at Netley, believing that such an attitude would emphasize the impermanence of seemingly intractable symptoms, then *War Neuroses* solicits this same feeling. Cast in this light, the comic artery of *War Neuroses* seems an act of almost maniacal ambition on Hurst's part. Through the medium of film, his curative 'atmosphere' could extend beyond the asylum walls and encourage an unflinching and cheerful response to the horrors of war-torn hysterical bodies among medical professionals and even in the public at large. To fully appreciate the extent to which Hurst may have understood

[71] Jean Epstein, 'Magnification' (1921), trans. Stuart Liebman, quoted in Rae Beth Gordon, 'From Charcot to Charlot: Unconscious Imitation and Spectatorship in French Cabaret and Early Cinema', *Critical Inquiry*, 27, 3 (2001), 515–49 (p. 523).

the audiences of his film as co-actors in the creation of an atmosphere of cure, it is vital to appreciate the style of cinematic spectatorship that he envisaged. In contrast to the late twentieth-century cinematic voyeur who Laura Mulvey imagines as sitting hidden in the dark, alone, with the 'illusion of looking in on a private world', the early twentieth-century cinema audiences were closer in kind to the *Schaulustige*, whose passionate, gestured acts of spectatorship were themselves a show.[72]

From its very inception, going to the 'electric theatre' was an activity associated with experiencing visceral, volatile emotions, and performing them too. It is, in fact, in the passionate and self-conscious audiences of sensation theatre in the 1860s and 1870s that early cinema audiences find their clearest parallel. One of cinema's founding myths famously involved an audience flinching en masse. In 1895, the Lumière Brothers' unveiled a short film entitled *L'Arrivée d'un train en gare de la Ciotat*, in which a steam engine draws into a crowded station, appearing to come full-throttle towards to viewer before disappearing off the bottom left hand corner of the screen. The audience of the earliest screenings of this film were, so the legend goes, so panicked upon seeing the fast-approaching train that they rose up and fled the theatre. The tale of the mass exit from the theatre—a story which emerged some ten or fifteen years later—was almost certainly apocryphal, exaggerated to provide an amusing anecdote about the naïvety of early audiences who had not yet come to understand film's astonishing verisimilitude. Nonetheless, the anecdote put the performances of flinching bodies at the centre of this new kind of audience. According to the *Boston Herald* in 1896, the Lumière Brothers film was 'so realistic as to give those in the front seats a genuine start'.[73] The following year, Georges Brunel explained 'you get the feeling that the train is going to hit you and run you over...I was in the front row of spectators, some of whom drew back instinctively'.[74] Recalling the sensation theatre of the 1860s, in which audiences recoiled when water threatened to splash over the edge of the stage, the 'train effect' created a moment of visceral shock that moved spectators, pinning them to the back of their seats.

It was not only in their flinches and starts that early twentieth-century cinemagoers can be connected to an already established tradition of demonstrative spectatorship. At the outbreak of war, the 'pictures', were regarded a 'poor man's theatre', and an opportunity for some passionate

[72] Mulvey, 'Visual Pleasure and Narrative Cinema', p. 17.

[73] *Boston Herald*, 26 May 1896, p. 7, quoted in Charles Musser, *The Emergence of Cinema* (New York and Oxford: Maxwell Macmillan International, 1990) p. 118.

[74] Georges Brunel, *La Photographie et la Projection du Mouvement* (Paris, 1897) p. 61, quoted in Sephen Bottomore, 'The Panicking Audience? Early Cinema and the "Train Effect"', *Historical Journal of Film, Radio and Television*, 19, 2 (1999), 177–216 (p. 186).

audience participation. With its piano accompanist, and projectionist who had to beg 'one minute, please' to change the roll of film, early cinema, even with its luminous screen, did not allow for a complete immersion into the fictional world. As historian Nicolas Hiley has pointed out, cinemagoers were 'part of the performance', and had to 'learn not only the conventions of the screen but also the running jokes of the audience, as when "some vulgar member of the audience smacks his lips to imitate the kissing of lovers" '.[75] Their palpable enjoyment made cinemagoers the latest repositories for moral anxieties about looking which were already freely circulated. When war broke out, increasingly graphic depictions of life on the front line started to appear alongside newsreels shown in cinemas. In October 1916, the controversial documentary *The Battle of the Somme* was released in over two thousand theatres nationwide. Many praised its verisimilitude: 'this is the real thing. This is war, rich with death', proclaimed *The Cinema* magazine.[76] Meanwhile, in *The Times*, H. Hensley Henson, the Dean of Durham Cathedral, complained bitterly about 'crowds of Londoners' who 'feel no scruple at feasting their eyes on pictures which present the passion and death of British soldiers'. Calling the film 'an entertainment which violates the very sanctities of bereavement,' the Dean warned with surprising prescience that soon 'it will, perhaps, be thought decent to introduce the film-maker into the wards of the hospitals or into the operation theatre, or into the death-chamber of one's relatives'.[77] Despite the fact that working-class Londoners were likely to be 'feasting their eyes' on the deaths of their own sons, brothers, and friends, the Dean of Durham imagined the audience as hungry for the pleasures of horror, the spectacle of injury. Like the kind of audiences hospitals tried to dissuade from visiting their pathology collections, Henson's 'crowds of Londoners' were linked to a visceral, sensational style of spectatorship, deemed grossly inappropriate and unedifying.

One might imagine Hurst courted an aloof and unemotional audience for his medical film, the sort of audience the Dean of Durham might have approved of. In fact *War Neuroses* solicited the kind of pleasure-seeking, even sensational, watching that audiences of war films were already being criticized for enjoying. Recalling the medical students who purportedly laughed at the squeals of a cat during a vivisection experiment, the audiences framed by *War Neuroses* were simultaneously imagined to be studious experts and audiences

[75] Nicholas Hiley, 'The British Cinema Auditorium', in *Film and the First World War*, ed. Karel Dibbets and Bert Hogenkamp (Amsterdam: Amsterdam University Press, 1995) 160–70 (p. 160; pp. 162–3).

[76] *The Cinema*, 21 August 1916. Quoted in Michael Paris, *The First World War and Popular Cinema* (New Jersey: Rutgers University Press, 2000) p. 37.

[77] H. Hensley Henson, 'A Contrast and A Protest', *The Times*, 1 September 1916.

at a farce, tickled by the quirky carnival of symptoms displayed before them. Through Hurst's use of competing visual languages and framing strategies, the film's expectations of its audience refuses to settle: one moment we are kept at arm's length, the next, we find ourselves encouraged to participate, drawn into the fictions of the 'atmosphere of cure' by colluding in Hurst's mockery of his patients' symptoms. Today, this conflation of comedy and illness in *War Neuroses* is profoundly uncomfortable, not least because it shines a spotlight on our own complicity as spectators in what Didi-Huberman has called the 'terrible attraction of hysteria'.[78] Like the nurses who dart out of sight, we discover that we too have stumbled onto the set to become part of the show. Perhaps it is the 'kinematographic record' of Pte. King which most vividly arouses self-consciousness about our own complicity, making us appear to ourselves. In their temporary auditorium on the steps of one of Netley's colonnades, the audience of convalescents laughs as King lopsidedly makes his way towards the camera, his legs shaking. With the audience giggling and guffawing behind his back, King points his trembling finger directly into the camera lens, catching us momentarily in a terrible self-reflection (06:48, Figure 26). As we watch the audience laughing at King, the invalid's own gesture reminds us that we also participate in this scene of looking. Perhaps it serves as an accusation too.

TURNING ASIDE, LOOKING ASKANCE

In 2004, the video artist Douglas Gordon called it 'the bedroom aesthetic'.[79] Watching a film taped off the TV, curled up in bed, most probably in the dark, most probably alone, at night, close enough to touch the screen, holding a remote that will switch the film off or fast forward it or pause it at will, 'the whole story of me in the room and the film in the room and the story of the film no more and no less important than the story of me watching the film and inseparable from the room itself'.[80] The first time I watched *War Neuroses* was in 2007. I wasn't in a bedroom, but in a secluded corner of the Wellcome Library on the Euston Road, not in a bed, but in a large bright orange armchair, a rack of glossy periodicals to one side of me, a large metallic bookcase on the other. In front of me was a small TV monitor that flickered into life when I loaded the video cassette and pressed 'play'. In my private corner of a public space, performing a solitary, and increasingly guilty act of spectatorship, the story of what I was

[78] Didi-Huberman, *The Invention of Hysteria.*
[79] Katrina M. Brown, *DG: Douglas Gordon* (London: Tate Publishing, 2004) p. 25.
[80] Douglas Gordon, *What Have I Done* (London: Haywood Gallery Publishing, 2002) p.18.

watching and story of me watching it were becoming woven together. We were becoming 'inseparable'. And I remember distinctly that, as the first of the soldiers to demonstrate their symptoms and rapid recoveries wobbled across the screen, my body began to sink back into the foam padding of the chair. It wasn't a sudden recoil, like the fearful, horrified starts of the soldiers, or the 'perception in the form of shocks' that Walter Benjamin ascribed to the experience of watching films.[81] It was more gradual than that. As the final cue card disappeared and the screen went blank, and after sitting very still for several moments, I noticed that my body had become folded in on itself. The shoulders hunched, face averted and screwed up in a sort of grimace, knees drawn into the torso, encircled by arms and angled away from the screen. My face averted. It was a kind of wince or cringe. I realized that I had turned aside and had been watching the film askance, over my right shoulder.

Gordon used small fragments of *War Neuroses*, slowed down to 10mm per second and looped, to create two video installations. *10ms-1* (1994) and *Trigger Finger* were, at the time I first saw *War Neuroses*, on display at the Tate Modern in London. He intended these works to confront viewers with an uncomfortable choice. 'You can see that what is happening on screen might be quite painful—both physically and psychologically', he argued. 'But it has a seductive surface. What do you do—switch off or face the possibility that a certain sadistic mechanism may be at work?'[82] In her important and passionate book *Regarding the Pain of Others*, Susan Sontag asked similar questions about the appeal of images which documented real suffering. Like Gordon, she characterizes the act of looking at pictures from medicine's past depicting etiologies and treatments as a profoundly ethically problematic. 'Perhaps the only people with the right to look at images of suffering of this extreme order', she wondered 'are those who could do something to alleviate it—say, the surgeons at the military hospital where the photograph was taken—or those who could learn from it'. 'The rest of us are voyeurs', she concludes, 'whether we mean to be or not'. The rest of '*us*', she says, folding herself into the category of the accused whose primary interest is not the accumulation of useful knowledge, but something else—curiosity, the frisson of an illicit encounter, the ambivalent fascination with a tortured body, or what Georges Bataille called a 'stirring nostalgia for death'. As Sontag knew, there is drama and excitement in the dilemma of whether or not to look. The wavering between

[81] Walter Benjamin, 'On Some Motifs in Baudelaire' (1939) repr. in *Illuminations*, trans. Harry Zorn (London: Pimlico, 1999) 152–96 (p. 171).

[82] Douglas Gordon, Artist Statement, <https://www.tate.org.uk/modern/exhibitions/cinema/gordon.htm> accessed 22 January, 2011.

repellence and attraction plays itself out in a choreography of recoiling bodies. 'There is the satisfaction of being able to look at the image without flinching', she wrote, and 'there is the pleasure in flinching'.[83] Though Sontag's primary subject is a late twentieth-century saturation of media imagery depicting the dead and dying, the questions she asks about her own looking feel like an echo chamber for anxieties which were already in place a hundred years earlier—the worry that the spectacle of pain may provide spine-tingling, toe-curling amusements.

Sontag is not alone to wonder out loud about the implications of her fascination with the medical archives. The historian Ruth Richardson, in her compelling account of wandering around the stacks at the Wellcome collection, writes of an experiencing an uncanny intimacy with objects of childbirth's past. She cannot help imagining the pain suffered by the women on whose bodies such instruments were used, whose lives they saved or whose deaths they hastened.[84] If a capacity for empathy seems a useful tool for a cultural historian, there is a wealth of scholarship from trauma studies, which calls into question the very possibility of remaining emotionally aloof when confronted with such devastating images. As Dori Laub has put it in his work on gathering testimonies of Holocaust survivors, becoming party to such horrors creates a 'crisis of witnessing'. 'No observer could remain untainted, that is, maintain an integrity—a wholeness and a separateness—that could keep itself uncompromised, unharmed, by his or her very act of witnessing.'[85] Yet, the impossibility of keeping our distance and maintaining 'integrity' is only half of the problem. It's not only that we are affected by what we see, but that we affect it too.

War Neuroses sits at a provocative angle to this debate, because to be an emotional audience of Hurst's film—to be seduced by its imagery—is not simply to be a voyeur who watches rather than does, but in fact the opposite. The ethical problem presented by Hurst's film is that we might accidentally end up doing as well as watching, and moreover, doing something we might not particularly want to do at all. To watch *War Neuroses* as it was meant to be watched, to laugh along with its witticisms, to catch its mood of levity, to read and respond appropriately to its theatricalized world of illness *as* a theatrical audience, is a form of playing along which finds us

[83] Sontag, *Regarding the Pain of Others*, p. 37.

[84] Ruth Richardson, 'Human Remains', in *Medicine Man: The Forgotten Museum of Henry Wellcome*, ed. Ken Arnold and Danielle Olsen (London: British Museum Press, 2003) pp. 319–45.

[85] Dori Laub, 'Truth and Testimony: The Process and the Struggle', in *Trauma: Explorations in Memory*, ed. Cathy Caruth (Baltimore: Johns Hopkins University Press, 1995) pp. 61–75 (p. 66).

not only legitimating, but more importantly, participating in a cure being enacted. While the nineteenth century's pursuit of objectivity might be read as an attempt to circumvent the impact of the observer on the field they observed, in the case of Hurst's experiment at Netley, these looping effects were deliberately called forth. For the soldiers who convalesced at Netley, their own acts of perception transformed, in very real ways, the world they encountered. Because of hypercuosis, the men heard noises others could not. Through their distorted flinch reflexes, they experienced danger where there was none, their bodies creating the world anew. As audience members in the wards and during the film-making process, they learnt to diminish the symptoms of others, remoulding their own bodies in the process. As spectators, then, the patients at Netley were simultaneously impressionable recipients of, and active participants in, its 'atmosphere of cure'. The audience of Hurst's film was similarly conceived. To be a 'good' spectator—that is, the kind of spectator Hurst requested—is to legitimate his 'atmosphere of cure' and give credence to the very idea that the malady of war neurosis was more than a little fictional. To laugh along with *War Neuroses*, in the manner of the giggling convalescents who attend Pte. King's kinematographic record, is to be cast in Hurst's immersive and transformative production: to act, to do, as well as to watch. At least part of what makes *War Neuroses* so disturbing to encounter at the beginning of the twenty-first century is precisely the experience of negotiating these solicitations, the demands the film makes upon us as its audience. As spectators we may find ourselves folded into the same regime of visibility the patients themselves have come to inhabit, our watching staged in Hurst's grand theatrical transformation.

There are many reasons why one might turn aside whilst watching *War Neuroses*. Looking away might be a gesture of resistance, a way of refusing the film's lure; or it might be an outward show of disgust, deliberately aimed to reassure any passer-by in the library that there is no pleasure in this horrifying duty, only work. At the same time, wincing may make the film easier to watch: by not meeting the eyes of the patients it depicts, it becomes easier to turn them into a spectacle. As did Leontius's flinches from the corpses outside Athens's city walls, our recoils might betray the illicit and conflicted pleasures of morbid fascination which turn the dead into entertainment. All the same, turning one's face aside can be an impulse born of fellow feeling when we find ourselves, like Hephaestus flinching and groaning as the humans meet defeat on the battlefields, unable to tolerate the spectacle of the suffering casualties of war. Or perhaps we might simply find ourselves embarrassed, and withhold our association—we speak, after all, of *giving audience*—from the desperately mugging figures on the screen before us. Delia, the dramatic critic's fiancée in H. G. Wells's story, is repelled by her husband-to-be's self-conscious posturing in the art gallery. 'Egbert,' Delia said, 'you are not yourself':

> 'Ah!' Involuntarily I clutched my diaphragm and averted my head (as is the way with them)
> 'There!' she said
> 'What do you mean?' I said, whispering in vocal italics.

Delia breaks off the engagement there and then, and Cummins responds with a ludicrous catwalk display of grimacing poses. One is a histrionic flinch: 'I clutched my diaphragm and averted my head.' Yet, rather than move empathetically towards the grief or misery of her ex-fiancée, his self-consciousness curdles Delia's feelings and squeamishly she turns aside: 'she looked into my working face and winced.'[86] If the earliest meanings attached to the word 'flinch' hint at betrayals of trust and secrets, at the severing of the bonds of criminal allegiance, then Delia's flinch, and my own, broke a tacit spectatorial pact—or what Kathy O'Dell has called the 'contract' the spectator makes—by withholding the kind of audience that the performance unashamedly courted.[87]

In wincing at *War Neuroses*, we might also turn away from the crowd of other spectators who appear in the film, and who are part of the film's attempts to coax its audience in. In his diaries, Guy de Maupassant described the experience of trying to resist becoming absorbed by a curious crowd. Seeing a wedding party emerge from a church, de Maupassant found himself among a group of passers-by who had all stopped to gawp. 'I at once experienced a curious and unbearable feeling of discomfort, a horrible unnerving sensation as though I were struggling with all my might against a mysterious and irresistible influence', he wrote. He tried to turn aside, to avoid looking with the rest of the passers-by who had stopped to stare, but 'in truth, I struggle with the spirit of the mob, which strives to take possession of me', he confessed.[88] Feeling oneself on the verge of being swallowed up in the 'spirit of the mob' was an anxious predicament which, as I have explored throughout this book, was already being worried about at the end of the nineteenth century, identified repeatedly as a distinctive experience of theatregoers. But if such audiences make a spectacle of themselves, like the German *Schaulustige* who gawped, laughed, and pointed at the humans in the compounds before them, those attempting to withdraw from the crowd are left even more exposed.

[86] Wells, 'The Sad Story of a Dramatic Critic', p. 526

[87] Kathy O'Dell, *Contract with the Skin: Masochism, Performance Art and the 1970s* (Minneapolis: University of Minnesota Press, 1998).

[88] Guy de Maupassant, *Afloat* (*Sur l'eau*, 1888), trans. Laura Ensor (London: Routledge, 1889) p. 158, quoted in Jaap van Ginneken, *Crowds, Psychology and Politics, 1871–1899* (Cambridge: Cambridge University Press, 1992) p. 1.

Like the nurses who darted out of view, attempting to hide ourselves can both be prompted by, and add fuel to, an excruciating experience of spectator's stage fright. We might cringe to minimize our presence, to shrink from view, to not be seen to look—but in doing so we become more conspicuous than ever; in hiding we become all the more part of the spectacle. Paying attention to these embodied encounters with the intolerable images of the last century may suggest a way to think about how emotions and gestures form part of the choreography of looking in the twenty-first. Rather than passive recipients of imagery, we find ourselves engaged in a reciprocal play wrought through the dynamic interactions of bodies in space.

By the end of the war, Arthur Hurst had treated hundreds of shell-shocked soldiers at Netley hospital, many of whom had arrived suffering exaggerated or inopportune flinch-reflex responses. Shunning both the physical punishments and talking therapies used by his colleagues, he relied on a treatment by immersive theatrics. At the heart of Hurst's treatment was the cultivation of an 'atmosphere of cure' in which the patients' spirits—and their belief in the possibility of recovery—were buoyed by the performances of the nurses and doctors, as well as by the demonstration of recovering and recovered patients to new arrivals. While *War Neuroses* might not at first glance appear to demonstrate the techniques Hurst used, it is clear that the process of film-making itself facilitated Hurst's theatre, making its cure through self-staging, watching, and imitation possible. Cultural historians such as Didi-Huberman and Showalter have rightly compared the exhibition of nineteenth-century asylum patients to actors in a theatre, but in Hurst's film the convalescing soldiers also appear as audience members, as highly pliable and susceptible to the emotions of others, at the same time as being self-conscious about their own performances. The film did not only depict this distinctive set of emotional and performing audience members, but also sought out active participation from those who watched it, folding them into the 'atmosphere of cure'. Through courting passionately performing spectators, Hurst's *War Neuroses* created its own theatrical and transformative exchange: audiences were not simply asked to gaze, but to join in, to become themselves part of the show.

Afterword: A Report to the Academy

In 1917, Franz Kafka published a short story, 'A Report to an Academy'. It is written in the form of a dramatic monologue, narrated by a monkey named Rotpeter, or Red Peter. To an audience of experts, the 'esteemed gentlemen of the academy', Rotpeter recounts his life story of how a wild animal, after being captured off the Gold Coast, 'penetrated into a human world and established himself there'. The first thing the monkey learnt from humans was how to shake hands. 'A handshake betokens frankness', he confides, with not a little irony, since he is a consummate performer, and the relationship between signifying gestures and the meanings they betoken is far from straightforward in his world. Over the next five years, the monkey's mimicry becomes increasingly sophisticated, until he attains 'the cultural level of the average European'. He takes up a place on the variety stage, attends dinners, and exhibits himself at scientific soirées. The lecture, given before an audience of experts, who silently gaze back, involves none of the invention of his theatrical career, or so Rotpeter claims. It simply narrates the facts. 'I wish only to spread knowledge, I am only reporting; to you, too, esteemed gentlemen of the academy', he insists at the end of his lecture. 'I have only made a report'.[1]

Rotpeter's emphatic insistence that his story is neither fiction nor contains subjective evaluations, but is impersonally a report, strikes a defensive note. Not least, because it follows on swiftly from a moment of accidental disclosure in his otherwise flawless performance. Reflecting at the end of the monologue on his current situation, Rotpeter describes his relationship with his female companion. He can only tolerate her in the darkness: 'by day, I have no wish to see her; for she has that wild, confused look of the trained animal in her eye; no one but me can recognize it, and it is more than I can bear.'[2] Rotpeter turns aside from his companion's obliging performances, unable to endure her confusion. For Rotpeter, witnessing his companion's puppet-like enactments, the repetition of learnt phrases, the

[1] Franz Kafka, 'A Report to An Academy', in *Metamorphosis and Other Stories*, trans. Malcolm Pasley (London: Penguin, 2000) pp. 187–95 (p. 188; p. 195).

[2] Kafka, 'A Report to An Academy', p. 195.

performance of tricks she will never understand, is a kind of humiliation for both monkeys. But crucially, this admission interrupts and betrays the monkey's smooth performance. Disclosing his own inability to look at his companion, Rotpeter reveals uncomfortable feelings about his own imposture. In turning aside, Rotpeter shows himself unable to bear the theatricality that has become an inevitable and ingrained part of his own being too.

At this moment in 'A Report to an Academy', readers are confronted with three nested audience-performer relationships, and are invited to compare them. At the centre is Rotpeter's encounter with his companion's awkward aping of humans: he cannot look at her, but turns aside in shame. The next is the relationship of the silently watching scientific gentlemen to Rotpeter. What are we to make of that? Do they also, at the moment of his confession, see the 'look of a wild confused trained animal' in Rotpeter's eyes, and embarrassed by their own proximity to the monkey, turn away? The scientific gentlemen mirror a third audience—the readers. On hearing of Rotpeter's flinch from his companion, do we also find ourselves confronted with the uncomfortable spectacle of our own imposture? Are we, like Rotpeter, punctured by the realization that the behaviour we have come to take for granted as human and civilized, may in fact be a mere performance grafted onto us over time? Kafka's story may be read straightforwardly as a tale about the ape in all of us, about the animal vestiges which linger beneath the apparently socialized exterior of the 'average cultivated European'.[3] Scratch the surface, and we are all trained creatures with confused looks in our eyes. But actually, Kafka's tale presents a far more troublesome relationship between theatrical performance and the animal 'real' than that. Rotpeter's animal instincts and his human behaviour are blended to such a degree that it is impossible to distinguish between what he has become and what he used to be. We are unable to tease apart the 'real' and the 'fictional' in the animal's body, and perhaps in the bodies of the 'esteemed gentlemen of the academy' too. In Kafka's story, theatricality and pretence are not so much second nature, as they have become part of nature itself.

This book has argued that theatricality remained deeply engrained in the late nineteenth century's flurry of interest in the physiology of emotions and sensations. Even in the context of an increasingly professionalized and codified scientific practice, theatrical techniques and problems remained an important experimental resource. Theatre did not only make appearances in dramatic displays of the latest scientific discoveries before an eager public. It was also an important experimental apparatus that made certain kinds of comparatively solitary acts of scientific enquiry possible. If experimenters drew on theatrical techniques to stage the emotional responses

[3] Kafka, 'A Report to An Academy', p. 195.

of their subjects for scrutiny, anxieties about theatricality and its disruptions also lingered in their conclusions, in particular, the conception of the reflex body as increasingly malleable and prey to deception which emerged in this period. Not entirely in command of itself or its affects, sliding between automatism and pretence and entangled in a web of relationships with other audiences and other performers, by the beginning of the twentieth century, the emotional and sensory body had been refashioned as a theatrical self in which the line between truth and fiction was smudged. In the 1870s, Darwin suggested that mimicry might be one of the mechanisms through which we develop emotional expressions and responses. By the beginning of the twentieth century, the perennial trouble with theatre—the impossibility of distinguishing between authentic emotions and their representations—not only haunted scientific observers in their act of looking, but had become ingrained in the structure of the body itself.

The nineteenth century has been identified as the age of objectivity, a time in which the human body was mapped and relentlessly categorized. Yet, even those who we most associate with the construction of this stable body of knowledge in the nineteenth century—and Darwin, Ferrier, and Head are certainly among them—were not immune from the disruptive and destabilizing effects of theatrical representation. Increasingly alert to their own performances and at pains to withdraw from the scene of looking so as not to disrupt the phenomena they sought to understand, at the same time these observers experienced the uncanny dislocations, self-consciousness, and 'ontological queasiness' familiar to theatrical audiences. In the four case studies discussed in this book, the relationships scientific observers staged with their subjects echoed similar encounters between audiences and performers in the theatre. Like the audiences of sensation theatre who went to the theatre to enjoy their feelings of shock and horror in the 1870s, Darwin's experiments left him alert to his own emotional performances. Just as, in the new vogue for theatrical naturalism, spectators hid under cover of darkness spying in on intimate scenes of domestic life in the 1880s, so Ferrier lurked behind doors acutely self-conscious of his own presence, hoping to avoid being caught watching by his experimental monkey. Henry Head's attempts to enter meditative states of reverie during his experiments in nerve-regeneration were, in the early twentieth century a common feature of the experience of theatre audiences who hoped to enjoy an unmediated sensory connection with the artist on stage. And in Arthur Hurst's experimental treatment at Netley hospital, both medical staff and patients took on the roles of audience members who were simultaneously impressionable, self-conscious, and capable of influencing others through their own passionately performed responses. Not only the audiences depicted on camera, but those imagined by Hurst as witnesses to the finished spectacle, highlighted the fact that practices previously associated with audiences of sensation theatre re-emerged among early cinemagoers. In each of these four examples, scientific experimenters enacted techniques of passionate and gestured looking usually attributed to theatrical audiences. At the same time, they shared the queasy frustrations of theatre-going when the physical world they sought to study became opaque and unstable, its emotional outsides and insides unreliably corresponding.

One of the conclusions we can draw from this study is that, though conventionally regarded as very different and incompatible fields of human endeavour, by the end of the nineteenth century forms of theatrical and scientific looking were mutually constitutive. Cultural historians have already recognized that the late nineteenth-century architects of theatrical naturalism drew on ideas about scientific looking for their self-legitimization, and that theatrical displays were also part of the creation of the period's scientific knowledge. Yet, in this period which emphasized the importance of experimentation and observation, which championed self-recording technologies for measuring the fickle, fleeting physiological human experiences, which demarcated an objective gaze as the stance of the professionally detached scientist, and which approached the question of human emotions and sensations in physiological, observable terms, scientific experimentation drew on theatrical practices too. In the last three decades, historians and philosophers of science have emphasized the heterogeneous spaces and practices of nineteenth-century science, drawing attention to the reciprocal relationship between theories and practices, between public demonstrations and private experiments, and between iterative laboratory performances and the knowledge they produced. The nineteenth century's innovations, many of which underpin much of our own scientific culture, were not dreamt up in heroic isolation, but rather institutions, available technologies, laboratory practices, and methods of communication irrevocably shaped the substance of scientific knowledge. What, then, might be at stake in arguing that, alongside the camera and cardiograph, theatre was one of technologies which shaped modern experimental practice, and in turn our own physiological conception of the emotional and sensory body? As Iwan Morus has recently suggested, it seems 'relatively passé' to talk of the politics of knowledge nowadays, but nonetheless, one of the implications of this kind of interdisciplinary work is to draw attention to the deep interdependence of disparate fields of knowledge, particularly at a time when the relative value of the humanities is under such scrutiny.[4]

[4] Iwan Morus, 'Placing Performance', *Isis*, 101 (2010), 775–8 (p. 777).

As the examples discussed in this book have shown, the relationship between theatre and scientific experiments in this period was not an entirely straightforward one. It was one shaped more by theatre's vicissitudes than its successes, coming to the foreground most readily when scientific observers found themselves attempting to negotiate the distinctive problems of theatre—its slippery tricksiness, its 'ontological queasiness', its uncoupling of emotional form and content, and its failures of transparency. Untrustworthy relationships between outward signs and inward feelings troubled both Darwin and Ferrier's looking, while Head found the self-consciousness of his own theatrical performance deeply distracting. Rather than simply approaching these sticking points as obstacles to scientific knowledge, the problems of looking experienced by Darwin, Ferrier, Head, and Hurst may be regarded as extremely revealing, as repositories for wider anxieties about the instability of the body raised by their experiments. Certainly, the untrustworthiness of theatre and its audiences became an important conceptual resource to articulate a vision of the emotional and sensory body which felt increasingly estranged, de-centred, and out of voluntary control. Darwin was amused by his own involuntary flinch from the puff adder, but there was something disturbing too about the idea of a body responding despite its own intentions, a body whose behaviours were always already imitations of those performed in other times and places. In his experiments to map the brain centres of sensory experience, the responses of monkeys were not always legible, the line between gestures which were spontaneous and those performed in imitation of others, hard to draw. For Henry Head, the discovery of wandering tactile sensations in his left arm drew attention to the untrustworthiness of sensory experience, a misperception built into the physiology of pain and pleasure itself. By 1918, the malleability of the body and its visceral responses had become so accepted that it also came to be deliberately manipulated for the purposes of a treatment. The defensive reflexes were no longer seen as reliable reactions to outer stimuli, but responses which could be transformed under the influence of imagination, sympathy, suggestion, experiences all made possible by the theatrical exchange of both being, and having, an audience. One of the questions this history of flinching raises, then, concerns the genealogy of what contemporary scholars in the humanities and social sciences have dubbed 'the affective turn'. This 'affective turn' emphasizes the dynamic and mutual relationships between minds and bodies, feelings and actions. Often with recourse to scientific models that emphasize forms of indeterminacy— the language of small particles, quantum physics, and information theory, among them—affect theorists have undermined cherished notions of autonomous, subjective human emotion by describing sensations hopping like parasites between subjects and bodies vibrating together. According to one of its leading theorists Patricia Clough, the model of individual emotional agency and subjectivity which the affect theory calls into question was one forged in the crucible of the nineteenth-century human sciences. 'What we are facing', she writes, 'is the necessity to rethink the relationship of the social sciences, the humanities, and the sciences of the nineteenth and early twentieth centuries, a relationship that for so long has informed what we take matter to be, what we take bodily forms of life to be, what we take technology to be, what we take sociality and subjectivity to be—or not to be'.[5] Yet, as the examples discussed in this book suggest, late nineteenth-century scientific practice also undermined the idea of a stable organism, calling into question the possibilities of individual intention and the ownership of emotions. In the questions they raised about the malleability of the body, the composite nature of emotional expressions, and the transmission of feelings in groups, late nineteenth-century psychologists, neurologists, and physiologists were not altogether out of step with today's theorists of the post-human and the destabilized bodily interactions they seek to articulate.

The scientific looking conventionally associated with nineteenth-century modernity is one modelled on mechanical objectivity and characterized by the self-restraint of a silent, still, and gazing witness who does not intervene. As I have argued in this book, in practice, observation in the late nineteenth-century human sciences was understood in diverse ways. This is not to deny that the rhetoric of a penetrating gaze was dominant in this period, but to argue that the concept was far from stable. Constituted through a range of often contradictory sites and practices, objective looking was not always incompatible with the emotional and theatrical performances of the scientific witnesses. While scientific observers may have intentionally flinched, for example, during self-experiments or in their attempts to shrink out of view, winces and starts also interrupted their sustained gaze and foregrounded the scientist's own choreography of looking, closing the gap between observer and the field he observed. The pursuit of objectivity required that efforts were made to minimize the disruptive effects of the observer's own emotional presence: Darwin was anxious that watching the emotions of others would rouse his own, causing him to detect feelings that may or may not be present; Head acknowledged that embarrassment and a desire to 'get it right' might cause him to distort his self-reports. Yet, the fact that they were eager to minimize

[5] Patricia Ticineto Clough, 'Afterword: The Future of Affect Studies', *Body and Society*, 16, 1 (2010), 222–30 (p. 223).

distortions certainly did not mean these scientific observers were naïve to the looping effects of their own presence. Rather, their strategies for looking contained an acceptance that as observers, they were very much *there*. In many ways, the simmering worries late nineteenth-century scientific observers expressed about their own presence found a clear resolution in the 1920s, in Werner Heisenberg's 'uncertainty principle'. At its simplest level, the 'uncertainty principle' acknowledged that the mere fact of observing and measuring changed the phenomena observers tried to quantify.

The examples discussed in this book, which span a period of fifty years remind us that scientific objectivity was not a separate category, but that experimental observation was deeply embedded in other cultural models of looking already in circulation during this period. Though self-recording machines have been identified as the dominant model for scientific looking, techniques of theatrical audiences were an important practical resource and conceptual reference point. Alongside the *flâneur*, the panopticon, the camera, the X-ray or the sphymograph, we can identify a self-consciously affective pattern of spectatorship in the practice of scientific observers, a motif typified by the demonstrative and emotional performances of theatrical audiences. And if theatregoers modelled this kind of looking, flinching was one of its most immediate expressions. It is a type of looking summed up by the German word *Schaulustige*—the excitable, impressionable spectator who looks as well as performs, who plays at watching but also plays at being seen. Recognizing this pattern of multi-sensory, gestured, and impassioned spectatorship, which straddled the worlds of theatre and science in the nineteenth century, expands our understanding of how Victorians thought about their acts of looking: they did not simply 'gaze' *at*, but became visible to themselves and each other as performing, participatory bodies. This recognition should contribute to our already rich understanding of the multiple and contrasting ways looking was thought and written about in a period whose concerns about spectatorship anticipate many of our own.

From Darwin's flinch in the Reptile House, to the audiences who recoiled from *L'Arrivée d'un train en gare de la Ciotat*, by the beginning of the twentieth century flinching, wincing, and starting was firmly embedded in the spectatorial repertoire. And whilst scientific experimenters sought to understand the movement as a physiological reflex, subject to external manipulation and leaving us open to self-deception, its 'thick' meanings continued to link the gesture to vacillation, cowardice, and untrustworthiness. In its exploration of flinching, this book has alighted on numerous instances of wincing and cringing, following the bodily movements of recoiling, shrinking, and turning aside as they move through diverse settings. Each brings into focus the gesture's many overlapping and complementary meanings, each aggregate adding further to the significance that this seemingly innocuous movement has for thinking about the social experience of spectatorship. Rather than providing a psychologizing, or even biologizing, account of these winces and cringes, the vignettes in which they appear serve to remind us that affects and sensations can also have a life of their own. Though flinches and winces might form part of illicit or fugitive language of the body, they can also become unmoored from the realm of the intentional subject, entering the social fabric, hopping between their hosts and stretching the potentials of their communication and meaning in unforeseen ways. My aim in this book has been to tell stories about this fragile network of flinches, winces, starts, and cringes, in a period when they came most under scrutiny. On the one hand, this book has explored the regimens of scientific knowledge through which the flinch became an evolved and involuntary reflex, and addressed the social and political networks that interpolated the gesture through which it accrued its thick meanings as a 'speck of behaviour, a fleck of culture'.[6] On the other, it has approached the task of writing a history of flinching through explorations of mutual intensifications, meanings unmade, and significations scrambled. As Brian Massumi has put it, 'feelings have a way of folding into each other, resonating together, interfering with each other, mutually intensifying, all in unquantifiable ways', and a history of them may echo this form.[7] My approach in this book has endeavoured to identify repeating patterns of emotional, gesturing, and self-conscious spectatorship, echoing across a broad cultural surface at the end of the long nineteenth century. But it has also aimed to draw attention to the interference in those patterns, and to moments when they crease or fold together in unexpected ways.

According to Walter Benjamin, in an essay he wrote on the tenth anniversary of Franz Kafka's death, transient bodily movements offer insights that language alone can not always provide. 'Each gesture is an event', he wrote, '—one might even say, a drama—in itself'. Bodily gestures accrue significance in Kafka's writing through their 'ever changing contexts and experimental groupings'. Less important is the 'motivation' of any gesture, than the way it breaks out or wanders, transcending accustomed behaviours, linking disparate people, times, and places loosely together in patterns.[8] Tracing the journeys of flinches, starts, cringes, recoils, and winces, through these strange constellations has been my aim in this book,

[6] Geertz, 'Thick Description', p. 3.
[7] Massumi, *Parables for the Virtual*, p. 1.
[8] Benjamin, 'Franz Kafka', p. 117.

a peripatetic endeavour which has taken circuitous routes and wandered over the boundaries between disciplines. Indeed, flinching seems aptly suited to such an approach. While the flinch gestures towards a delicate fabric of fine connections—of sympathetic resonances, contagious imitations, and viscerally felt complicities—it also speaks of shirking, avoiding, wandering off, and looking askance.

APPENDIX

Transcription of Ferrier's Notebooks Regarding Experiment F

A NOTE ON THE TRANSCRIPTION

Every effort has been made to transcribe the notebooks as accurately as possible. Where the handwriting was hard to read, I searched for comparisons in the following two published accounts of the experiments: David Ferrier and Gerald F. Yeo, 'A Record of Experiments on the Effects of Lesion of Different Regions of the Cerebral Hemispheres'; David Ferrier, 'Schäfer on the Temporal and Occipital Lobes'. Where no comparisons were available, I have omitted the illegible sentences and replaced them with bracketed ellipses. David Ferrier's experimental notebooks are kept at the Royal College of Physicians Heritage Centre, London (full details can be found in the bibliography).

Experiment F, 22 June 1881

Small monkey
Exposed the region of the superior tempero–sphenoidal convolution on both sides . . . and both were destroyed by means of the actual cautery directed along their course with the aid of a director.

3.35pm
Placed in cage alone, it dozed for some minutes then suddenly lurched up wide awake. Came to bars of cage and climbed up hand on hand, clinging properly with hands . . . now hanging on to the bars. . . . His companion in next cage is making plaintive howls but not the slightest sign of reaction is given by F who does not turn his head.

3.45pm
Touching its hands or feet with the point of a pencil causes the animal to withdraw its hands sharply as if from pain. It lurches about and places its hands on the bars of cage clearly without sight.

5.30pm
Animal well—moves about. . .. Companion allowed in cage with it, went to it when it saw it. Not the slightest indication of hearing it. Various sounds made, whistle, tapping the bars . . . No attention to whistling . . . the companion always started. So other monkeys with same sounds.

23 June 1881

5.30pm
F is today very dull and drowsy-looking. Some oedema of face and eyelids. Right eye partially closed. Left eye open. Put out its hand and took hold of its companion sitting near it and eating a piece of bread. Pays no attention, does not even open its eyes when the loudest sounds [are made] which startle all the other monkeys... whistling, tapping close to its ear &c.... Oil of Bergamot 'placed on a rod and held at its nostrils' causes it to apparently smell and make movements with his lips. Acetic acid causes it to sneeze and make signs of irritation, retracting its head sharply. Acetic acid placed on lips causes it to lick and make movements of tongue and mouth of tasting. Salt does the same. After observing its actions for half an hour there is no doubt that it sees perfectly well, as it can see its companion and goes about from one cage to the other through small door... Pays no attention whatever to whistling in its ear. Does not even open its eyes when this was done repeatedly. Turned away its head from whistling close to its ear.

25 June 1881

4.30pm
F is quite bright and active. Runs about, picks up pieces of food. Peers eagerly through bars at what is going on. Seizes hold of things offered. Took a piece of date, smelt it and threw it down; so also a piece of bread. Took, smelt and ate apparently with relish a cold boiled potato. It is very quiet... Pays no attention to sounds which caused the others to look startled, failed to excite the attention of F. Scratching sound which caused F's neighbours to be always very frightened caused not the slightest semblance of hearing in the part of F. This done on both sides of cage... with precisely similar results.

5.30pm
Have spent an hour testing in various ways F's hearing, certainly this is not absolutely established. The animal is... running about, climbing, hitting things on its cage, and always comes eagerly towards the bars of cage when I was in sight. Going down to the place where the animals are kept, sets all the others on the *qui vive*. No sign of this on the part of F.

7 July 1881

F is well and active. Experiments made with percussive caps. Occasionally seems to start, but other times pays no attention. After numerous experiments by Dr Yeo, still in doubt as to any sign of hearing. The dressings removed today; all aseptic; wound perfectly healed. The ears are now mobile and seem to twitch at sounds?

On 7 July, Ferrier and Yeo operated on F's companion, monkey G, another small probably Macacque, monkey. In this experiment the middle temporo–sphenoidal convolution was exposed in its upper half on both sides, and both were similarly operated on.

8 July 1881

Hearing tested and not the slightest difference observable. Animal well.

12 July 1881

A percussive cap applied caused G to start, while F paid no attention. The other monkeys also very much startled. G answers calls I make, F never. F only grunts. When it starts it is to anything in sight, never in reply to sounds.

25 July 1881

Have made numerous experiments now to test the hearing of F. G and F are together, but as to the response of G to sounds no question whatsoever.... This afternoon, at six, made an interesting experiment while sitting in the cage with its companion (G), and both quite still and engaged in examining each other. I made repeatedly a scraping sound on floor with foot as if going up to cage. The companion G invariably opened its eyes and looked up, whereas there was never any sign on the part of F. Made several experiments with electric bell placed against side of cage. On ringing it, the companion was at first very anxious about the sound, while F paid no attention, but after a time it ceased to regard it. Cannot be sure whether the animal hears at all, but certainly is not at all disturbed by sounds which make the others start, twitch ears, wink &c. No twitching of the ear in F. Otherwise perfectly well. Runs about; is very expert in catching flies, which it watches carefully and pursues skilfully. Very much on the alert to all that goes on, and occasionally utters a grunt if it sees anything like water, food, &c. which it wants. Never, however, replies by grunts to those of its companions, and is generally perfectly silent. Formerly it was continually in the habit of grunting &c. in reply to name &c.

27 July 1881

Owing to the death of G, F, which has been disconsolate, and occasionally uttering plaintive cries, was transferred yesterday to the cage of C (hemiplegic). The two seemed to agree tolerably well, with the exception of squabbles as to food—C being very indignant and occasionally attacking F for seizing the food first. Made various experiments as to hearing, and it seems that the signs of reaction (which have caused so much doubt) to sounds are less evident. The electric bell was transferred to the side of its cage. Ringing it suddenly caused C to be very much disturbed and annoyed, whereas F. paid no attention whatever. Coming downstairs to the place where the animals are kept, I observed C looking out attentively, but F remained in back of cage, not coming forward until such signs on the part of C as to attract notice. Repeated percussion cap experiment several times. C invariably started, but today I failed to detect any unequivocal indication of this on the part of F. As to other sounds—calling, whistling &c.—F pays no attention whatever, whereas the attention of the other monkeys is at once excited. The animal is excessively on the alert, and it follows every movement, and is with difficulty surprised.

29 July 1881

The percussion cap experiment repeated today several times in the presence of Dr Yeo and J. G. Romanes, was every time negative, causing no reaction or starting, while its companion was invariably much startled and annoyed.

> *4 August 1881*
>
> The animal was exhibited today before the Physiological section of the International Medical Congress. A percussion cap was exploded close to it several times before the audience, and it gave no sign whatever of starting; whereas C started very emphatically.
>
> *12 December 1881*
>
> The animal has kept in excellent health, and is most lively, and continually engaged in active gymnastics. Many experiments were made with the view of testing its hearing. Sometimes it appears to start when a pistol cap is exploded, so that occasionally it is judged to hear. Today tried the experiment of calling from the top of stairs. The other monkeys are both on the alert, looking eagerly and making sounds of expectation; but F pays no attention whatever and goes on with its own occupation quite unheeding. It does not pay any attention to scratching on cage as others do, and in general does not respond to sound-calls &c.... It does not utter sounds in reply to calls. Occasionally, when left all alone, it utters a short cry of loneliness.
>
> *31st March 1882*
>
> While sitting today having its back scratched, a pistol cap was exploded close to cage; not the slightest start, thought the others, and Mr N. who was scratching the monkey, made a sudden start.
>
> *27 July 1882*
>
> The animal has remained well and lively without showing any new symptom, and still to all appearances exactly in the same condition as before as regards hearing. Today, made another series of observations of the animal while in its cage, and also after it was removed and placed in a small cage on table. Loud whistling, knocking, ringing electric bells in the neighbourhood failed to elicit any sign of attention. Occasionally, as before, there was an appearance of a start, or a look round, apparently conditioned by the noise, but repeated experimentation showed that this was pure coincidence.

Although I was unable to find a record of this in the notebooks, Ferrier and Yeo's description of the experiment in the Philosophical Transactions of the Royal Society, source reveals:

> Six months after the operation the animal was in the same condition, in excellent health and spirits, and deficient in nothing but hearing. Sounds which always attracted the attention of the monkeys failed to elicit any signs of perception. When the experiment was tried of one person going to a distance out of sight, while another watched, and the one in the distance called the monkeys as if coming with food, &c., all the others would go to the bars of the cage and watch eagerly, while this animal would go on with its occupation quite unheedingly.
>
> Thirteen months after the operation the condition was unchanged. The animal was perfectly well, in full possession of its other faculties, but manifestly totally deaf.
>
> It was killed with chloroform.

Bibliography

ARCHIVES

Cambridge University Library, Cambridge, *Darwin Papers*, DAR59.2 DAR53.

Royal College of Physicians Heritage Centre, London, *David Ferrier Notebooks*, 1873–1883, GB 0113 MS–FERRD.

Wellcome Library for the History of Medicine, London, *Henry Head Papers*, PP/HEA.

PRIMARY PRINTED SOURCES

Anon., 'The Fatal Accident in the Zoological Gardens', *The Times*, 23 October 1852.

Anon., *The Eclectic Magazine of Foreign Literature, Science and Art*, 31 (New York: Bidwell, 1854)

Anon., *A Journal of Medical Science Literature, Criticism and News*, 2 vols. (London: John Churchill, 1864).

Anon., 'Theatre Royal', *Birmingham Daily Post*, 12 November 1867.

Anon., 'The Tichborne Case. Advertisements and Notices', *Daily News*, 8 July 1871

Anon., 'Drama', *Daily News*, 6 May 1872.

Anon. 'Correspondence. The Royal Bull Hunt at Chillingham', *The Examiner*, 26 October 1872.

Anon., 'Darwin in the Drawing-Room', *The Globe*, 7 November 1872.

Anon., 'The Expression of the Emotions in Man and Animals', *The Times*, 13 December 1872.

Anon., 'An Act to Amend the Law Relating to Cruelty to Animals', *Public General Statutes Passed in the Thirty-Ninth and Fortieth Years of the Reign of Her Majesty Queen Victoria, 1876* (London: Queen's Printing Office, 1876) pp. 459–64.

Anon., 'Sensation Science', *Funny Folks*, 28 September 1878.

Anon., 'Hengler's Cirque', *The Era*, 1 January 1881.

Anon., 'Public Amusements', *Reynold's Newspaper*, 2 January 1881.

Anon., 'Sensational Dramas', *The Era*, 22 January 1881.

Anon., 'Theatres', *The Graphic*, 19 March 1881.

Anon., 'The Decay of Drama', *The Times*, 17 June 1881.

Anon., 'An Gnattempted Sensation', *Judy*, 26 October 1881.

Anon., 'The Court Theatre', *The Times*, 9 November 1881.

Anon., 'The Charge against a Vivisectionist', *The Daily News*, 18 November 1881.

Anon., 'The Charge against Professor Ferrier', *The Times*, 18 November 1881.

Anon., 'The Vivisection Case', *Glasgow Herald*, 18 November 1881.

Anon., 'The Vivisection Case', *The Leeds Mercury*, 18 November 1881.

Anon., 'The Charge against Professor Ferrier under the Vivisection Act: Dismissal of the Summons', *The British Medical Journal*, 2, 836 (1881).

Anon., 'Obituary, Gerald Yeo', *Nature*, 80 (1909), 314–15.

Anon. 'The Heroism of the British Army', *The Times*, 31 August 1914.

Anon. 'News from the Front', *The Times*, 7 September 1914.

Archer, William, *Henry Irving, Actor and Manager* (London: Routledge, 1883)

—— *Masks or Faces? A Study in the Psychology of Acting* (London: Longmans, 1888).

—— (ed.) *Three Plays By Maurice Maeterlinck* (London and Glasgow: Gowans & Gray, 1911).

Balance, Charles, 'The Thomas Vicary Lecture: Being a Glimpse into the History of the Surgery of the Brain', *The Lancet*, 1 (1922), 111–16.

Baldwin, James Mark, *The Story of the Mind* (London: George Newnes, 1899).

Barrett Browning, Elizabeth, *Poetical Works* (London: Elder, 1897).

Beard, G., 'Experiments with the Jumpers or Jumping Frenchmen of Maine', *The Journal of Nervous and Mental Disease*, 7 (1880), 487–90.

Bennett, Hughes, Rickman J. Godlee, 'Hospital for Epilepsy and Paralysis, Regent's Park: Excision of a Tumour from the Brain', *The Lancet*, 2, 3199 (1884) 1090–1.

Bergson, Henri, *Laughter: An Essay on the Meaning of the Comic* (1900), trans. Cloudesley Brereton and Fred Rothwell (London: MacMillan, 1911).

Boring, Edwin G., 'Cutaneous Sensation after Nerve-Division', *Quarterly Journal of Experimental Physiology*, 10 (1916), 1–95.

Boucicault, Dion, *The O'Dowd* (London and New York: Samuel French, 1908).

Braddon, Mary Elizabeth, *Belgravia*, vol. 66 (London: Willmer and Rogers, 1888).

Browne, W. A. F., *What Asylums Were, Are and Ought to Be* (Edinburgh: Black, 1837).

—— 'The Moral Treatment of the Insane; A Lecture', *British Journal of Psychiatry*, 10 (1864), 309–37.

Bunn, Alfred, *The Stage: Both Before and Behind the Curtain*, 3 vols. (London: Bentley, 1840).

Burdon Sanderson, J., *A Handbook for the Physiological Laboratory* (Philadelphia: Blackiston, 1884).

Carlyle, Thomas, *Critical and Miscellaneous Essays* (Boston: Phillips, Sampson and Company, 1858).

Cobbe, Frances Power, 'Vivisection and its Two-Faced Advocates', *Contemporary Review*, 41 (1882), 610–26.

Cook Eliza, *Eliza Cook's Journal*, 12 vols. (London: John Owen Clarke, 1850).

Cunningham, Peter, *Handbook of London Past and Present* (London: Murray, 1850).

Darwin, Charles, *On the Origin of Species* (London: John Murray, 1859).

—— 'Review of Contributions to an Insect Fauna of the Amazon Valley. By Henry Walter Bates, Esq.', *Natural History Review*, 3 (April 1862), 219–24.

—— *The Descent of Man, and Selection in Relation to Sex* (London: John Murray, 1871).

—— *The Expression of the Emotions in Man and Animals* (London: Murray, 1872).

Diamond, H. W., 'On the Application of Photography to the Physiognomic and Mental Phenomena of Insanity', *Proceedings of the Royal Society*, 8 (1856), 117.

Diderot, Denis, *The Paradox of Acting* (1773/1830) trans. Walter Herries Pollock (London: Chatto & Windus, 1883).

Dudgeon, R. E., *The Pathogenetic Cyclopaedia: A Systematic Arrangement and Analysis of the Homeopathic Materia Medica* (London: Samuel Highley, 1850).

Engel, Johann Jacob, and Henry Siddons, *Practical Illustrations of Rhetorical Gesture and Action, Adapted to the English Drama*, trans. Henry Siddons (London: Richard Phillips, 1807).

Ferrier, David, 'Experimental Research in Cerebral Physiology and Pathology', *West Riding Lunatic Asylum Reports*, 3 (1873), 30–96.

——'Pathological Illustrations of Brain Function', *West Riding Lunatic Asylum Reports*, 4 (1874), 30–62.

—— 'Cerebral Localisation. The Marshall Hall Prize Oration', *Medico-Chirurgical Transactions*, 67, 3 (1884), 33–49.

—— *The Functions of the Brain*, 2nd edn. (London: Smith, Elder and Co., 1886).

—— 'Schäfer on the Temporal and Occipital Lobes', *Brain*, 11, 1 (April 1888), 7–30.

—— and Gerald F. Yeo, 'A Record of Experiments on the Effects of Lesion of Different Regions of the Cerebral Hemispheres', *Philosophical Transactions of the Royal Society of London*, 175 (1884), 479–564.

Godwin, William, *Fleetwood, or, the New Man of Feeling* (1805), (London: Bentley, 1853).

Hall, Marshall, 'On The Reflex Function of the Medulla Oblongata and Medulla Spinalis', *Philosophical Transactions of the Royal Society of London*, 123 (1833), 635–65.

Hamilton, Clayton, *Theory of the Theatre: And Other Principles of Dramatic Criticism* (New York: Henry Holt and Company, 1910).

Head, Henry, 'On Disturbances of Sensation with Especial Reference to the Pain of Visceral Disease' *Brain* 16 (1893), 1–130.

—— 'Sensation and the Cerebral Cortex', *Brain*, 41, 2 (1918), 58–202.

—— *Studies in Neurology*, 2 vols. (London: Hodder & Stoughton, 1920).

—— and Gordon Holmes, 'Sensory Disturbances From Cerebral Lesions', *Brain*, 34, 2–3 (1911), 102–254.

—— and James Sherren, 'The Consequences of Injury to the Peripheral Nerves in Man', *Brain*, 28, 2 (1905), 116–338.

Henson, H. Hensley, 'A Contrast and A Protest', *The Times*, 1 September 1916.

HM Stationery Office (HMSO), *Report of the War Office Committee of Enquiry Into 'Shell-Shock'*, (London: HMSO, 1922).

Hobhouse, John, *Recollections of a Long Life* (London: W. Clowes & Sons, 1865).

Howard, George Elliott, 'Psychology of the Spectator', *The American Journal of Sociology*, 18, 1 (1912), 33–50.

Hughlings Jackson, John, 'A Study of Convulsions', *Transactions of the Saint Andrews Medical Graduate Association*, 3 (1870), 162–204.

—— *Clinical and Physiological Researches on the Nervous System* (London: Churchill, 1875).

Hurst, A. F., 'Cinematograph Demonstration of War Neuroses', *Proceedings of the Royal Society of Medicine*, 11 (1918), 39–42.

—— *War Neuroses*, Netley Hospital, Seale Hayne, *Pathé Frères*, 1918.

—— *Medical Diseases of the War*, 2nd edn. (London: Edward Arnold, 1918).
—— and J. L. M. Symns, 'The Rapid Cure of Hysterical Symptoms in Soldiers', *The Lancet*, 192 (1918), 139–41.
Irving, Henry, *The Drama* (London: Heinemann, 1893).
James, William, 'What is an Emotion?' *Mind*, 9 (1884), 188–205.
—— *The Principles of Psychology*, 2 vols. (New York: Holt, 1890).
—— *Psychology: A Briefer Course* (London: Macmillan, 1892).
Lewes, George Henry, *Sea-Side Studies* (London: Blackwood and Sons, 1858).
—— *On Actors and the Art of Acting* (London: Smith, Elder & Co., 1875).
—— *Problems of Life and Mind*, 5 vols. (London: Trübner, 1879).
Lewis, Leopold, *The Bells: A Drama in Three Acts* (London: Samuel French, 1871).
MacCormac, William, *Transactions of the International Medical Congress, Seventh Session*, 4 vols. (London: J. W. Kolckmann, 1881).
Marey, Etienne Jules, *La Méthode Graphique dans les Science Expérimentales* (Paris: Masson, 1878).
de Maupassant, Guy, *Afloat* (*Sur l'eau*, 1888), trans. Laura Ensor (London: Routledge, 1889).
Meige, Henry and Eugene Clement Louis Feindel, *Tics and Their Treatment*, trans. S. A. K. Wilson (London: Sidney Appleton, 1907).
Mogg, Edward, *Mogg's New Picture of London and Visitor's Guide to its Sights* (London: Mogg, 1848).
Morley, Henry, *The Journal of a London Playgoer* (London: Routledge, 1891).
Mosso, Angelo, *Fear* (1884), trans. E. Lough and Frederich Kiesow (London and New York: Longmans, 1896).
Mott, Frederick W., 'The Effects of High Explosives on the Central Nervous System', *The Lancet*, 187, (1916), 331–8.
Myers, C. S., 'A Contribution to the Study of Shell-Shock', *The Lancet*, 1, 13 (February 1915), 316–20.
Paget, James, 'President's Address', *British Medical Journal*, 2, 1075 (6 August 1881), 195–8.
Parsons, J. H., 'The Psychology of Traumatic Amblyopia Following Explosions of Shells', *Proceedings of the Royal Society of Medicine (Neurological Section)* 8, 2 (1915), 55–65.
Ribot, T. H., *The Diseases of the Will*, trans. Merwin-Marie Snell (Chicago and London: Open Court, 1896).
Rivers, W. H. R *Instinct and the Unconscious* (Cambridge: Cambridge University Press, 1920).
—— and Henry Head, 'A Human Experiment in Nerve Division', *Brain*, 31 (1908), 323–450.
Romanes, George, *Mental Evolution in Animals* (New York: Appleton, 1884).
Sherrington, Charles Scott, *Integrative Action of the Nervous System*, (New Haven: Yale University Press, 1906).
Sully, James, *Studies of Childhood* (New York: Appleton, 1896).
Tarde, Gabriel, *Laws of Imitation* (1890) trans. Elsie Clews Parsons (New York: Holt, 1903).

Trotter, Wilfred and H. Morriston Davies, 'Experimental Studies in the Innervation of the Skin', *Journal of Physiology*, 38 (1909), 134–246.

Walkley, A. B., *Dramatic Criticism* (London: John Murray, 1903).

—— 'Eleonora Duse in *La Dame aux Camélias*', *The Times* (16 June 1900).

Watson, John B. and Rosalie Rayner, 'Conditioned Emotional Reactions', *Journal of Experimental Psychology*, 3, 1 (1920), 1–14.

Wells, H. G., *The Plattner Story and Others* (London: Methuen, 1897).

Whewell, William, 'Mary Somerville's *On the Connexion of the Physical Sciences*', *Quarterly Review*, 51, 101 (1834), 54–68.

Yeo, Gerald, 'The Practice of Vivisection in England', *Fortnightly Review*, 37 (1882) 352–68.

SECONDARY SOURCES

Anon., dir. *The Battle of the Somme* (1916) (Trustees of the Imperial War Museum, ADTSTW004, 2008).

Anon., dir. *'Crocked' But Cheerful* (1916) British Pathé Archives, 1860.39). Available at <http://www.britishpathe.com/video/crocked-but-cheerful/query/crocked+but+cheerful> accessed 4 November 2013.

Anon., dir. *Dr Thames Begins His Summer Treatment* (1918) (British Pathé Archives, 1894.47). Available at < http://www.britishpathe.com/video/dr-thames-begins-his-summer-treatment-river-trip/query/189447> accessed 4 November 2013.

Anon. 'Obituary—Sir David Ferrier', *British Medical Journal*, 1, 3407 (1928), 525–6.

Anon., 'Obituary—Sir David Ferrier', *The Lancet*, 211, 5456 (1928), 627–9.

Anon. 'Obituary, Sir Arthur Hurst', *British Medical Journal*, 2, 292 (1944), 292–3.

Alberti, Fay Bound ed., *Medicine, Emotion and Disease, 1700–1950* (Basingstoke: Palgrave Macmillan, 2006).

Altman, Lawrence K., *Who Goes First? The Story of Self-Experimentation in Medicine* (Berkley and London: University of California Press, 1998).

Armstrong, Isobel, *Victorian Glassworlds: Glass Culture and the Imagination 1830–1880* (Oxford: Oxford University Press, 2008).

Arnold, Ken and Danielle Olsen, *Medicine Man: The Forgotten Museum of Henry Wellcome* (London: British Museum Press, 2003).

Babington, Anthony, *Shell Shock: A History of the Changing Attitudes to War* (London: Cooper, 1997).

Baer, Marc, *Theatre and Disorder in Late Georgian London* (Oxford and New York: Oxford University Press, 1992).

Barham, Peter, *Forgotten Lunatics of the Great War* (London and New Haven: Yale University Press, 2007).

Barish, Jonas A., *The Antitheatrical Prejudice* (Berkeley and London: University of California Press, 1981).

Barthes, Roland, *Camera Lucida* (1982) trans. Richard Howard (London: Vintage, 1993).

Beer, Gillian, *Darwin's Plots: Evolutionary Narrative in Darwin, George Eliot and Nineteenth-Century Fiction* (London: Routledge & Kegan Paul, 1983).

——*Open Fields: Science in Cultural Encounter* (Oxford: Clarendon Press, 1996).

Bell, Charles, *Anatomy and Philosophy of Expression* (London: Longmans, 1806).

Bending, Lucy, *The Representation of Bodily Pain in Late Nineteenth-Century English Culture* (Oxford: Clarendon, 2000).

Benjamin, Walter, *Illuminations*, trans. Harry Zohn (London: Pimlico, 1999).

Bennett, Susan, *Theatre Audiences: A Theory of Production and Reception* (London: Routledge, 1990).

Bentham, Jeremy, *The Panopticon Writings*, ed. Miran Bozovic (London: Verso, 1995).

Bentley, Eric ed., *The Theory of the Modern Stage: An Introduction to Modern Theatre and Drama* (Harmondsworth: Penguin, 1976).

Bettelheim, Bruno, *Freud and Man's Soul* (London: Chatto & Windus, 1982).

Brown, Katrina M., *DG: Douglas Gordon* (London: Tate Publishing, 2004).

Biesenbach, Klaus, *Douglas, Gordon, Timeline* (New York: MOMA, 2006).

Blanchard, Pascal et al. eds., *Human Zoos: Science and Spectacle in the Age of Colonial Empires* (Liverpool: Liverpool University Press, 2008).

Blau, Herbert, *The Audience* (Baltimore and London: Johns Hopkins University Press, 1990).

von Bonin, Gerhardt, trans. and ed., *Some Papers on the Cerebral Cortex* (Springfield, IL: C. C. Thomas, 1960).

Borch-Jacobsen, Mikkel, *Making Minds and Madness: From Hysteria to Depression* (Cambridge: Cambridge University Press, 2009).

Boring, E. G., 'A History of Introspection', *Psychological Bulletin*, 50, 3 (1953), 169–89.

Bottomore, Stephen, 'The Panicking Audience? Early Cinema and the "Train Effect"', *Historical Journal of Film, Radio and Television* 19, 2 (1999), 177–216.

Bourke, Joanna, *Dismembering the Male: Men's Bodies, Britain and the Great War*, (London: Reaktion Books, 1996).

Brecht, Bertolt, *The Messingkauf Dialogues* (1942) trans. John Willett (London: Methuen, 1977).

Brennan, Teresa, *The Transmission of Affect* (Ithaca: Cornell University Press, 2004).

Brontë, Charlotte, *Villette* (1853), (Oxford: Oxford University Press, 2008).

Brown, G. H. ed. *Lives of the Fellows of the Royal College of Physicians of London*, 4 vols. (London: Royal College of Physicians, 1955).

Bunn, Geoffrey C., A. D. Lovie, and G. D. Richards eds., *Psychology in Britain: Historical Essays and Personal Reflections* (Leicester: BPS Books, 2001).

Burdett, Carolyn, 'Is Empathy the End of Sentimentality?' *Journal of Victorian Culture*, 16, 2 (2011), 259–274.

—— '"The subjective inside us can turn into the objective outside": Vernon Lee's Psychological Aesthetics', *19: Interdisciplinary Studies in the Long Nineteenth Century*, 12 (Spring 2011), 1–31.

Burke, Edmund, *A Philosophical Enquiry* (1757) (Oxford: Oxford University Press, 1998).

Burrows, Jon, *Legitimate Cinema: Theatre Stars in Silent British Films, 1908–1918* (Exeter: University of Exeter Press, 2003).

Bynum, W. F., *Science and the Practice of Medicine* (Cambridge: Cambridge University Press, 1994).

—— R. Porter and M. Shepherd eds., *The Anatomy of Madness: Essays in the History of Psychiatry*, 2 vols. (London and New York: Tavistock, 1985).

Camp, Pannill, 'Theatre Optics: Enlightenment Theatre Architecture in France and the Architectonics of Husserl's Phenomenology', *Theatre Journal*, 59 (2007), 615–33.

Carson, Peter trans. and ed., *Anton Chekhov, Plays* (London and New York: Penguin, 2002).

Cartwright, Lisa, *Screening the Body: Tracing Medicine's Visual Culture* (Minneapolis: University of Minnesota Press, 1995).

Clarke, Edwin and L. S. Jacyna, *Nineteenth-Century Origins of Neuroscientific Concepts* (Berkley and London: University of California Press, 1987).

—— and Charles Donald O'Malley, *The Human Brain and Spinal Cord: A Historical Study Illustrated by Writings from Antiquity to the Twentieth Century* (Berkeley: University of California Press, 1996).

Claude Bernard, *An Introduction to the Study of Experimental Medicine* (1865) trans. H. Copley Greene (London: Macmillan, 1927).

Clough, Patricia Ticineto, 'Afterword: The Future of Affect Studies', *Body and Society*, 16, 1 (2010), 222–30.

Colligan, Colette and Margaret Linley, *Media, Technology and Literature and the Nineteenth Century: Image, Sound, Touch* (Farnham: Ashgate, 2011).

Collins, Wilkie, *Man and Wife* (1870), (Oxford: Oxford University Press, 1995).

—— *Heart and Science*, (1883), ed. Steve Farmer (Peterborough: Broadview, 1997).

Conan Doyle, Arthur, *The Sign of Four* (1890) (London: Penguin, 2001).

Connor, Steven, *The Book of Skin* (London: Reaktion Books, 2004).

—— 'The Shakes: Conditions of Tremor', *The Senses and Society*, 3 (2008) 205–20.

Cooke, Lynne and Karen Kelly eds., *Double Vision: Stan Douglas and Douglas Gordon*, (New York: Dia, 2000).

Cottingham, John, Robert Stoothoff, and Dugald Murdoch trans. and eds., *The Philosophical Writings of Descartes*, 2 vols. (Cambridge: Cambridge University Press, 1985).

Crary, Jonathan, *Techniques of the Observer: On Vision and Modernity in the Nineteenth Century* (Cambridge, MA and London: MIT Press, 1992).

—— *Suspensions of Perception: Attention, Spectacle and Modern Culture*, (Cambridge, MA and London: MIT Press, 2000).

Darwin, Charles, *The Expression of the Emotions in Man and Animals* (1872) ed. Paul Ekman (Oxford and New York: Oxford University Press, 1998).

Daston, Lorraine and Peter Galison, 'The Image of Objectivity', *Representations*, 40 (1992), 81–128.

—— and Gregg Mitman eds., *Thinking with Animals: New Perspectives on Anthropomorphism* (New York: Columbia University Press, 2005).

Davis, Jim and Victor Emeljanow, *Reflecting the Audience* (Iowa City: University of Iowa Press, 2001).

Davis, Tracy and Thomas Postlewait eds., *Theatricality* (Cambridge: Cambridge University Press, 2003).

Dekker, Thomas, *The Honest Whore* (1604), (London: Nick Hern, 1998).

Deleuze, Gilles, *The Logic of Sense*, ed. Constantin V. Boundas, trans. Mark Lester with Charles Stivale (London: Continuum, 2004).

—— and Félix Guattari, *A Thousand Plateaus: Capitalism and Schizophrenia*, trans. Brian Massumi, new edn. (London: Continuum, 2004).

Diamond, Michael, *Victorian Sensation, or, the Spectacular, the Shocking, and the Scandalous in Nineteenth-Century Britain* (London: Anthem Press, 2003).

Dibbets, Karel and Bert Hogenkamp eds., *Film and the First World War* (Amsterdam: Amsterdam University Press, 1995).

Dickens, Charles, *Oliver Twist* (1838), (London: Penguin, 2003).

—— *The Old Curiosity Shop* (1841), (London: Penguin, 1972).

—— *Bleak House* (1853) (London: Penguin, 1996).

Didi-Huberman, Georges, *The Invention of Hysteria. Charcot and the Photographic Iconography of the Salpêtrière*, (1982) trans. Alisa Hartz (Cambridge, MA and London: MIT Press, 2003).

Dixon, Thomas, *From Passions to Emotions: The Creation of a Secular Psychological Category* (Cambridge and New York: Cambridge University Press, 2003).

—— 'The Tears of Mr Justice Willes', *Journal of Victorian Culture*, 17, 1 (2012), 1–23.

Dobson, George, *Dobsons Drie Bobbes: A Story of Sixteenth Century Durham*, ed. Ernest Alan Horsman (London: Oxford University Press, 1955).

Dror, Otniel E., 'The Affect of Experiment, The Turn of Emotions in Anglo-American Physiology, 1900–1940', *Isis*, 90 (1999), 205–37.

Eliot, George, *Daniel Deronda* (1876), (London: Penguin 1995).

Finger, Stanley, *Minds Behind the Brain: A History of the Pioneers and their Discoveries* (Oxford: Oxford University Press, 2000).

—— *Origins of Neuroscience: A History of Explorations into Brain Function* (Oxford and New York: Oxford University Press, 2001).

Fischer-Lichte, Erika, 'Theatricality: A Key Concept in Theatre and Cultural Studies', *Theatre Research International*, 20, 2 (1995), 85–9.

Flint, Kate, *The Victorians and the Visual Imagination* (Cambridge: Cambridge University Press, 2000).

Foucault, Michel, *Madness and Civilization*, trans. Richard Howard (London and New York: Routledge, 2002).

——*The Birth of the Clinic* trans. A. M. Sheridan (London and New York: Routledge, 2009).

Freud, Sigmund, *The Standard Edition of the Complete Psychological Works of Sigmund Freud*, ed. James Strachey, 24 vols. (London: Hogarth Press, 1955).

Fried, Michael, *Absorption and Theatricality: Painting and Beholder in the Age of Diderot* (Berkley: University of California Press, 1980).

—— *Art and Objecthood: Essays and Reviews* (Chicago: University of Chicago Press,1998).

Fyfe, Aileen and Bernard Lightman eds., *Science in the Marketplace, Nineteenth-Century Sites and Experiences* (Chicago and London: University of Chicago Press, 2007).

Gaines, Jane M. and Michael Renov eds., *Collecting Visible Evidence* (Minneapolis, University of Minnesota Press, 1999).

Garner, Stanton B., Jr., 'Artaud, Germ Theory, and the Theatre of Contagion', *Theatre Journal*, 58, 1 (2006) 1–14.

—— 'Introduction: Is there a Doctor in the House? Medicine and the Making of Modern Drama', *Modern Drama*, 51, 3 (2008), 311–28.

Gebauer, Gunter and Christoph Wulf, *Mimesis: Culture, Art, Society* (Berkeley and London: University of California Press, 1995).

Geertz, Clifford, *The Interpretation of Cultures* (New York: Basic Books, 1973).

Gilman, S. L., *The Face of Madness: Hugh W. Diamond and the Origin of Psychiatric Photography* (New York: Brunner-Mazel, 1976).

van Ginneken, Jaap, *Crowds, Psychology and Politics, 1871–1899* (Cambridge: Cambridge University Press, 1992).

Glenn, Penny H. and Matti Buzi Bruckner eds. *Worldly Provincialism: German Anthropology in the Age of Empire* (Ann Arbor: University of Michigan Press, 2003).

Goffman, Erving, *The Presentation of the Self in Everyday Life* (1959), (New York and London: Penguin, 1990).

Goldstein, Jan, *Console and Classify: The French Psychiatric Profession in the Nineteenth Century* (Chicago and London: University of Chicago Press, 2001).

Gordon, Douglas, *What Have I Done*, (London: Haywood Gallery Publishing, 2002).

Goodall, Jane, *Performance and Evolution in the Age of Darwin: Out of the Natural Order* (London: Routledge, 2002).

Gooding, David, Trevor Pinch, and Simon Schaffer eds., *The Uses of Experiment: Studies in the Natural Sciences* (Cambridge: Cambridge University Press, 1989).

Gordon, Rae Beth, 'From Charcot to Charlot: Unconscious Imitation and Spectatorship in French Cabaret and Early Cinema', *Critical Inquiry*, 27, 3 (2001), 515–49.

Green-Lewis, Jennifer, *Framing the Victorians: Photography and the Culture of Realism* (Ithaca: Cornell University Press, 1996).

Gunning, Tom, 'The Cinema of Attraction: Early Film, it's Spectator and the Avant-Garde', *Wide Angle*, 6, 2 (1986), 63–70.

Hacking, Ian, *Representing and Intervening: Introductory Topics in the Philosophy of Natural Science* (Cambridge: Cambridge University Press, 1983).

Hadley, Elaine, *Melodramatic Tactics: Theatricalized Dissent in the English Marketplace, 1800–1885* (Stanford: Stanford University Press, 1995).

Hamilton, Susan ed., *Animal Welfare and Anti–Vivisection 1870–1910: Nineteenth -Century Woman's Mission*, 3 vols. (New York: Routledge, 2004).

Harpin, A. and J. L. H. Foster eds., *Considering Performance, Madness and Psychiatry: Isolated Acts* (Basingstoke: Palgrave, 2014) (in press).

Hardy, Thomas, *Far from the Madding Crowd* (1874), (London: Penguin, 2003).

—— *The Return of the Native* (1878), (London: Penguin, 1999).

Harrison, Charles and Paul Wood eds., *Art in Theory, 1900–1990: An Anthology of Changing Ideas* (London: Blackwell, 1993).

Hartley, Lucy, *Physiognomy and the Meaning of Expression in Nineteenth-Century Culture* (Cambridge: Cambridge University Press, 2001).

Hoare, Philip, *Spike Island: The Memory of a Military Hospital* (London: Fourth Estate, 2001).

Holmes, Gordon, 'Henry Head, 1861–1940', *Obituary Notices of Fellows of the Royal Society*, 3, 10 (1941) 665–89.

Holzapfel, Amy Strahler, 'Strindberg as Vivisector: Physiology, Pathology, and Anti-Mimesis in *The Father* and *Miss Julie*', *Modern Drama*, 51, 3 (2008), 329–52.

Huxley, T. H., *Prolegomena, Evolution and Ethics* (1894), (Princeton: Princeton University Press), 1989.

Hyman, Stanley Edgar, *The Tangled Bank : Darwin, Marx, Fraser, Freud as Imaginative Writers* (New York: Atheneum, 1962).

Jacyna, L. S., *Medicine and Modernism: A Biography of Henry Head* (London: Pickering and Chatto, 2008).

Jones, Edgar, 'War Neuroses and Arthur Hurst: A Pioneering Medical Film about the Treatment of Psychiatric Battle Casualties', *Journal of the History of Medicine and Allied Sciences*, 67, 3 (2012), 345–73.

Kaes, Anton, *Shell Shock Cinema: Weimar Culture and the Wounds of War* (Princeton, NJ and Oxford: Princeton University Press, 2009).

Kafka, Franz, *Metamorphosis and Other Stories*, trans. Malcolm Pasley (London: Penguin, 2000).

Kittler, Friedrich A., *Discourse Networks 1800/1900* (Stanford: Stanford University Press, 1990).

Knowles, Ric, Joanne Tompkins, and W. B. Worthen, eds., *Modern Drama: Defining the Field* (Toronto, Buffalo, and London: University of Toronto Press, 2003).

Kroker, Kenton, 'The Progress of Introspection in America, 1896–1938', *Studies in History and Philosophy of Biomedical Sciences*, 34, 1 (2003), 77–108.

Kusch, Martin, *Knowledge by Agreement: The Programme of Communitarian Epistemology* (Oxford and New York: Oxford University Press, 2002).

Landecker, Hanna, 'Microcinematography and the History of Science and Film', *Isis*, 97 (2006), 121–32.

Lanzoni, Susan, 'Practising Psychology in the Art Gallery: Vernon Lee's Aesthetics of Empathy', *Journal of the History of the Behavioral Sciences*, 45, 4 (2009), 330–54.

Larson, Barbara and Fae Brauer eds., *The Art of Evolution: Darwin, Darwinisms and Visual Culture* (Lebanon: Dartmouth College Press, 2009).

Latour, Bruno and Steve Woolgar, *Laboratory Life: The Construction of Scientific Facts* (Beverly Hills: Sage, 1979).

Laub, Dori, 'Truth and Testimony: The Process and the Struggle', in *Trauma: Explorations in Memory*, ed. Cathy Caruth (Baltimore: Johns Hopkins University Press, 1995) pp. 61–75.

Lawrence, Christopher and Steven Shapin eds., *Science Incarnate: Historical Embodiments of Natural Knowledge* (Chicago and London: University of Chicago Press, 1988).

Ledger, Sally and Roger Luckhurst eds., *The Fin de Siècle: A Reader in Cultural History, c.1880–1900* (Oxford: Oxford University Press, 2000).

Lee, Vernon and C. Anstruther-Thomson, *Beauty and Ugliness and Other Studies in Psychological Aesthetics* (London: John Lane, 1912).

Leese, Peter, *Shell Shock: Traumatic Neurosis and the British Soldiers of the First World War* (New York: Palgrave, 2002).

Lerner, Paul, 'Hysterical Cures: Hypnosis, Gender and Performance in World War I and Weimar Germany', *History Workshop Journal*, 45 (1998), 79–101.

Lewis, Leopold, *The Bells: A Drama in Three Acts* (London: Samuel French, 1871).

Leys, Ruth, *From Sympathy to Reflex: Marshall Hall and His Opponents* (New York and London: Garland, 1990).

Lightman, Bernard, *Victorian Popularizers of Science* (Chicago and London: University of Chicago Press, 2007).

Locke, John, *Some Thoughts Concerning Education* (1693), (London: Churchill, 1712).

Loughran, Tracey, 'Shell Shock and Psychological Medicine in First World War Britain', *Social History of Medicine*, 22, 1 (2009), 79–95.

Luckhurst, Roger. *The Invention of Telepathy: 1870–1901* (Oxford: Oxford University Press, 2002).

Lyly, John, *Euphues, The Anatomy of Wit; Euphues and his England*, (1578), ed. Leah Scragg (Manchester: Manchester University Press, 2003).

MacIntyre, C. F. trans. and ed., *Selected Poems, Paul Verlaine* (Berkeley and London: University of California Press, 1948).

Macmillan, M., 'Localization and William Macewen's Early Brain Surgery', *Journal of the History of Neuroscience*, 14, 1 (2005) 24–56.

Marshall, David, *The Figure of Theater: Shaftesbury, Defoe, Adam Smith, and George Eliot* (New York: Columbia University Press, 1986).

Marshall, Gail eds., *The Cambridge Companion to the Fin de Siècle* (Cambridge: Cambridge University Press, 2007).

Massumi, Brian, *Parables for the Virtual: Movement, Affect, Sensation* (Durham: Duke University Press, 2002).

du Maurier, George, *Trilby*, (London: Osgood, 1895).

Mayer, Jed, 'The Expression of the Emotions in Man and Laboratory Animals', *Victorian Studies*, 50, 3 (2008), 399–417.

Mayhew, Henry, *London Labour and the London Poor* (1851) (Oxford: Oxford University Press, 2010).

Micale, Mark S., *Approaching Hysteria: Disease and its Interpretations* (Princeton: Princeton University Press, 1995).

Mitchell, W. J. T. *Picture Theory: Essays on Verbal and Visual Representation* (Chicago: University of Chicago Press, 1995).
Morus, Iwan Rhys, *Frankenstein's Children: Electricity, Exhibition, and Experiment in Early Nineteenth-Century London* (Princeton: Princeton University Press, 1998).
—— 'Worlds of Wonder: Sensation and the Victorian Scientific Performance', *Isis*, 101 (2010), 806–16.
—— 'Placing Performance', *Isis*, 101 (2010), 775–8.
Mulvey, Laura, *Visual and Other Pleasures* (London: Macmillan, 1989).
Musser, Charles, *The Emergence of Cinema: The American Screen to 1907* (New York and Oxford: Maxwell Macmillan International, 1990).
Nashe, Thomas, *The Unfortunate Traveller, and Other Works* ed. John Barry Steane (Harmondsworth: Penguin, 1972).
Newton-Smith, W. H. ed., *A Companion to the Philosophy of Science* (Oxford: Blackwell, 2000).
Nicoll, Allardyce and F. Theodore Cloak eds., *Dion Boucicault, Forbidden Fruit and Other Plays* (Bloomington: Indiana University Press, 1964).
North, Helen, *Sophrosyne: Self-Knowledge and Self-Restraint in Greek Literature* (New York: Cornell University Press, 1966).
O'Dell, Kathy, *Contract with the Skin: Masochism, Performance Art and the 1970s* (Minneapolis: University of Minnesota Press, 1998).
Otis, Laura ed., *Literature and Science in the Nineteenth Century: An Anthology*, (Oxford: Oxford University Press, 2002).
—— *Networking: Communicating with Bodies and Machines in the Nineteenth Century* (Ann Arbor: University of Michigan Press, 2001).
Otter, Chris, *The Victorian Eye* (Chicago: University of Chicago Press, 2008).
Parker, Patricia and Geoffrey Hartman eds., *Shakespeare and the Question of Theory*, (London: Methuen, 1985).
Paris, Michael, *The First World War and Popular Cinema* (New Brunswick: Rutgers University Press, 2000).
Pater, Walter, *The Works of Walter Pater* (Cambridge: Cambridge University Press, 2011).
Pauli, Lori ed., *Acting the Part: Photography as Theatre* (London: Merrell, 2006).
Pavlov, Ivan Petrovich, *Conditioned Reflexes: An Investigation of the Physiological Activity of the Cerebral Cortex*, trans. G. V. Anrep (London: Oxford University Press, 1927).
Picker, John M., *Victorian Soundscapes* (Oxford and London: Oxford University Press, 2003).
Pickering, Andrew, *Science as Practice and Culture*, ed. Andrew Pickering (Chicago: University of Chicago Press, 1992)..
——*The Mangle of Practice: Time, Agency and Science* (Chicago: University of Chicago Press, 1995).
Plato, *The Republic*, ed. Andrea Tschemplik, trans. John Llewelyn Davies and David James Vaughan (Oxford: Rowman and Littlefield, 2005).
—— *The Republic*, trans. A. D. Lindsay (London: Dent and Sons, 1906).

—— *The Republic*, trans. Desmond Lee (Harmondsworth: Penguin, 1988).

Pocock, Stephanie J., 'The Judicial and the Melodramatic Stage: Trial Scenes in Boucicault's *Arrah-na-Pogue and The Octoroon*', *Theatre Journal*, 60 (2008), 545–61.

Powell, Kerry ed., *The Cambridge Companion to Victorian and Edwardian Theatre*, (Cambridge: Cambridge University Press, 2004).

Prodger, Phillip, *An Annotated Catalogue of the Illustrations of Human and Animal Expression from the Collection of Charles Darwin: An Early Case of the Use of Photography in Scientific Research* (New York: Edwin Mellen, 1998).

Proust, Marcel, *In Search of Lost Time*, trans. Mark Treharne et al., 6 vols. (London: Penguin, 2002).

Rancière, Jacques, *The Emancipated Spectator*, trans. Gregory Elliott (London and New York: Verso, 2009).

Rees, Terence, *Theatre Lighting in the Age of Gas* (London: Society for Theatre Research, 1978).

Ridout, Nicholas, *Stage Fright, Animals, and Other Theatrical Problems* (Cambridge: Cambridge University Press, 2006).

Rivers, W. H. R. and Henry Head, 'A Human Experiment in Nerve Division', *Brain*, 31 (November 1908), 323–450.

Roach, Joseph R., *The Player's Passion: Studies in the Science of Acting* (Ann Arbor: University of Michigan Press, 2001).

Rose, Clifford, *Twentieth-Century Neurology: The British Contribution* (London: Imperial, 2001).

Rubery, Matthew, 'Play It Again, Sam Weller: New Digital Audiobooks and Old Ways of Reading', *The Journal of Victorian Culture*, 13, 1 (2008), 58–79.

Ryan, Andrew H., 'History of the British Act of 1876: An Act to Amend the Law Relating to Cruelty to Animals', *Journal of Medical Education*, 38 (1963), 182–94.

Salisbury, Laura and Andrew Shail, *Neurology and Modernity: A Cultural History of Nervous Systems 1800–1950* (Basingstoke: Palgrave Macmillan, 2010).

Sartre, Jean-Paul, *Being and Nothingness* (1943) trans. Hazel E. Barnes (London: Routledge, 2000).

Sassoon, Siegfried, *Collected Poems, 1908–1956* (London: Faber and Faber, 1984).

Scarry, Elaine, *The Body in Pain: The Making and Unmaking of the World* (Oxford: Oxford University Press, 1985).

Schoch, Richard W., *Queen Victoria and the Theatre of Her Age* (Basingstoke: Palgrave Macmillan, 2004).

Schwartz, Vanessa R. and Jeannene M. Przyblyski eds., *The Nineteenth-Century Visual Culture Reader* (London: Routledge, 2004).

Shakespeare, William, *The Complete Works of William Shakespeare*, ed. Stanley Wells and Gary Taylor (Clarendon Press, Oxford: 1988).

Shephard, Ben, *A War of Nerves: Soldiers and Psychiatrists 1914–1994* (London: Jonathan Cape, 2000).

Shepherd-Barr, Kirsten, *Science on Stage: From Doctor Faustus to Copenhagen* (Princeton, NJ: Princeton University Press, 2006).

Showalter, Elaine, *The Female Malady: Women, Madness and English Culture 1830–1980* (London: Virago Press, 1985).
Shuttleworth, Sally, *The Mind of the Child: Child Development in Literature, Science and Medicine 1840–1900* (Oxford: Oxford University Press, 2010).
Simons, Ronald C., *Boo!: Culture, Experience and the Startle Reflex* (New York and Oxford: Oxford University Press, 1996).
Smith, Adam, *The Theory of Moral Sentiments* (1759), (London: Millar, 1761).
Smith, Jonathan, *Charles Darwin and Victorian Visual Culture* (Cambridge: Cambridge University Press, 2006).
Smith, Roger, *Inhibition* (London: Free Association Books, 1992).
Sontag, Susan, *Regarding the Pain of Others* (London: Hamish Hamilton, 2003).
Stedman, Gesa, *Stemming the Torrent: Expression and Control in the Victorian Discourses on Emotion, 1830–1872* (Aldershot: Ashgate, 2002).
Stevenson, Robert Louis, *Strange Case of Dr. Jekyll and Mr. Hyde*, (London: Longmans, 1886).
Stiles, Anne, *Popular Fiction and Brain Science in the Late Nineteenth Century* (Cambridge: Cambridge University Press, 2012).
Strachey, James, 'Obituary of Joan Riviere, 1883–1962', *International Journal of Psycho-analysis*, 44, (1963), 228–30.
Strindberg, August, *Miss Julie* (1888) trans. Michael Robinson (Oxford: Oxford University Press, 2008).
Symonds, Charles, *Studies in Neurology* (Oxford: Oxford University Press, 1970).
Tait, A. C., 'History of Crichton Royal', *Medical History*, 16, 2 (1972), 178–84.
Taylor, George, *Players and Performances in Victorian Theatre* (Manchester: Manchester University Press, 1989).
Tennyson, Alfred, *The Poetical Works of Alfred Tennyson* (Boston: Ticknor and Fields, 1860).
Thurschwell, Pamela, Carolyn Burdett, and Nicola Brown eds., *The Victorian Supernatural* (Cambridge: Cambridge University Press, 2004).
Tjoa, Hock Guan, *George Henry Lewes: A Victorian Mind* (Cambridge, MA and London: Harvard University Press, 1977).
Voskuil, Lynn M., 'Feeling Public: Sensation Theatre, Commodity Culture, and the Victorian Public Sphere', *Victorian Studies* 44 (2002), 245–72.
Ward, Graham ed., *The Certeau Reader* (Oxford: Blackwell, 2000).
Watt Smith, Tiffany, 'Cardboard, Conjuring and "A Very Curious Experiment" ', *Interdisciplinary Science Reviews*, 38, 4 (2013), 306–20.
Wells, H. G., *The Island of Doctor Moreau* (1896) (London: Penguin, 2005).
van Wyhe, John, *Phrenology and the Origins of Victorian Scientific Naturalism* (Aldershot: Ashgate, 2004).
White, Paul, 'Introduction: The Emotional Economy of Science', *Isis*, 100 (2009) 792–7.
—— 'Darwin's Emotions: The Scientific Self and the Sentiment of Objectivity', *Isis*, 100 (2010), 811–26.
Wilde, Oscar, *The Picture of Dorian Gray* (1891), ed. Isobel Murray (London: Oxford University Press, 1974).

Willis, Martin, *Vision, Science and Literature, 1870–1920: Ocular Horizons* (London: Pickering and Chatto, 2011).

Winter, Alison, *Mesmerized: Powers of Mind in Victorian Britain* (Chicago: University of Chicago Press, 2000).

DIGITAL DATABASES

19th Century British Library Newspapers, <http://newspapers.bl.uk/blcs/> accessed 16 October 2013 (available only within British Library Reading Rooms).

BFI ScreenOnline, <http://www.screenonline.org.uk/film/id/440553/> accessed 16 September 2013.

The Complete Works of Darwin Online, <http://darwin-online.org.uk/> accessed 16 September 2013.

Pathé Archives, <http://www.britishpathe.com/> accessed 16 September 2013.

Tate Online, <https://www.tate.org.uk/modern/exhibitions> accessed 16 September 2013.

Wellcome Library <http://catalogue.wellcome.ac.uk/record=b1667864~S8%29> accessed 15 October 2013.

Index

Note: Page numbers in *italics* indicate illustrations